Gambling Disorder

A Clinical Guide to Treatment

SECOND EDITION

Edited by

Jon E. Grant, M.D., M.P.H., J.D.

Marc N. Potenza, M.D., Ph.D.

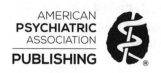

AMERICAN
PSYCHIATRIC
ASSOCIATION
PUBLISHING

Copyright © 2022 American Psychiatric Association Publishing

ALL RIGHTS RESERVED

Second Edition

Manufactured in the United States of America on acid-free paper
25   24   23   22   21   5   4   3   2   1

American Psychiatric Association Publishing
800 Maine Avenue SW, Suite 900
Washington, DC 20024-2812
www.appi.org

Library of Congress Cataloging-in-Publication Data
Names: Grant, Jon E., editor. | Potenza, Marc N., editor. | American Psychiatric Association Publishing, issuing body.
Title: Gambling disorder : a clinical guide to treatment / edited by Jon E. Grant, Marc N. Potenza.
Other titles: Pathological gambling (Grant)
Description: Second edition. | Washington, DC : American Psychiatric Association Publishing, [2022] | Preceded by Pathological gambling : a clinical guide to treatment. 1st ed. c2004. | Includes bibliographical references and index.
Identifiers: LCCN 2021016174 (print) | LCCN 2021016175 (ebook) | ISBN 9781615373031 (paperback : alk. paper) | ISBN 9781615373987 (ebook)
Subjects: MESH: Gambling—therapy | Behavior, Addictive—therapy
Classification: LCC RC569.5.G35 (print) | LCC RC569.5.G35 (ebook) | NLM WM 192 | DDC 616.85/841—dc23
LC record available at https://lccn.loc.gov/2021016174
LC ebook record available at https://lccn.loc.gov/2021016175

British Library Cataloguing in Publication Data
A CIP record is available from the British Library.

Contents

Appendix A

Appendix B

Appendix C

Appendix D

Appendix E

Contributors

Donald W. Black, M.D.
Professor Emeritus of Psychiatry, University of Iowa Roy J. and Lucille A. Carver College of Medicine, Iowa City, Iowa

Austin W. Blum, M.D., J.D.
Resident Physician in Psychiatry, Department of Psychiatry and Behavioral Neuroscience, University of Chicago, Chicago, Illinois

Brad W. Brazeau, B.Sc.
Graduate Student, Department of Psychology, University of Calgary, Calgary, Alberta, Canada

Samuel R. Chamberlain, M.B./B.Chir., Ph.D., MRCPsych
Professor of Psychiatry, Department of Psychiatry, University of Southampton, College Keep, Southampton, United Kingdom

Linda B. Cottler, Ph.D.
Associate Dean for Research & Dean's Professor, Department of Epidemiology, College of Public Health and Health Professions and College of Medicine, University of Florida, Gainesville, Florida

Paul H. Delfabbro, Ph.D.
Professor, School of Psychology, University of Adelaide, SA, Australia

Jeffrey L. Derevensky, Ph.D.
James McGill Professor; Director, McGill University International Centre for Youth Gambling Problems and High-Risk Behaviors, Montreal, Quebec, Canada

Luis C. Farhat, M.D.
Ph.D. Candidate, Departamento de Psiquiatria, Faculdade de Medicina FMUSP, Universidade de São Paulo, São Paulo, SP, Brazil

Sally M. Gainsbury, Ph.D.
Director, Gambling Treatment and Research Clinic, Brain and Mind Centre, School of Psychology, University of Sydney, NSW, Australia

Lynette Gilbeau, B.Ed.
Research Coordinator, McGill University International Centre for Youth Gambling, Problems and High-Risk Behaviors, Montreal, Quebec, Canada

ix

Jon E. Grant, M.D., M.P.H., J.D.
Professor, Department of Psychiatry and Behavioral Neuroscience, University of Chicago, Chicago, Illinois

Georgina M. Gross, Ph.D.
Clinical Psychologist, Northeast Program Evaluation Center, PTSD Program Evaluation; Associate Research Scientist, Yale University School of Medicine, New Haven, Connecticut

David C. Hodgins, Ph.D.
Professor, Department of Psychology, University of Calgary, Calgary, Alberta, Canada

Rani A. Hoff, M.P.H., Ph.D.
Director, Northeast Program Evaluation Center, Office of Mental Health and Suicide Prevention, Veterans Affairs Central Office; Professor of Psychiatry, Yale University School of Medicine, New Haven, Connecticut

Daniel L. King, Ph.D.
Senior Research Fellow, College of Education, Psychology, and Social Work, Flinders University, Adelaide, SA, Australia

Elijah Otis, B.A.
Ph.D. Student (Clinical Psychology), Department of Psychology and Neuroscience, Dalhousie University, Halifax, Nova Scotia, Canada

Marc N. Potenza, M.D., Ph.D.
Professor, Department of Psychiatry, Child Study Center, and Department of Neuroscience, Yale School of Medicine, New Haven, Connecticut; Senior Scientist, Connecticut Council on Problem Gambling, Wethersfield, Connecticut

Nathan D. L. Smith, A.B.D.
Ph.D. Candidate, Department of Epidemiology, College of Public Health and Health Professions and College of Medicine, University of Florida, Gainesville, Florida

Sherry H. Stewart, Ph.D.
Professor, Departments of Psychology and Neuroscience and Psychiatry, Dalhousie University, Halifax, Nova Scotia, Canada

Randy Stinchfield, Ph.D.
Retired Clinical Psychologist, Department of Psychiatry, University of Minnesota, Minneapolis, Minnesota

Igor Yakovenko, Ph.D.
Assistant Professor, Department of Psychology and Neuroscience, Department of Psychiatry, Dalhousie University, Halifax, Nova Scotia, Canada

Introduction

It has been 16 years since the first edition of this text, *Pathological Gambling* (Grant and Potenza 2004). During the intervening years, not only has the volume of research on gambling disorder grown significantly, but the name of the disorder has officially changed from pathological gambling to gambling disorder (American Psychiatric Association 2013). Thus, as a textbook devoted exclusively to gambling disorder, this volume reflects an exciting moment in the history of gambling research. Because of this research, clinicians now have available an array of treatment options that can appreciably improve the lives of patients with gambling disorder.

The study of gambling disorder is important from both clinical and research perspectives. Gambling disorder is a common disorder that is associated with significant morbidity (decreased self-esteem, comorbid substance use disorders, financial and legal difficulties, stress on relationships and families, and suicidality). Over the past 16 years, our understanding of the phenomenology, epidemiology, neurobiology, psychology, and treatment of this disorder has increased. Unfortunately, although many clinicians encounter individuals with gambling disorder (elevated rates of gambling disorder are observed in patients with other mental health disorders), clinicians often do not diagnose gambling disorder and are frequently unaware of the treatment options for the disorder.

Many clinicians are also unaware of the personal and social consequences of gambling disorder. This lack of awareness in turn often leads physicians to ignore gambling evaluations in both psychiatric and primary care settings. Gambling disorder has significant public health implications, and Smith and Cottler (Chapter 1, "Epidemiology: The Good, the Bad, and the Ugly") examine the effects of gambling on societal, familial, and individual health and well-being. Assessment instruments that are useful in diagnosing gambling disorder and monitoring symptom change are discussed by Randy Stinchfield later in this volume (Chapter 9, "Screening and Assessment Instruments").

The primary purpose of this book is to document the clinical phenomenology, etiology, and treatment of gambling disorder. Current clinical approaches that are most likely to lead to early identification, symptom remission, and maintenance of improvement are highlighted. Donald Black (Chapter 2, "Clinical Characteristics") provides a comprehensive description of the symptoms and sequelae of gambling disorder. The book also provides contributions on how gambling disorder differs in older adults (Chapter 3, "Older Adults") and between men and women (Chapter 4, "Gender Differences").

Gambling behavior takes multiple forms today and has expanded far beyond casinos. Daniel King et al. provide an important overview of the complex interplay between gambling and technology (Chapter 5, "Online Gambling and Gambling-Gaming Convergence"). In addition, this volume includes a chapter, new to this edition, on the always evolving field of gambling and criminal and legal issues (Chapter 6, "Legal and Forensic Aspects").

To enhance treatment options, both clinicians and researchers look to possible psychological and behavioral etiologies, as well as to a deeper understanding of possible neurobiological underpinnings. Therefore, these two important realms of explanations for the behavior of gambling disorder are examined. Elijah Otis et al. (Chapter 7, "Cognitive and Behavioral Underpinnings") discuss behavioral, cognitive, and dispositional theories of the etiology of gambling disorder and provide an association between psychological models and neurobiological systems that have been linked to gambling disorder. To augment the psychological basis for gambling disorder, Farhat and Potenza (Chapter 8, "Neurobiology") examine the neurochemical, cognitive, genetic, and brain imaging data in gambling disorder. The psychological and biological understanding of gambling disorder may be useful in understanding a range of addictive and impulsive disorders.

Although effective treatments for gambling disorder currently exist, with this book we seek to enhance clinicians' abilities to identify and provide early intervention for individuals with gambling disorder. Adolescents and young adults have been consistently found to exhibit relatively high rates of gambling disorder. To address this issue, Derevensky and Gilbeau provide a prevention strategy tailored specifically for this age group (Chapter 10, "Understanding Youth Gambling Problems: Prevention and Treatment Strategies").

Tremendous advances in the treatment of gambling disorder have been made over the past 16 years. As a result, clinicians caring for patients with gambling disorder have many treatment options at their disposal. Brazeau and Hodgins (Chapter 11, "Psychosocial Treatments") discuss the current understanding of the behavioral treatment approaches and their effectiveness in helping individuals with gambling disorder. They evaluate the rationale behind, empirical support for, and practical aspects of a variety of behavioral interventions, including participation in 12-step programs, financial counseling, motivational interviewing, motivational enhancement, brief interventions, and cognitive-behavioral treatment. Furthermore, these authors discuss self-help–based and professional-based interventions targeting family members. In a related chapter, Grant and Chamberlain (Chapter 12, "Pharmacological Treatments") discuss the rationale of the various pharmacological approaches to gambling disorder and review the current status of drug treatments.

In summary, gambling disorder is an important clinical condition that often results in significant personal difficulties for patients. As the chapters of this volume eloquently attest, extraordinary progress has been made regarding the epidemiology, phenomenology, comorbidity, and possible etiology of this disorder.

Prevention and treatment interventions—including cognitive, behavioral, and pharmacological treatments—have made it possible for patients with gambling disorder to often find relief from this disabling disorder.

Jon E. Grant, M.D., M.P.H., J.D.
Marc N. Potenza, M.D., Ph.D.

References

American Psychiatric Association: Diagnostic and Statistical Manual of Mental Disorders, 5th Edition. Arlington, VA, American Psychiatric Association, 2013

Grant JE, Potenza MN (eds): Pathological Gambling: A Clinical Guide to Treatment. Washington, DC, American Psychiatric Publishing, 2004

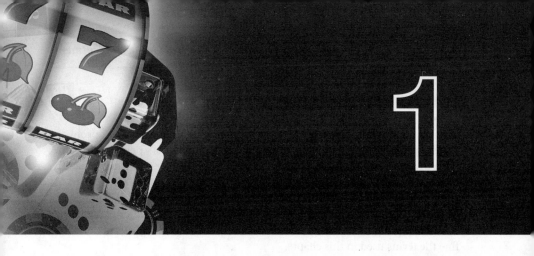

Epidemiology

The Good, the Bad, and the Ugly

Nathan D. L. Smith, A.B.D.

Linda B. Cottler, Ph.D.

Measuring gambling-related problems is an important, but complicated, endeavor. How are "gambling-related problems" defined? What population was assessed? How was the sample derived? Is the sample representative of the population?

In this chapter, each of these epidemiological fundamentals is detailed to show how gambling disorder has been studied in the past and to provide ideas for the future. We begin with a section on nomenclature to establish clear definitions for use throughout the chapter, and then explore the good, the bad, and the ugly in the history and present reality of the epidemiology of gambling disorder. By the end of this chapter, the reader should be familiar with the fundamental components of the epidemiology of gambling disorder and understand how to evaluate the strengths and weaknesses of these components in an epidemiological study.

Nomenclature

What is a gambling disorder? Is it the same as gambling addiction, problem gambling, problematic gambling, or compulsive gambling? Is a person with gambling disorder a compulsive gambler, pathological gambler, or probable pathological gambler? Understanding and differentiating between the words used to study gambling problems is the first step toward understanding its epidemiology. In this section, we define terms commonly used in recent studies of gambling disorder, highlight the strengths and weaknesses of a few notable terms, and define the terms used in this chapter.

DSM

DSM-5 Gambling Disorder: The Gold Standard

The term *gambling disorder* is used in the fifth edition of the *Diagnostic and Statistical Manual of Mental Disorders* (DSM-5), published in 2013 (American Psychiatric Association 2013a). For many clinicians and researchers, the definitions included in the most recent edition of DSM are the de facto "current" definitions of the included mental disorders. This is because of the central role DSM has played in psychiatric research since it was published in 1952, the rigorous process used to write the manual (Petry et al. 2014), and the practical reality that DSM often dictates how insurance companies reimburse treatment providers for their work (American Psychiatric Association 2013b).

For many, the DSM-5 definition is the gold standard (Frances and Nardo 2013; Wakefield 2015). The value of the DSM-5 definition is not that it is perfect, but that its imperfections are knowable and testable. That is, because DSM publishes exactly how it determines diagnoses, the diagnoses can be replicated by other research teams. This then gives DSM a broad base of users and tests of the definition that can be used to make adjustments to the current version and improve later versions. All of this happens openly in the scientific literature for anyone to see and learn from.

When a study uses the DSM-5 definition of gambling disorder, the field knows exactly what definition is being examined, what criteria characterize the definition, and how many criteria make up the diagnosis. This is the value of the DSM-5 definition and why it is considered the gold standard.

The main criteria for a DSM-5 gambling disorder (American Psychiatric Association 2013a; emphasis added) are given below:

Persistent and recurrent problematic gambling behavior **leading to clinically significant impairment or distress**, as indicated by the individual exhibiting **four** (or more) of the following **in a 12-month period**:

1. Needs to gamble with increasing amounts of money in order to achieve the desired excitement.
2. Is restless or irritable when attempting to cut down or stop gambling.
3. Has repeated unsuccessful efforts to control, cut back, or stop gambling.
4. Is often preoccupied with gambling (e.g., having persistent thoughts of reliving past gambling experiences, handicapping or planning the next venture, thinking of ways to get money with which to gamble).
5. Often gambles when feeling distressed (e.g., helpless, guilty, anxious, depressed).
6. After losing money gambling, often returns another day to get even ("chasing" one's losses).
7. Lies [to family members, therapist, or others] to conceal the extent of involvement with gambling.
8. Has jeopardized or lost a significant relationship, job, or educational or career opportunity because of gambling.
9. Relies on others to provide money to relieve desperate financial situations caused by gambling.

DSM-IV

DSM-5 changed the nomenclature published in 1994 in DSM-IV (American Psychiatric Association 1994), *pathological gambling*, and moved the disorder from the section Impulse-Control Disorders Not Otherwise Classified to the chapter Substance Use and Related Disorders. This move made gambling disorder the first and only behavior categorized alongside more traditional substance use disorders such as cocaine use disorder and opioid use disorder.

DSM-IV was the state-of-the-art diagnostic guide for mental disorders until 2013, when DSM-5 was published. At that time, DSM-IV had all of the same benefits of the current DSM. That is, it was publicly available, widely used by both clinicians and researchers, and had clearly laid out criteria backed up by a body of theory and supporting research. Studies published between 1994 and 2013 (and even after) may use the term "pathological gambling" for what is now described as gambling disorder. This term was state-of-the-art at the time and reflected the most up-to-date thinking of scholars at that time.

"Problem Gambling" in the DSM-IV Era

During the DSM-IV era, the term "pathological gambling" was used for people who reported 5 or more of 10 DSM-IV criteria. However, in many studies, there were people whose gambling did not meet this threshold who were of interest to researchers. For this reason, it became common practice to group people reporting 3 or 4 DSM-IV criteria of pathological gambling together under the heading of "problem gambling." Problem gambling (or "problem gamblers") was never recognized in DSM, but the category was commonly used, and there is extensive literature that describes the people in this group.

When DSM-5 lowered the number of criteria needed to meet the clinical threshold from 5 to 4, it created a problem for researchers using the construct of problem gambling. To address this problem, researchers could 1) continue recognizing those with three criteria as "problem gamblers," 2) redefine "problem gambling" to include people with 2 or 3 criteria, 3) broaden the definition to include people with 1–3 criteria, or 4) discontinue the use of the term "problem gambling." Each option has benefits and drawbacks. At this time, no answer to this problem has emerged as the standard of the field.

Beyond DSM

DSM does not include every question of interest related to gambling disorder. This is not a bug, but a feature. DSM is meant as a reference for clinical diagnosis and a standard for the field to use at a moment in time. There are many other interesting and useful questions that can be asked about gambling disorder beyond the scope of DSM.

Into this void have arisen many instruments designed to study these questions. Among these are a small number of well-established and widely used instruments such as the Canadian Problem Gambling Index (CPGI; Ferris and Wynne 2001) and the South Oaks Gambling Screen (SOGS; Lesieur and Blume 1987) and shorter screening instruments such as the Brief Biosocial Gambling Screen (BBGS; Gebauer et al. 2010). This section is meant not to discuss the many measures and screens that exist in the field (see Chapter 9, "Screening and Assessment Instruments," for a more detailed discussion), but rather to demonstrate how to interact with the nomenclature of such instruments.

We use as our example the CPGI, which was developed by Jackie Ferris and Harold Wynne. The CPGI is notable because its stated goal was to measure negative outcomes of gambling behavior over and above what was measured by DSM. Specifically, the authors of the CPGI were interested in what kinds of gambling activities a person participated in, how often they did each activity, and what family or community consequences gambling caused (Ferris and Wynne 2001). These questions are important and not addressed in DSM. Thus, the CPGI was created to fill an important gap in knowledge in the field.

Since its creation, the CPGI has been use dozens of times in high-quality studies carried out all over the world. These studies provide a broad body of reference material for understanding what a CPGI score means in various contexts. To be useful in measuring gambling problems, an instrument needs to be clear in what it is trying to measure and well calibrated through psychometric testing. An instrument that is very similar to DSM has less utility than a measure that is more unique, because most studies would get more benefit from producing an actual DSM diagnosis than from using an instrument that is similar to DSM but not the same.

Within the CPGI is a problem gambling screen sometimes separated out from the whole, called the Problem Gambling Severity Index (PGSI). The PGSI consists of nine questions scored from 0 to 3 for a scoring range of 0 to 27 points. A score of 0 indicates a nongambler or nonproblem gambler. A score of 1–2 indicates a low-risk gambler, 3–7 a moderate-risk gambler, and 8 or more a problem gambler (Jackson et al. 2010).

These terms are only valuable when used as the authors intended, because their meaning derives from the theory and testing of the authors and the body of research generated by others who used the instrument as intended. That is to say, a study that purports to use the PGSI but changes the criteria cut points for the categories is not using the instrument as intended and is producing data that have no knowable meaning.

Nomenclature in This Chapter

In this chapter, we set an example of how to use clear nomenclature. We use "gambling disorder" as it is used in DSM-5, "pathological gambling" as it is defined in DSM-IV, and "problem gambling" as it was commonly used in the DSM-IV era. We use "gambling-related problems" to mean the full spectrum of problems related to gambling, including gambling disorder and all other problems. Anytime we use a term that comes from a specific non-DSM instrument, we identify that instrument, the cutoff score proposed by the instrument's creator, and the cutoff score used by the author. It is our belief that this type of complete reporting of the measures used is the only way to ensure that the field moves toward consistent and proper use of measurement instruments.

The Good

First, the population prevalence of gambling disorder has been thoroughly researched and has been stable at approximately 1% for the past 40 years. This stability has also provided reliable information on other important topics such as demographics, comorbidities, and pathways. Second, there have been several very high quality studies of gambling disorder that can serve as exemplars for best practices of methodology. We discuss each of these points in greater detail next.

Prevalence

Prevalence refers to the percentage of people in the population who have a particular disorder at any time. This is different from *incidence,* which is the rate of new cases of a disorder that occur in a certain time period.

Gambling disorder is a conditional disorder. That is, it can only be present among people who have gambled. This is similar to other psychiatric disorders such as PTSD, which can only be found in individuals who have experienced trauma (Smith and Cottler 2018). It is best practice to only report prevalence of conditional disorders among those who meet the conditions of having the disorder. In the case of gambling disorder, this practice has generally not been followed. Although it is our preference that prevalence rates be reported in groups that have met the conditions, because this has generally not been the case in research on gambling disorder, we report population percentages in this chapter to reflect the work done in the field as a whole.

Overall Findings

The percentage of the U.S. population with gambling disorder is around 1%. This finding has been surprisingly durable for the past 40 years, going all the way back to the Epidemiologic Catchment Area (ECA) study finding in 1980 of 0.9%. In one notable example of the collection of prevalence data on gambling disorder, researchers collated nearly every prevalence survey on gambling-related problems conducted all over the world between 1975 and 2011 (Williams et al. 2012). Of these studies, the 57 studies that included DSM-IV data produced 72 measures of gambling disorder (either past year or lifetime). Of these 72 measures, 69 were between 0.1% and 1.8%, and all 72 were between 0.0% and 2.2%. These findings show the remarkable durability of prevalence rates regardless of differences in the location, year, methodology, or quality of the research study.

Exemplar Studies

Although the majority of studies have found an approximately 1% population prevalence of gambling disorder, a handful are truly outstanding (Table 1–1). These studies are highlighted next.

Epidemiologic Catchment Area.   The ECA study was the first truly modern psychiatric epidemiological study and probably the most influential study of population mental health in the past 50 years. The ECA took place in 1980 in five cities: New Haven, St. Louis, Los Angeles, Baltimore, and Durham, NC. The ECA used the Diagnostic Interview Schedule (Robins et al. 1981) created by Robins and colleagues at Washington University and used trained raters to produce accurate psychiatric diagnoses in a large population survey. This method of collecting psychiatric data has come to dominate the research field over the past 40 years, along with several other novel methodologies first put together in the ECA study (Robins and Regier 1992). Gambling disorder in the ECA was studied only in St. Louis, where the population prevalence rate was found to be approximately 0.9% (Cunningham-Williams et al. 1998).

The Harvard Medical School meta-analysis.   In 1999, a team at the Division on Addictions at Harvard Medical School completed a meta-analysis of the existing research on gambling disorder in the United States and Canada (Shaffer et al. 1999). The meta-analysis was significant because there were many studies on the subject at the time, but the quality of many of these studies was

TABLE 1–1. Exemplar studies of gambling disorder in the United States and Canada

Study	Authors	Sample size	Location	Measure	Rate of gambling disorder
ECA study	Cunningham-Williams et al. 1998	3,004	St. Louis, MO	DIS	0.9%
Harvard Medical School meta-analysis	Shaffer et al. 1999	N/A	U.S. and Canada	N/A	1.6%
NCS-R	Kessler et al. 2008	9,282	U.S.	CIDI	0.6%

Note. CIDI=World Health Organization Composite International Diagnostic Interview; DIS=Diagnostic Interview Schedule; ECA=Epidemiologic Catchment Area; NCS-R= National Comorbidity Survey—Replication.

questionable. The meta-analysis found lifetime prevalences of 1.6% in adults, 3.9% in adolescents, and 14.2% in incarcerated individuals (Shaffer et al. 1999). This meta-analysis became the benchmark study of gambling disorder prevalence for the decade after its publication.

National Comorbidity Survey—Replication. The National Comorbidity Survey (NCS) (Kessler et al. 1994) and the later National Comorbidity Survey—Replication (NCS-R) (Kessler and Merikangas 2004) were intended to provide detailed information about how comorbid mental illnesses occur in the population. The NCS-R was a representative survey of 9,282 English-speaking Americans interviewed between 2001 and 2003. The survey asked questions about mental health conditions, including age at onset, and provided considerable information on psychiatric comorbidity in people with gambling disorder. The NCS-R found a lifetime prevalence of pathological gambling of 0.6%, with the vast majority (97%) of people with the disorder having additional comorbid mental health conditions (Kessler et al. 2008).

Demographics

It used to be that gambling disorder was considered a disorder of older men. Even up to the 1990s, the stereotypical person with gambling disorder was often portrayed as a man older than 60 years who spent most of his time at a racetrack or card table. However, in recent years, the demographics of gambling disorder have not fit this profile. In the United States, although there are still more men than women who report behaviors meeting the criteria for gambling disorder, surveys of treatment-seeking samples show no gender difference (Grant et al. 2012; Kessler et al. 2008; Merkouris et al. 2016). This could be because women are more apt than men to seek treatment, or it might reflect the shift of gambling disorder toward a more equal gender balance in the population.

In terms of race/ethnicity, gambling disorder is less prevalent among whites (1.2%) than among African Americans (2.2%), but there are no significant differences between Hispanics and whites (Alegria et al. 2009). However, conditional rates of gambling disorder are much higher among African Americans, who gamble at lower rates than whites (75% vs. 83%) but experience higher rates of disorder (Welte et al. 2002). This pattern of less overall use but higher conditional rates of disorder among African Americans has been found at times with potentially harmful substances, such as cocaine (John and Wu 2017), but not others, such as alcohol (Vaeth et al. 2017).

Comorbidities

Comorbid disorders are other physical and mental illnesses that occur in individuals who have gambling disorder. Mental health comorbidities are highly prevalent among those with gambling disorder, although rates vary. The NCS-R found that about 64% of people with a gambling disorder also had three or more mental health comorbidities (Kessler et al. 2008), whereas the rate for persons without gambling disorder was 6% (Kessler et al. 2005). In about 75% of people, the onset of gambling disorder occurred after another disorder; in the remaining 25% of cases, gambling disorder preceded the onset of comorbid disorders (Kessler et al. 2008). In either case, the idea that gambling disorder very rarely appears without other mental health comorbidities is an a very important reality for both treatment providers working with individuals with gambling disorder and public health and policy workers designing programs for people with gambling disorder.

Pathways Model

People with gambling disorder are a very heterogeneous group. Several theories and studies have examined symptom clusters and subtypes of people with gambling disorder. Perhaps the most supported theory is the "Pathways Model" published by Blaszczynski and Nower in 2002. The model suggests that there are three distinct subgroups of people with gambling disorder: 1) "behaviorally conditioned" problem gamblers (i.e., heavy gamblers who oscillate between gambling problematically and gambling only heavily based on behavioral conditioning and habituation); 2) "emotionally vulnerable" problem gamblers who have premorbid anxiety, depression, or other mental health conditions and experiences that can be moderated by gambling; and 3) "antisocial impulsivist" problem gamblers who often have a premorbid impulse-control disorder or personality disorder that causes significant dysfunction (Blaszczynski and Nower 2002). Some additional studies have found support for the general principles of this model (Milosevic and Ledgerwood 2010), but others have presented a more complicated pattern of symptoms (Alvarez-Moya et al. 2010).

The Bad

The "bad" in the epidemiology of gambling disorder includes methodological issues that hamper the effectiveness of the field in answering its most pressing issues. Many of the issues that we address in this section are common across all survey research.

Inadequate Response Rates

A response rate is the percentage of people who completed the survey divided by the number of people in the total sample (Table 1–2). It is one of the most important metrics in survey research. As previously discussed, surveys are intended to provide information about a particular population, but they can only do so if the sample included in the survey is representative of the population it purports to represent.

In general, as response rates decrease, our confidence that the sample represents the population should also decrease. This is important to understand because studies of addiction are particularly vulnerable to selection bias. *Selection bias* occurs when the sample selected does not represent the population it is drawn from. People who are experiencing gambling disorder (or other addictive or mental health disorders) are often more difficult to reach via commonly used methods of survey recruitment than those without such disorders. It may be that they are less likely to answer calls from an unknown number or less likely to be home when their phone is called, or there may be any number of other reasons why they cannot be reached.

In one classic example from the ECA, one author of this chapter (L.B.C.) analyzed the effort used to recruit the sample itself (Cottler et al. 1987). One of the disorders assessed in the ECA was alcohol use disorder. The research team continued to call members of the sample without limiting the number of times each individual could be called. The data showed that if researchers stopped after five calls, the prevalence of alcohol use disorder was 3.9; if they stopped after 9 calls, it increased to 4.3%, and if they called 10–57 times, the rate was 4.6%. The study demonstrated that people with addictive disorders may need more contact attempts than those without such disorders.

This study demonstrates the importance of insisting on very high response rates in studies of all addictive disorders, including gambling disorder. Simply hoping that survey respondents include the same proportion of people with gambling disorder as the general population is not good enough. This hypothesis is not supported by theory, previous experience, the scientific literature, or simple logic. Therefore, as a field we must insist on the highest possible response rates.

TABLE 1–2.　Building blocks of an epidemiological study

Concept	Definition	Examples
Population	The entire defined group that researchers are interested in learning about	Adults living in Massachusetts
Sample	The people from the population selected for inclusion in the research study	1,000 adult survey respondents
Measure	The instrument used to measure the variables of interest	Diagnostic Interview Schedule
Response rate	The percentage of people who were invited to complete the survey who actually complete the survey	75%

Inadequate Understanding of Assumptions and Biases in Study Design

The scientific method is, fundamentally, a process of making and testing hypotheses. For epidemiologists, this means that we do not go into the field simply with the goal of counting numbers of cases. We always work from our previous knowledge, the extant literature, and our own questions to form hypotheses.

For example, before we began collecting data for a recent study, the authors of this chapter sat with the research team and discussed a number of factors: What theory drives this research? What does the existing literature suggest we will find? What are our a priori assumptions? What do we hypothesize we will find in this sample? Do we need to add any additional questions to be able to test these hypotheses before data collection? These questions must be carefully considered and answered before any part of the practical process of research can begin.

Working without understanding one's own assumptions and biases can lead to the biases being built into the study design, and after the study is designed and executed, it is often too late for these fundamental problems to be fixed. The consequences of unexamined research bias are outlined in the next section.

Problems With Nomenclature: Defining "At Risk"

At the beginning of this chapter, we discussed nomenclature. It is worth highlighting one particularly problematic piece of nomenclature in this section: "at risk." The term deserves particular criticism for two reasons. First, "at risk" is already used in public health and epidemiology to mean every person who is able to contract a disorder. For example, any person with a prostate is at risk for prostate cancer. If a person with a prostate has it removed, that person is no longer at risk of prostate cancer. Using a phrase with an existing public health definition to mean something different when in the context of gambling is unnecessary and confusing.

Second, the definition of what "at risk" means is not clear. The phrase is defined and used differently by researchers, government employees, journalists, and advocates, with little consistency or clarity as to what it means. That said, it is hard to fault people for not having a clear understanding of what "at risk" means when it has no agreed-upon meaning among epidemiologists. In one example, a 2018 study makes the claim that "[l]ongitudinal studies have found that at-risk gambling is one of the strongest predictors of future problem gambling" (Mazar et al. 2018), citing three studies in support (Billi et al. 2015; el-Guebaly et al. 2015; Williams et al. 2015). However, the three studies cited each define "at-risk gamblers" in different, and at times contradictory, ways.

In this way, the term "at risk" becomes a Rorschach test on which people project their personal feelings about gamblers, gambling, and people living with addiction. At this time, the concept of "at-risk gamblers" is doing more harm than good and should be replaced with a better-defined term, such as the well-defined terms discussed earlier (see above subsection "Nomenclature in This Chapter").

The Ugly

In the previous sections, we have discussed what has been done well in the field (the good) and what has been done poorly and needs improvement (the bad). Now we must turn our attention to the great failings of the field over the previous 40 years (the ugly).

To be clear, this section is not intended to single out particular researchers of gambling disorder. That said, there is no way to address the serious methodological and ethical concerns that have plagued the field over the past 40 years without a willingness to discuss what the problems are. We believe that the ultimate goal of challenging the field to do better in the future is worth the discomfort and risk that having this discussion may bring.

The Healthy People: 2020 public health goals put out by the U.S. government emphasize the importance of addressing health disparities that impact minority groups as part of a comprehensive plan for improving public health (Koh et al. 2011). In a recently published chapter on the impacts of culture and race on responsible gambling, Ortiz and Hernandez argued for the importance of considering differences in culture and race related to gambling, gambling disorder, and responsible gaming (Ortiz and Hernández 2019). In response to the important health goals of the U.S. government and the example of Ortiz and Hernandez, in this section we examine the epidemiology of gambling disorder through the health disparities lens.

You recall that the goal of any epidemiological study is to draw a sample that is representative of the population under investigation. That is, to understand the health of residents of a particular state, the sample must reflect the population of that state. The more divergence between the sample and the population, the less confidence we have in the research findings on that sample. Previously in this chapter, we noted that response rates for traditional research methods have been declining, with researchers having increasing difficulty reaching participants with lower socioeconomic status, certain racial and ethnic minorities, and those with unstable housing.

These factors have combined in such a way that samples meant to be representative of states, provinces, or nations have tended to be representative of only the most highly resourced groups within those localities. In this way, the very groups most at risk for gambling disorder (low-income individuals, individuals with comorbid mental health conditions, individuals with unstable housing, and so on) have been systematically excluded from the vast majority of epidemiological studies of gambling disorder (Ortiz and Hernández 2019).

This exclusion has two main negative consequences. The first is the obvious ethical problem of excluding the most vulnerable people from research. This means that the work produced is not based on the vulnerable and thus is unlikely to benefit this group. In research ethics, this violates the principle of justice: the conscious balancing of how the risks and benefits of a research project are distributed in the population (National Commission for the Protection of Human Subjects of Biomedical and Behavioral Research 1978). Exclusion of vulnerable populations breaks the research ethics principle of fair subject selection and is overtly unethical (National Institutes of Health 2015). The second negative consequence of exclusion is the methodological problem that arises because the groups most likely to report a gambling disorder are being excluded from samples. It is possible that this systematic exclusion has led to an underreporting of the prevalence of gambling disorder in most studies over the past 30 years. This reality must temper the good news discussed in the first part of this chapter regarding the consistency of the rate of gambling problems; pervasive systematic exclusion must be overcome if the field is to move forward with confidence in prevalence estimates.

The exclusion of incarcerated and homeless populations is often conscious and overt. For many reasons, it is more difficult, time consuming, and expensive to get the population prevalence data from some groups than from others. In particular, studying persons in the criminal justice system or those who are homeless is particularly logistically difficult. There are some good reasons for this, such as the additional protections these groups are granted by institutional review boards; some neutral reasons, such as the simple difficulty of getting a representative sample of people with unstable housing; and some problematic reasons such as the fact that incarcerated or homeless people may be viewed with disdain or indifference and the improvement of their lives is not valued by the politicians, research funders, and researchers who are commissioning or conducting the study.

Conclusion

The population prevalence of gambling disorder has been stable at 1% for the past 40 years, providing reliable information on the demographics, comorbidities, and pathways of the disorder. However, the lowering of response rates, the lack of effort put into the pre-research process, and the use of confusing and meaningless nomenclature have weakened many more recent prevalence studies. The field must also grapple with a history of the exclusion of vulnerable populations, including racial and ethnic minorities and people who are incarcerated or homeless. For the field to move ahead, a culture of inclusion is needed. Moving forward, researchers should consider how their studies can include racial and ethnic minorities and vulnerable populations and ensure that the research principle of justice is central to the design of the study from the start.

References

Alegria AA, Petry NM, Hasin DS, et al: Disordered gambling among racial and ethnic groups in the US: results from the National Epidemiologic Survey on Alcohol and Related Conditions. CNS Spectr 14(3):132–143, 2009

Alvarez-Moya EM, Jiménez-Murcia S, Aymamí MN, et al:Subtyping study of a pathological gamblers sample. Can J Psychiatry 55(8):498–506,.2010

American Psychiatric Association: Diagnostic and Statistical Manual of Mental Disorders, 4th Edition. Arlington, VA, American Psychiatric Association, 1994

American Psychiatric Association: Diagnostic and Statistical Manual of Mental Disorders, 5th Edition. Arlington, VA, American Psychiatric Association, 2013a

American Psychiatric Association: Insurance implications of DSM-5. Psychiatr News, May 3, 2013b. Available at: https://psychnews.psychiatryonline.org/doi/full/10.1176/appi.pn.2013.5a27. Accessed July 28, 2020.

Billi R, Stone CA, Abbott M, Yeung K: The Victorian Gambling Study (VGS), a longitudinal study of gambling and health in Victoria 2008–2012: design and methods. Int J Ment Health Addict 13(2):274–296, 2015

Blaszczynski A, Nower L: A pathways model of problem and pathological gambling. Addiction 97(5):487–499, 2002

Cottler LB, Zipp JF, Robins LN, Spitznagel EL: Difficult-to-recruit respondents and their effect on prevalence estimates in an epidemiologic survey. Am J Epidemiol 125(2):329–339, 1987

Cunningham-Williams RM, Cottler LB, Compton III WM, Spitznagel EL: Taking chances: problem gamblers and mental health disorders—results from the St. Louis Epidemiologic Catchment Area Study. Am J Public Health 88(7):1093–1096, 1998

el-Guebaly N, Casey DM, Currie SR, et al: The Leisure, Lifestyle, and Lifecycle Project (LLLP): a longitudinal study of gambling in Alberta. Calgary, Alberta, Canada, Alberta Gambling Research Institute, 2015

Ferris JA, Wynne HJ: The Canadian Problem Gambling Index. Ottawa, ON, Canadian Centre on Substance Abuse, 2001

Frances AJ, Nardo JM: ICD-11 should not repeat the mistakes made by DSM-5. Br J Psychiatry 203(1):1–2, 2013

Gebauer L, LaBrie R, Shaffer HJ: Optimizing DSM-IV-TR classification accuracy: a brief biosocial screen for detecting current gambling disorders among gamblers in the general household population. Can J Psychiatry 55(2):82–90, 2010

Grant JE, Chamberlain SR, Schreiber LRN, Odlaug BL: Gender-related clinical and neurocognitive differences in individuals seeking treatment for pathological gambling. J Psychiatr Res 46(9):1206–1211, 2012

Jackson AC, Wynne H, Dowling NA, et al: Using the CPGI to determine problem gambling prevalence in Australia: measurement issues. Int J Ment Health Addict 8(4):570–582, 2010

John WS, Wu L-T: Trends and correlates of cocaine use and cocaine use disorder in the United States from 2011 to 2015. Drug Alcohol Depend 180:376–384, 2017

Kessler RC, Merikangas KR: The National Comorbidity Survey Replication (NCS-R): background and aims. Int J Methods Psychiatr Res 13(2):60–68, 2004

Kessler RC, McGonagle KA, Zhao S, et al: Lifetime and 12-month prevalence of DSM-III-R psychiatric disorders in the United States: results from the National Comorbidity Survey. Arch Gen Psychiatry 51(1):8–19, 1994

Kessler RC, Chiu WT, Demler O, Walters EE: Prevalence, severity, and comorbidity of 12-month DSM-IV disorders in the National Comorbidity Survey Replication. Arch Gen Psychiatry 62(6):617–627, 2005

Kessler RC, Hwang I, LaBrie R, et al: DSM-IV pathological gambling in the National Comorbidity Survey Replication. Psychol Med 38(9):1351–1360, 2008

Koh HK, Piotrowski JJ, Kumanyika S, Fielding JE: Healthy People: a 2020 vision for the social determinants approach. Health Educ Behav 38(6):551–557, 2011

Lesieur HR, Blume SB: The South Oaks Gambling Screen (SOGS): a new instrument for the identification of pathological gamblers. Am J Psychiatry 144(9):1184–1188, 1987

Mazar A, Williams RJ, Stanek EJ, et al: The importance of friends and family to recreational gambling, at-risk gambling, and problem gambling. BMC Public Health 18(1):1080, 2018

Merkouris SS, Thomas AC, Shandley KA, et al: An update on gender differences in the characteristics associated with problem gambling: a systematic review. Curr Addict Rep 3(3):254–267, 2016

Milosevic A, Ledgerwood DM: The subtyping of pathological gambling: a comprehensive review. Clin Psychol Rev 30(8):988–998, 2010

National Commission for the Protection of Human Subjects of Biomedical and Behavioral Research: The Belmont Report: Ethical Principles and Guidelines for the Protection of Human Subjects of Research, Vol 2. Washington, DC, U.S. Department of Health and Human Services, 1978

National Institutes of Health: Guiding principles for ethical research. June 3, 2015. Bethesda, MD, National Institutes of Health. Available at: www.nih.gov/health-information/nih-clinical-research-trials-you/guiding-principles-ethical-research. Accessed July 28, 2020.

Ortiz V, Hernández H: Responsible gambling: public health and social justice considerations to inform research, policy, and practice, in Responsible Gambling: Primary Stakeholders Perspective. Edited by Shaffer HJ, Blaszczynski A, Ladouceur R, et al. New York, Oxford University Press, 2019, pp 111–131

Petry NM, Blanco C, Auriacombe M, et al: An overview of and rationale for changes proposed for pathological gambling in DSM-5. J Gambl Stud 30(2):493–502, 2014

Robins LN, Regier DA: Psychiatric disorders in America: The Epidemiologic Catchment Area Study. J Psychiatry Neurosci 17(1):34–36, 1992

Robins LN, Helzer JE, Croughan J, Ratcliff KS: National Institute of Mental Health Diagnostic Interview Schedule: its history, characteristics, and validity. Arch Gen Psychiatry 38(4):381–389, 1981

Shaffer HJ, Hall MN, Vander Bilt J: Estimating the prevalence of disordered gambling behavior in the United States and Canada: a research synthesis. Am J Public Health 89(9):1369–1376, 1999

Smith NDL, Cottler LB: The epidemiology of post-traumatic stress disorder and alcohol use disorder. Alcohol Res Curr Rev 39(2):113–120, 2018

Vaeth PAC, Wang-Schweig M, Caetano R: Drinking, alcohol use disorder, and treatment access and utilization among U.S. racial/ethnic groups. Alcohol Clin Exp Res 41(1):6–19, 2017

Wakefield JC: Psychological justice: DSM-5, false positive diagnosis, and fair equality of opportunity. Public Aff Q 29(1):32–75, 2015

Welte JW, Barnes GM, Wieczorek WF, et al: Gambling participation in the U.S.—results from a national survey. J Gambl Stud 18(4):313–337, 2002

Williams RJ, Volberg RA, Stevens RMG: The Population Prevalence of Problem Gambling. Guelph, Ontario, Canada, Ontario Problem Gambling Research Centre, 2012

Williams RJ, Hann R, Schopflocher D, et al: Quinte Longitudinal Study of Gambling and Problem Gambling. Guelph, Ontario, Canada, Ontario Problem Gambling Research Centre, 2015

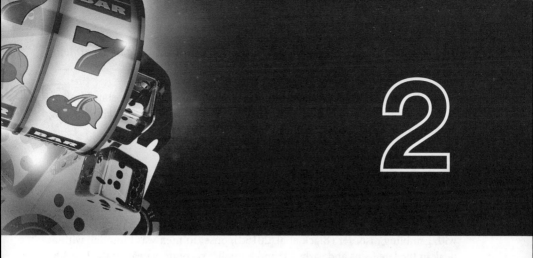

Clinical Characteristics

Donald W. Black, M.D.

Mary, a 42-year-old accountant, had gambled recreationally for years. At age 38 years, for reasons she cannot explain, she became hooked on casino slot machines. Her interest in gambling gradually escalated, and within a year Mary was gambling during most business days. She also gambled most weekends, telling her husband she was at work. To acquire money for gambling, Mary created a fake company to which she transferred nearly $300,000 from her accounting firm. The embezzlement was eventually detected, and Mary was arrested. After her arrest and the associated public humiliation, Mary became severely depressed and attempted suicide by drug overdose. After a brief hospital stay, Mary entered counseling and was prescribed paroxetine. In a plea bargain, she agreed to perform 400 hours of community service.

Like Mary in the case vignette above, many individuals struggle with gambling disorder and its consequences. Gambling led her to commit criminal acts that never would have occurred but for the disorder. Mary's case also illustrates the tendency of women to start recreational gambling later in life than men, often in their early 30s (Black et al. 2015d; Grant and Kim 2002; Tavares et al. 2001). Women tend to have a more rapid progression from recreational gambling to disorder, a phenomenon known as *telescoping*. In one study, the time interval from recreational gambling to disorder averaged 1 year in women and 4.6 years in men (Tavares et al. 2001). Gender differences are discussed more fully in Chapter 4 ("Gender Differences").

In this chapter, I describe gambling disorder and its many important clinical aspects, including onset, course, suicidality, phenomenology, illegal behavior, emotional consequences, and comorbidity.

Age at Onset

Age at onset for gambling disorder usually ranges from the mid-20s to the late 30s but can occur for the first time in older adults. In a study of 255 participants with gambling disorder (Black et al. 2015d), onset in men was bimodal, with a peak in the late teens and early 20s and a smaller secondary peak in the late 30s and early 40s. For women, the higher peak occurred in the 40s, with the smaller secondary peak in the 20s. Mean age at onset was 34 years, with men having an earlier onset than women (28 years vs. 42 years), a finding consistent with a large body of work on gambling disorder and gender differences. Fifty percent of the sample had an onset by age 30 years, 70% by age 40 years, and 84% by age 50 years. These data are compatible with clinical data reported by other investigative teams. For example, whereas Grant and Kim (2001) reported a mean age at onset of 36.8 years among 131 treatment-seeking people with gambling disorder, Grant et al. (2006) found that 207 gambling disorder participants assigned to one of four treatment cells in a medication trial had a mean age at onset ranging from 34.2 to 36.9 years.

Epidemiological surveys tend to report an earlier onset. In a general population study in Edmonton, Alberta, Bland et al. (1993) reported a mean age at onset of 25 years for people with "heavy betting." Blanco et al. (2006), in reporting data from the National Epidemiologic Study of Alcohol and Related Conditions (NESARC), calculated an earlier mean age at onset for men (29.6 years) compared with women (34.9 years). Kessler et al. (2008), reporting data from the National Comorbidity Survey—Replication, indicated that gambling disorder has a bimodal distribution, with a peak in the late teens to early 20s and a smaller secondary peak in the late 30s to early 40s.

Course

Although often considered chronic and deteriorating (American Psychiatric Association 2013), gambling disorder, as data show, has a natural ebb and flow, with many individuals moving toward reduced gambling involvement over time or even experiencing spontaneous remission. In a review of five follow-up studies (Abbott et al. 2004; DeFuentes-Merillas et al. 2004; Shaffer and Hall 2002; Slutske et al. 2003; Winters et al. 2002), LaPlante et al. (2008) concluded that most individuals with gambling disorder and at-risk gamblers move toward a lower (or less intensive) level of gambling behavior over time, but those who gamble recreationally—or do not gamble—are unlikely to move to a more severe level of gambling activity or to take up gambling. Slutske (2006) found that more than one-third of persons reporting lifetime gambling disorder in the Gambling Impact and Behavior (National Opinion Research Center 1999) and NESARC (Petry et al. 2005) studies had no gambling-related problems in the past year. The absence of past-year symptoms in one-third of the individuals was characterized as "natural recovery," leading Slutske to conclude that gambling disorder is not always chronic. Sartor et al. (2007) evaluated gambling characteristics retrospectively in 1,343 men from the Vietnam Era Twin Registry; in this sample, 268 developed symptoms suggestive of gambling disorder, and 35 had symptoms that met criteria for gambling disorder. Those with gambling disorder first met criteria at age 21 years and first sought treatment at age 29 years. They experienced five or more gambling "phases" (defined as a "consistent pattern of gambling behavior"); whereas 17% of these individuals also reported periods of abstinence, 43% reported five or more symptom-free gambling phases.

In a systematic follow-up study, Black et al. (2017) rated the gambling behaviors of three groups of participants every 6 months for up to 5 years (mean= 2.6 years), including individuals with gambling disorder age 60 years or older, individuals with gambling disorder younger than 40 years, and individuals age 60 years or older who had no evidence of gambling problems. Week-by-week gambling activity showed a significant downward trend for older and younger individuals with gambling disorder. Older adult control participants without gambling problems had no change in their level of gambling activity. Nearly 50% of persons with gambling disorder experienced periods of spontaneous remission.

Other follow-up data suggest that individuals with gambling disorder who have comorbid disorders, impaired decision-making, or poor social support have a more severe course. Russo et al. (1984) reported that 1-year remission rates following a treatment program for veterans were associated with less depression. Taber et al. (1987) conducted a 6-month follow-up of 57 of 66 patients (86%) who completed a comprehensive treatment program; 56% reported total abstinence and had improved on measures of alcohol abuse, suicidal behavior, and overall distress. Goudriaan et al. (2008) compared a group of persons with gambling disorder who had relapsed and a group who had not and found that those who relapsed performed worse on indicators of disinhibition (stop-signal reaction time) and decision-making (card playing task), suggesting that neurocognitive measures may be important tools in predicting progression and relapse.

Suicidal Ideations and Behaviors

People with gambling disorder tend to consider suicide and attempt suicide at rates much higher than in the general population, with completed suicide perhaps the most worrisome outcome (Black et al. 2015c; Blaszczynski and Farrell 1998). Much evidence supporting a link to suicide comes from clinical samples. In a sample of 114 consecutive admissions to a Veterans Administration gambling treatment program, Kausch (2003) reported that nearly 40% of participants had past suicide attempts, two-thirds of the attempts prompted by gambling-related problems. Ledgerwood and Petry (2004) found that of 125 persons, 48% had a history of gambling-related suicidal ideation, and 12% reported a past gambling-related suicide attempt. In another treatment-seeking sample, Battersby et al. (2006) reported even higher rates of suicidal ideation and attempts among 43 treatment-seeking people with gambling disorder (81% and 30%, respectively).

Data from a recent study show that suicidal ideation and suicide attempts occur at rates substantially greater in people with gambling disorder than among control participants (Black et al. 2015c). Ninety-five participants with gambling disorder and 91 control participants were assessed as part of a family study. There were significant differences in the prevalence of lifetime suicidal ideation (27% vs. 9%) and lifetime suicide attempts (36% vs. 4%) between participants with gambling disorder and control participants. Whereas half of those who attempted suicide made a single attempt, the other half made more than one attempt.

Phenomenology

Early descriptions of addictive gambling were influenced by the observations of Custer (1984), who described gambling disorder as a progressive, multistage illness that began with a winning phase that was followed by a losing phase and finally a desperation phase. The initial, or "winning," phase conferred feelings of status, power, and omnipotence. Fantasies of winning and thoughts of great successes were proposed to be common in this phase.

A string of bad luck or an unexpected loss was proposed to then lead to the second, or "losing," phase. For some, the development of gambling disorder might be precipitated by a major life stressor (Lesieur and Rosenthal 1991). The losing phase centers on the behavior known as "chasing," in which the gambler desperately attempts to recover lost money. Wagering is more frequent and often involves larger amounts. The uncontrollable spiraling of losing and chasing losses was proposed to lead the gambler to the third, or "desperation," phase. Here, the gambler may engage in illegal activities such as fraud, embezzlement, writing bad checks, or stealing to support his gambling problem. Illegal behaviors are rationalized, often with the intent to pay back what is taken after the "big win" that is thought by the gambler to be in their imminent and eminent future. Fantasies of escape and thoughts of suicide are reported to be common during this phase (Lesieur and Rosenthal 1991).

Data-based descriptions have confirmed many of these early observations. Grant and Kim (2001) described the clinical characteristics of a sample of 131 treatment-seeking pathological gamblers. Mean age was 31 years; mean length of time from initial gambling to onset of pathological gambling was 6 years, with a range from 0 to 33 years. Nearly 50% of the participants progressed to gambling disorder within 1 year of beginning gambling; later onset of gambling disorder and the acknowledgment of gambling urges triggered by advertisements correlated with rapid progression. On average, participants gambled about 16 hours per week and had lost nearly 45% of their income to gambling during the previous year. Their mean South Oaks Gambling Screen score (Lesieur and Blume 1987) was 14 (a score of 5 or higher indicates probable gambling disorder). All but one participant reported unsuccessful attempts to quit gambling, and 87% reported chasing their losses. More than 80% reported gambling to escape dysphoria. Gamblers frequently reported lying to family and friends (44%), borrowing money to pay bills or buy food (30%), and reaching maximum credit limits (64%).

Illegal Behavior

Although complicated, an association between crime and gambling disorder is well established (Rosenthal and Lorenz 1992). The prevalence of criminal activity among persons with gambling disorder has been estimated to be between 20% and 80% (Blaszczynski et al. 1989; Brown 1987). In a sample of 109 treatment-seeking problem gamblers, 55% reported having committed gambling-related offenses, and 21% reported having been charged with a crime (Blaszczynski et al. 1989). The authors found a fourfold increase in gambling-related illegal behaviors (e.g., offenses designed to obtain money for gambling purposes). Illegal behaviors reported include writing bad checks and engaging in embezzlement, larceny, tax fraud, or prostitution in women (Rosenthal 1992).

Despite the existence of a relationship between criminality and gambling, a causal nature of the relationship is still unclear. In the progression of gambling disorder, some gamblers (including Mary in the vignette presented earlier) resort to illegal acts to finance gambling or to pay outstanding debts. The addictive nature of gambling disorder may represent an important criminogenic factor (Meyer and Stadler 1999). Other work suggests that the need to maintain gambling is the primary motivation for criminal behavior (Lesieur 1979). As the gambler chases losses and exhausts legitimate sources of money, he or she often resorts to criminal behavior. As losses increase, the pressure to offend increases (Blaszczynski et al. 1989). In fact, gambling-related offenses may be associated with severity of gambling disorder, as demonstrated by involvement with multiple forms of gambling, owing debts to acquaintances, acknowledging gambling-related suicidality, reporting excessive substance use, and having received mental health treatment (Potenza et al. 2000).

Although an association exists between criminality and gambling disorder, personality features might mediate the relationship. Antisocial personality disorder (ASPD) is more frequently found in pathological gamblers than in the general population (Black et al. 2015a; Cunningham-Williams et al. 1998). Problem gamblers reporting gambling-related arrest or incarceration were more likely to have features consistent with ASPD (Potenza et al. 2000). High rates of gambling disorder have been reported in prison settings. In a study of prison inmates in Nevada, 26% were considered to be probable pathological gamblers (Templer et al. 1993).

Emotional Consequences

Gambling disorder can adversely influence multiple life domains, including social, financial, professional, and personal (National Opinion Research Center 1999). Persons may begin gambling as an enjoyable pastime or as a means of socialization. As gambling progresses, people with gambling disorder may isolate themselves. Many persons with gambling disorder experience a loss of control or feelings of guilt or shame related to their gambling. A study of 131 pathological gamblers found that more than 15% reported gambling-related marital problems (Grant and Kim 2001). Gambling disorder can contribute to an erosion of the trust of family members, particularly that of the spouse, leading to diminished intimacy (Moody 1990). Gambling disorder is well documented to contribute to chaos and dysfunction within the family unit; can disrupt marriages, leading to high rates of separation and divorce; and is associated with child abuse and neglect. Divorce rates are high, which is not surprising considering reports that these marriages are often abusive (Shaw et al. 2007).

Gambling disorder often leads to work-related problems. Gambling urges may be frequent and difficult to control, resulting in absenteeism, poor performance, and job loss (National Opinion Research Center 1999). The loss of financial support associated with job loss can lead to desperate attempts to obtain funds, including exhausting one's own savings while chasing. Bankruptcy filings are relatively common (Potenza et al. 2000). In one study, 44% of persons with gambling disorder reported having no savings or retirement funds, and 22% described losing their homes or automobiles or pawning valuables to cover gambling losses (Grant and Kim 2001).

Psychiatric Comorbidity

Psychiatric comorbidity is the rule for persons with gambling disorder. In community surveys and clinic-based reports, mood and anxiety disorders, substance use disorders (SUDs), ADHD, impulse-control disorders (ICDs), and personality disorders are frequently comorbid with gambling disorder (Black et al. 2014; Crockford and el-Guebaly 1998). Findings from research studies are reported in Tables 2–1 and 2–2.

TABLE 2–1. Comorbid major psychiatric disorders in persons with gambling disorder

Study	Sample size (n)	Assessment method	Mood disorders	Psychotic disorders	ADHD	OCD	SUDs	Eating disorders	ICDs	Anxiety disorders	No disorder
McCormick et al. 1984	50	RDC	76%	N/A	N/A	N/A	36%	N/A	N/A	N/A	N/A
Linden et al. 1986	25	SCID-III	72%	N/A	N/A	20%	48%	N/A	N/A	28%	N/A
Bland et al. 1993	30	DIS	33%	0%	N/A	17%	63%	N/A	N/A	27%	N/A
Specker et al. 1995	40	Operationalized Diagnostic Interview for ADHD; MIDI	N/A	N/A	20%	N/A	N/A	N/A	35%	N/A	N/A
Specker et al. 1996	40	SCID-III-R	78%	3%	N/A	3%	60%	N/A	N/A	38%	8%
Black and Moyer 1998	30	DIS	60%	3%	40%	10%	63%	7%	43%	40%	N/A
Cunningham-Williams et al. 1998	161	DIS	MDD (9%); dysthymia (4%)	4%	N/A	1%	Alcohol (45%); illicit drugs (40%)	N/A	N/A	PD (23%); GAD (8%); phobias (15%)	N/A
Hollander et al. 1998	10	N/A	30%: bipolar I and II*	*	20%	10%	Current*	N/A	N/A	N/A	50%

TABLE 2–1. Comorbid major psychiatric disorders in persons with gambling disorder (*continued*)

Study	Sample size (*n*)	Assessment method	Mood disorders	Psychotic disorders	ADHD	OCD	SUDs	Eating disorders	ICDs	Anxiety disorders	No anxiety disorder
Hollander et al. 2000	10	N/A	50%	N/A	N/A	10%	10%	N/A	N/A	20%	N/A
Grant and Kim 2001	131	SCID-IV	34%	N/A	N/A	0%	35%	N/A	18%	9%	N/A
Zimmerman et al. 2002	15	SCID-IV; DID; BDI	53% mania*	*	N/A	N/A	Current*	N/A	N/A	20%	N/A
Petry et al. 2005	195	AUDADIS-IV	50%	N/A	N/A	N/A	73% AUD	N/A	N/A	41%	N/A
Zimmerman et al. 2006	40	SCID-IV	62.5% MDD	5%	5%	10%	67.5%	17.5%	20%	42.5% PD	N/A
Kessler et al. 2008	21	CIDI	56%	N/A	13%	N/A	76%	N/A	42%	60%	N/A
Park et al. 2010	43	DIS	12%	N/A	N/A	N/A	70%	N/A	N/A	14%	N/A
Black et al. 2014	95	SCID-IV	72%	N/A	N/A	13%	68%	14%	N/A	51%	N/A

Note. AUD=alcohol use disorder; AUDADIS-IV=Alcohol Use Disorder and Associated Disabilities Interview Schedule–IV; BDI=Beck Depression Inventory; CIDI=Composite International Diagnostic Interview; DID=dissociative identity disorder; DIS=Diagnostic Interview Schedule; GAD=generalized anxiety disorder; ICD=impulse-control disorder; MDD=major depressive disorder; MIDI=Minnesota Impulse Disorders Interview; OCD=obsessive-compulsive disorder; PD=panic disorder; RDC=Research Diagnostic Criteria; SCID-III=Structured Clinical Inventory for DSM-III; SCID-III-R=Structured Clinical Inventory for DSM-III-R; SCID-IV=Structured Clinical Interview for DSM-IV; SUD=substance use disorder.
*Excluded condition.

TABLE 2–2. Comorbid personality disorders in persons with gambling disorder

Study	Sample size	Assessment method	Any PD	Paranoid	Schizoid	Schizotypal	BPD
Blaszczynski et al. 1989	109	DSM-III criteria	N/A	N/A	N/A	N/A	14%
Lesieur and Blume 1990	7	N/A	71%	N/A	N/A	28%	N/A
Bellarie and Caspari 1992	51	N/A	N/A	N/A	N/A	N/A	N/A
Bland et al. 1993	30	DIS	N/A	N/A	N/A	N/A	N/A
Specker et al. 1996	40	SCID-P, SCID-II	25%	3%	3%	0%	3%
Black and Moyer 1998	30	PDQ-R	87%	26%	33%	30%	23%
Blaszczynski and Steel 1998	82	PDQ-R	93%	40%	21%	38%	70%
Fernandez-Montalvo and Echeburua 2004	50	IPDE	32%	8%	0%	0%	16%
Petry et al. 2005	195	AUDADIS-IV	N/A	24%	15%	N/A	N/A
Bagby et al. 2008	61	SCID-II-PQ/SCID-II	92%/23%	30%/5%	15%/3%	20%/0%	62%/10%
Pelletier and Ladaceur 2008	100	SCID-II	64%	18%	4%	3%	10%
Odlaug et al. 2012	77	SCID-II	46%	3%	1%	0%	7%
Black et al. 2015a	93	SIDP	41%	7%	1%	1%	19%

TABLE 2–2. Comorbid personality disorders in persons with gambling disorder *(continued)*

Study *(continued)*	Histrionic	Narcissistic	Avoidant	OCPD	ASPD	Dependent	Unspecified
Blaszczynski et al. 1989	N/A	N/A	N/A	N/A	N/A	N/A	14%
Lesieur and Blume 1990	N/A	N/A	N/A	N/A	N/A	N/A	49%
Bellarie and Caspari 1992	N/A	N/A	N/A	N/A	15%	N/A	N/A
Bland et al. 1993	N/A	N/A	N/A	N/A	40%	N/A	N/A
Specker et al. 1996	0%	5%	13%	5%	0%	5%	3%
Black and Moyer 1998	7%	20%	50%	59%	17%	7%	N/A
Blaszczynski and Steel 1998	66%	57%	37%	32%	29%	49%	N/A
Fernandez-Montalvo and Echeburua 2004	0%	8%	0%	0%	8%	0%	8%
Petry et al. 2005	13%	N/A	14%	28%	23%	3%	N/A
Bagby et al. 2008	26%/0%	53%/0%	26%/5%	64%/5%	35%/5%	3%/0%	N/A
Pelletier and Ladaceur 2008	1%	15%	10%	16%	29%	3%	27%
Odlaug et al. 2012	4%	5%	10%	27%	3%	4%	0%
Black et al. 2015a	2%	6%	6%	10%	15%	6%	N/A

Note. ASPD=antisocial personality disorder; AUDADIS-IV = Alcohol Use Disorder and Associated Disabilities Interview Schedule–IV; BPD=borderline personality disorder; DIS=Diagnostic Interview Schedule; IPDE=International Personality Disorder Examination; OCPD=obsessive-compulsive personality disorder; PDQ-R = Personality Diagnostic Questionnaire—Revised; PD=personality disorder; SCID-P=Structured Clinical Interview for DSM-III-R–Personality Disorders; SCID-II=Structured Clinical Interview for DSM-IV Personality Disorders; SCID-II-PQ=Structured Clinical Interview for DSM-IV Personality Disorders—Personality Questionnaire; SIDP=Structured Interview for DSM-IV Personality.

Substance Use Disorders

Lifetime alcohol or drug dependence is the best-documented group of comorbid disorders in persons with gambling disorder. Two large studies have addressed this issue, showing a strong association between gambling disorder and SUDs. Welte et al. (2001) found that 28% of persons with gambling disorder had current alcohol dependence, compared with a rate of 1% for people without gambling disorder. The National Opinion Research Center study found that among persons with gambling disorder, the rate of alcohol or drug abuse was nearly seven times higher than that among nongamblers or recreational gamblers (National Opinion Research Center 1999). Other surveys have shown that rates of alcohol abuse and dependence are four or more times higher among persons identified as having a gambling disorder compared with those without gambling disorder (Bland et al. 1993; Cunningham-Williams et al. 1998). In a nationally representative sample, almost three-quarters (73.2%) of individuals with gambling disorder had an alcohol use disorder (Petry et al. 2005). As many as 30%–50% of persons with gambling disorder seeking treatment were reported to have lifetime histories of alcohol or other substance abuse (Lesieur et al. 1986). Rosenthal (1992) observed that the use of alcohol or illicit drugs while a person gambles can lead to deterioration in cognitive abilities and judgment, which, Rosenthal believes, may cause gambling disorder to progress more rapidly. Although in some cases gambling disorder may predate the onset of substance misuse, psychopathology typically precedes the onset of gambling disorder (Kessler et al. 2008).

The National Opinion Research Center (1999) study found that 8.1% of persons with gambling disorder and 16.8% of persons with problem gambling reported illicit drug use in the past year, compared with 4.2% of recreational gamblers and 2% of nongamblers. Bland et al. (1993) similarly found that the prevalence of illegal drug abuse and dependence for individuals with gambling disorder was about four times higher than for people who do not gamble. In the study by Cunningham-Williams et al. (1998), 15.5% of individuals with gambling disorder evidenced illegal drug use disorders, compared with 7.8% of recreational gamblers and 3.5% of nongamblers. Among NESARC respondents with gambling disorder, the lifetime prevalence rate for any drug use disorder was 38.1% (Petry et al. 2005). Conversely, 9% to 16% of substance abusers are likely to have gambling disorder (Lesieur et al. 1986; Spunt et al. 1998).

The frequency of addictions is also high in treatment-seeking individuals with gambling disorder. Zimmerman et al. (2002) found that 67.5% of treatment-seeking individuals with gambling disorder had a SUD, compared with 40.1% of psychiatric outpatients without gambling disorder. Among research subjects, Black et al. (2014) reported that 68% of treatment-seeking individuals with gambling disorder had a lifetime SUD, compared with 27% of control participants. Several differences emerge from looking at treatment-seeking individuals with gambling disorder with and without a history of substance misuse. Those with a history of a SUD have greater psychiatric distress, experience more frequent gambling, have more years of disordered gambling, and are more likely to receive mental health treatment (Ladd and Petry 2003).

Cunningham-Williams et al. (1998) reported, on the basis of data from the Epidemiologic Catchment Area survey, that problem gambling occurred within 2 years of the onset of alcoholism in 65% of gambling cases. Individuals with gambling disorder may use alcohol or other drugs when they stop gambling; similarly, gambling may serve as a substitute for alcohol and other drugs to prolong feelings of exhilaration from gambling or ameliorate the dysphoria that develops during gambling abstinence (Lesieur and Blume 1990).

Mood Disorders

Multiple general population surveys have investigated the association between specific psychiatric comorbidities and disordered gambling, including major depression, dysthymia, bipolar disorder, and suicidality. Bland et al. (1993) found elevated rates of mood disorders in individuals with gambling disorder (33.3%) compared with nongamblers (14.2%). Rates of major depression were also higher for individuals with gambling problems in the sample reported by Cunningham-Williams et al. (1998). Interestingly, these investigators also found that recreational gamblers appear to be at greater risk for major depression and dysthymia than those who have never gambled. Neither of these two surveys found a significant association between gambling disorder and mania. In the NESARC survey, 49.6% of persons with gambling disorder had a mood disorder (Petry et al. 2005). Furthermore, the investigators in this study showed that mania was the mood disturbance most strongly related to gambling disorder, with an odds ratio (OR) of 8. ORs for major depression and dysthymia were each 3.3, and hypomania was 1.8.

Clinical studies also show a relationship between mood disorders and gambling disorder. In an early study, 76% of an inpatient sample admitted for treatment of gambling disorder had symptoms that met criteria for a current major depressive disorder (McCormick et al. 1984). In a sample of 25 problem gamblers recruited from a Gamblers Anonymous chapter, Linden et al. (1986) found that 72% of subjects had experienced at least one episode of major depression. Bipolar disorder has also been reported at high rates in persons with gambling disorder. Whereas Linden et al. (1986) reported a lifetime prevalence of 24% in persons with gambling disorder, McCormick et al. (1984) found current hypomania in 38% of an inpatient sample. Mood disorders are also relatively common in the treatment-seeking segment of the gambling disorder population. Stinchfield and Winters (2001), for example, found that 12% of their 592 gambling disorder treatment seekers also had a current mood disorder. Black et al. (2014) systematically assessed gambling disorder subjects for a family study and found that 72% had a lifetime history of a mood disorder, compared with 30% of control participants. The most common mood disorders were major depression (61%) and bipolar disorder (9%).

Anxiety Disorders

Persons with gambling disorder also report high rates of lifetime anxiety disorders, such as panic disorder, phobias, obsessive-compulsive disorder (OCD), generalized anxiety disorder (GAD), and PTSD. General population surveys show a strong association between gambling disorder and anxiety disorders. Kessler et al. (2008) found that 60.3% of their sample had any anxiety disorder, with 52.2% having phobias, 21.9% panic disorder, 16.6% GAD, and 14.8% PTSD. Furthermore, these authors found that gambling disorder is temporally predicted by panic disorder, GAD, and phobia. Petry et al. (2005) reported that panic disorder with and without agoraphobia was most strongly related to gambling disorder; the odds of having phobias or GAD were significant but less so. Cunningham-Williams et al. (1998) also found the highest percentage of subjects experiencing panic disorder (23.3%), followed by phobias (14.6%), GAD (7.7%), and OCD (7.7%). Likewise, Bland et al. (1993) found that persons diagnosed with gambling disorder had high rates of anxiety disorders. These authors reported lifetime rates of 26.7% for GAD, 17.7% for phobias, 3.3% for panic disorder, and 16.7% for OCD.

In their sample of 43 treatment-seeking outpatients, Ibáñez et al. (2001) reported a lifetime rate for GAD of 7.2%, much lower than the 40% reported by Black and Moyer (1998) or 37.5% reported by Specker et al. (1996). Black and Moyer (1998) also reported rates of panic disorder and OCD at 10% each, but Specker et al. (1996) reported 20% and 2.5%, respectively. Although samples and rates differ somewhat, there remains little doubt that gambling disorder and anxiety disorders share a relationship, although the relationship with OCD seems less clear.

Some investigators (Blaszczynski 1999; Hollander 1993) believe that gambling disorder falls within the obsessive-compulsive spectrum. They point to similarities between gambling disorder and OCD, as exemplified by persistent thoughts and urges followed by repetitive behaviors. Differences include the person's attitude toward the behavior; with OCD, the person reports that obsessions and compulsions are unwanted, yet with gambling disorder, the behavior is generally perceived as pleasurable. Comorbidity studies suggest that from 2.5% (Specker et al. 1996) to 20% (Linden et al. 1986) of persons with gambling disorder also have OCD. In two family studies of OCD in which gambling disorder was also assessed (Bienvenu et al. 2000; Black et al. 2013b), the findings did not support a relationship between the disorders.

Attention-Deficit/Hyperactivity Disorder

Gambling disorder has several attributes in common with ADHD, and clinical data suggest substantial syndromal overlap. Carlton and Manowitz (1992) compared persons with gambling disorder with persons with alcoholism and reported excessive and comparable levels of ADHD-related behaviors in child-hood for these two groups compared with control subjects. Rugle and Melamed (1993) compared 33 non-substance-abusing persons with gambling disorder with 33 nonaddicted control subjects on nine attention measures and childhood behavior questionnaires. They reported that individuals with gambling disor-der performed significantly worse than control subjects on higher-order atten-tional measures and had more childhood behaviors consistent with ADHD. They concluded that attentional deficits and the behavior problems associated with them are long-standing and may be a risk factor for the development of gambling disorder.

Specker et al. (1995) reported that 8 of 40 (20%) people with gambling dis-order met criteria for ADHD, and another 7 (17.5%) had symptoms that were considered subthreshold. These authors hypothesized that ADHD may predis-pose individuals to either substance abuse or gambling disorder and that gam-blers with attentional deficits might chose gambling activities that do not require sustained attention or concentration. Finally, Kessler et al. (2008) found in their general population survey that 13.4% of persons with gambling disor-der also had ADHD. Black et al. (2013a) showed that among 54 individuals with gambling disorder, ADHD symptoms were significantly more common than in 65 control subjects. The most pronounced differences observed for individual items from the ADHD Checklist (Achenbach 1991) were "difficulty sustaining attention" and "blurts out answers." In a series of medication trials, these inves-tigators also showed that ADHD symptoms subside when gambling disorder is successfully treated (Black et al. 2007a, 2007b).

Impulsivity, an important attribute of ADHD, is also reportedly common among persons with gambling disorder. Castellani and Rugle (1995) evaluated 843 subjects admitted to an inpatient addictions unit having a primary diagno-sis of gambling disorder, alcohol dependence, or cocaine abuse. In contrast to individuals with alcoholism and cocaine abuse, those with gambling disorder scored significantly higher on measures of impulsivity, such as coming to quick decisions, moving quickly from impulse to action, and lack of future planning. In the study of Black et al. (2013a), one-third of individuals with gambling dis-order were highly impulsive and had a total Barratt Impulsiveness Scale (BIS; Barratt 1959) score of ≥72, compared with 8% of control subjects. The BIS total score among individuals with gambling disorder was highly correlated with gambling severity.

Impulse-Control Disorders

Lifetime rates of ICDs also appear to be higher in persons with gambling dis-order than seen in the general population. Investigators have reported rates ranging from 18% to 43% for one or more of the ICDs (Black and Moyer 1998; Grant and Kim 2001, 2002; Specker et al. 1995). Specker et al. (1995) examined frequencies of ICDs in a treatment-seeking sample and found increased levels of compulsive shopping and sexual behaviors, intermittent explosive disorder, and kleptomania. Black and Moyer (1998) also found high frequencies of compulsive buying (23%), compulsive sexual behavior (17%), and intermittent explosive disorder (13%) in their sample. Grant and Kim (2002) reported lower frequencies with a larger sample, with 9% having compulsive sexual behavior, 8% having compulsive shopping, and just 2% reporting intermittent explosive disorder.

Compulsive shopping appears to be the most frequent comorbid ICD in persons with gambling disorder (Black et al. 2015b; Grant and Kim 2001, 2002; Specker et al. 1995), perhaps because, as Specker et al. suggest, both compulsive shopping and gambling disorder share characteristics of focused attention, monetary gratification, and monetary exchange. In their recent family study, Black et al. (2015b) found that the presence of gambling disorder increased the odds of having compulsive shopping nearly 12-fold.

Personality Disorders

Personality disorders are relatively common in persons with gambling disorder (Table 2–2), but prevalence is highly dependent on the study population and assessment method (Vaddiparti and Cottler 2017). Studies that use self-report instruments often yield higher rates for personality disorders than studies using structured or semi-structured interviews. For example, the prevalence estimates for personality disorders among people with gambling disorder assessed with self-report instruments ranged from 87% to 93%, compared with 25% to 61% for those assessed with a structured or semistructured interview (Bagby et al. 2008).

Data from the NESARC (Petry et al. 2005) showed a robust association between gambling disorder and all the personality disorders studied; the odds of having any personality disorder if one also has gambling disorder were 8.3 times greater than for the general population. The OR of having histrionic personality disorder was 6.9; avoidant personality disorder, 6.5; paranoid personality disorder, 6.1; ASPD, 6.0; dependent personality disorder, 5.5; schizoid personality disorder, 5.0; and obsessive-compulsive personality disorder, 4.6.

ASPD, characterized by a pervasive pattern of poor social conformity, deceitfulness, and lack of remorse, occurs at relatively high rates among those with gambling disorder, perhaps because the two are associated with criminality (Brown 1987). In studies using structured assessments, rates of ASPD have ranged from 3% to 40% (Black and Moyer 1998; Bland et al. 1993; Blaszczynski and Steel 1998; Blaszczynski et al. 1989). In a large community-based study examining this relationship, Slutske et al. (2001) reported that 15% of their sample of persons with gambling disorder also had ASPD, compared with 2% of the comparison sample without gambling disorder, leading to an OR of 6.4. Pietrzak and Petry (2005) compared treatment-seeking individuals with gambling disorder with and without ASPD. Those with ASPD had more severe gambling, more medical and drug-related problems, and higher scores on symptom measures of somatization, paranoid ideation, and phobic anxiety. They were also more likely to be younger, male, less educated, and divorced or separated and to have a history of substance abuse treatment than their non-ASPD counterparts.

In a controlled study, Black et al. (2015a) reported that when structured interviews were used, personality disorders were present in over 40% of those with gambling disorder assessed. Those with a personality disorder compared with those without had more severe gambling symptoms, earlier age at gambling disorder onset, more suicide attempts, more psychiatric comorbidity, and a more robust family history of psychiatric illness. The antisocial, borderline, dependent, and paranoid types were all significantly more frequent in those with gambling disorder than in control subjects. The most common comorbid personality disorders were the borderline, antisocial, and obsessive-compulsive types.

Bagby et al. (2008) used both a self-report and a semistructured interview in their study of 204 individuals with gambling disorder. As expected, personality disorder prevalence estimates with the self-report measure were high (92%), and much lower using a structured interview (23%). These investigators found that only borderline personality disorder had consistently high and significant prevalence rates in their non-treatment-seeking samples across both types of measures. Fernandez-Montalvo and Echeburua (2004) used a structured interview in their study of 50 non-treatment-seeking individuals with gambling disorder. These authors reported that borderline personality disorder was the most prevalent personality disorder at 16%, followed by antisocial, paranoid, narcissistic, and nonspecified, which were each observed in 8% of cases. They also reported that the presence of a personality disorder was associated with greater gambling severity and more severe symptoms of anxiety, depression, and alcohol abuse.

Gambling Disorder Subtypes

There is little disagreement that gambling disorder is heterogeneous, and attempts to identify subtypes of gambling disorder have generally been unsuccessful. Moran (1970) identified five subtypes based on work with 50 individuals with gambling disorder: 1) subcultural gambling (14%), in which a person gambles to fit in with a group of his peers but later exhibits difficulty controlling gambling; 2) neurotic gambling (34%), in which gambling is motivated in response to a strained situation or an emotional problem, such as marital conflict, and subsides when the problem is resolved; 3) impulsive gambling (18%), in which gambling is accompanied by poor behavioral control; 4) psychopathic gambling (24%), in which gambling appears as an antisocial behavioral pattern; and 5) symptomatic gambling (10%), in which gambling is associated with some other mental illness, such as depression, and is considered a secondary phenomenon. Although Moran's typology is clinically useful, it has not been empirically validated, and the different subtypes are not discrete.

Steel and Blaszczynski (1996) used principal components analysis to investigate the factorial structure of gambling disorder. They identified four primary factors: psychological distress, sensation seeking, crime and liveliness, and impulsive-antisocial. The psychological distress factor was associated with female gender, suicidal ideation and behavior, and family psychiatric history, the sensation-seeking factor with a history of alcohol abuse, the crime and liveliness factor with criminal activity, and the impulsive-antisocial factor (which was described as clinically most useful) with early onset of gambling, poor job history, separation or divorce due to gambling, and highly impulsive gambling-related illegal acts. The investigators concluded that gamblers exhibiting features of impulsivity and ASPD are at greatest risk for developing adverse personal and emotional consequences.

Blaszczynski and McConaghy (1989) described those with gambling disorder as either "escape seekers" or "sensation seekers." The former tends to include older persons who gamble out of loneliness or boredom, to seek relief from depression, or to fill time, and who choose passive forms of gambling (e.g., slot machines). Often women, they gamble to relieve negative affects (e.g., anxiety, depression). In these individuals, gambling may serve as an analgesic by providing an escape from unpleasant situations. The latter group includes persons who seek stimulation and arousal to alleviate boredom or hyperarousal. For these individuals, gambling provides an intense thrill or feeling of excitement (Custer 1984).

Blaszczynski and Nower (2002) provide a conceptual framework that integrates biological, developmental, cognitive, and other determinants of disordered gambling. They identified three distinct subgroups of individuals with gambling disorder: 1) behaviorally conditioned gamblers, 2) emotionally vulnerable gamblers, and 3) antisocial, impulsive gamblers. The behaviorally conditioned gamblers have no specific predisposing psychopathology and develop gambling disorder as a result of distorted cognitions and poor judgments regarding gambling. Depression, alcohol abuse, and anxiety may result from gambling but are not causal. The emotionally vulnerable gamblers have premorbid depression or anxiety and have a history of poor coping, frequent life events, and adverse developmental experiences (e.g., childhood abuse or neglect). For these individuals, gambling serves to modulate affective states or meet other psychological needs. Finally, the antisocial, impulsive gambler is highly disturbed with features of ASPD and impulsivity, suggestive of neurological or neurochemical dysfunction. For these persons, gambling begins early in life and escalates rapidly. This subtyping scheme has received some empirical support (Ledgerwood and Petry 2006; Nower et al. 2012).

References

Abbott MW, Williams MM, Volberg RA: A prospective study of problem and regular non-problem gamblers living in the community. Subst Use Misuse 39:855–884, 2004

Achenbach TM: Manual for the Child Behavior Checklist/4-18 and 1991 Profile. Burlington, Department of Psychiatry, University of Vermont, 1991

American Psychiatric Association: Diagnostic and Statistical Manual of Mental Disorders, 5th Edition. Washington, DC, American Psychiatric Association, 2013

Bagby RM, Vachon DD, Bulmash E, Quilty LC: Personality disorders and pathological gambling: a review and re-examination of prevalence rates. J Person Disord 22:191–207, 2008

Barratt EE: Anxiety and impulsiveness related to psychomotor efficiency. Perceptual Motor Skills 9:191–198, 1959

Battersby M, Tolchard B, Scurrah M, Thomas L: Suicide ideation and behavior in people with pathological gambling attending a treatment service. Int J Ment Health Addict 4:233–246, 2006

Bellarie W, Caspari D: Diagnosis and therapy of male gamblers in a university psychiatric hospital. J Gambl Stud 8:143–150, 1992

Bienvenu OJ, Samuels JF, Riddle MA, et al: The relationship of obsessive-compulsive disorder to possible spectrum disorders—results from a family study. Biol Psychiatry 48:387–393, 2000

Black DW, Moyer T: Clinical features and psychiatric comorbidity of subjects with pathological gambling behavior. Psychiatr Serv 49:1434–1439, 1998

Black DW, Arndt S, Coryell WH, et al: Bupropion in the treatment of pathological gambling: a randomized, placebo-controlled, flexible-dose study. J Clin Psychopharmacol 27:143–150, 2007a

Black DW, Shaw M, Forbush KT, Allen J: An open-label study of escitalopram in the treatment of pathological gambling. Clin Neuropharmacol 30:206–212, 2007b

Black DW, Smith MM, Forbush KT, et al: Neuropsychological performance, impulsivity, symptoms of ADHD, and Cloninger's personality traits in pathological gambling. Addict Res Ther 21:216–226, 2013a

Black DW, Stumpf A, McCormick B, et al: A blind re-analysis of the Iowa family study of obsessive-compulsive disorder. Psychiatry Res 209:202–206, 2013b

Black DW, Coryell WC, Crowe RR, et al: A direct, controlled, blind family study of pathological gambling. J Clin Psychiatry 75:215–221, 2014

Black DW, Coryell WH, Crowe RR, et al: Personality disorders, impulsiveness, and novelty seeking in persons with DSM-IV pathological gambling and their first-degree relatives. J Gambl Stud 31:1201–1214, 2015a

Black DW, Coryell WH, Crowe RR, et al: The relationship of DSM-IV pathological gambling to compulsive buying and other possible spectrum disorders: results from the Iowa PG family study. Psychiatry Res 226:273–276, 2015b

Black DW, Coryell WH, Crowe RR, et al: Suicide ideation, suicide attempts, and completed suicide in persons with DSM-IV pathological gambling and their first-degree relatives. Suicide Life Threat Behav 45:700–709, 2015c

Black DW, Shaw M, Coryell WH, et al: Age at onset of DSM-IV pathological gambling in a non-treatment sample: early- versus later-onset. Compr Psychiatry 60:40–46, 2015d

Black DW, Coryell W, McCormick B, et al: A prospective follow-up study of younger and older subjects with pathological gambling. Psychiatry Res 256:162–168, 2017

Blanco C, Hasin DS, Petry N, et al: Sex differences in subclinical and DSM-IV pathological gambling: results from the National Comorbidity Survey on Alcohol and Related Conditions. Psychol Med 36:943–953, 2006

Bland RC, Newman SC, Orn H, Stebelsky G: Epidemiology of pathological gambling in Edmonton. Can J Psychiatry 38:108–112, 1993

Blaszczynski A: Pathological gambling and obsessive-compulsive spectrum disorders. Psychol Rep 84:107–113, 1999

Blaszczynski A, Farrell E: A case series of 44 completed gambling-related suicides. J Gambl Stud 14:93–109, 1998

Blaszczynski A, McConaghy N: Anxiety and/or depression in the pathogenesis of addictive gambling. Int J Addict 24(4):337–350, 1989

Blaszczynski A, Nower L: Pathways model of problem and pathological gambling. Addiction 97:487–499, 2002

Blaszczynski A, Steel Z: Personality disorders among pathological gamblers. J Gambl Stud 14:51–71, 1998

Blaszczynski A, McConaghy N, Frankova A: Crime, antisocial personality, and pathological gambling. J Gambl Behav 5:137–152, 1989

Brown RIF: Pathological gambling and associated patterns of crime: comparisons with alcohol and other drug addictions. J Gambl Behav 3:98–114, 1987

Carlton PL, Manowitz P: Behavioral restraint and symptoms of attention deficit disorder in alcoholics and pathological gamblers. Neuropsychobiology 25:44–48, 1992

Castellani B, Rugle L: A comparison of pathological gamblers to alcoholics and cocaine misusers on impulsivity, sensation seeking, and craving. Int J Addict 30:275–289, 1995

Crockford ND, el-Guebaly N: Psychiatric comorbidity in pathological gambling: a critical review. Am J Psychiatry 43:43–50, 1998

Cunningham-Williams RM, Cottler LB, et al: Taking chances: problem gamblers and mental health disorders—results from the St. Louis Epidemiologic Catchment Area Study. Am J Public Health 88:1093–1096, 1998

Custer RL: Profile of the pathological gambler. J Clin Psychiatry 45:35–38, 1984

DeFuentes-Merillas L, Koeter MW, Schippers GM, van den Brink W: Temporal stability of pathological scratchcard gambling among adult scratchcard buyers two years later. Addiction 99:117–127, 2004

Fernandez-Montalvo J, Echeburua E: Pathological gambling and personality disorder: an exploratory study with the IPDE. J Person Disord 18:500–505, 2004

Goudriaan AE, Oosterlaan J, de Beurs E, van den Brink W: The role of self-reported impulsivity and reward sensitivity versus neurocognitive measures of disinhibition and decision-making in the prediction of relapse in pathological gamblers. Psychol Med 38:41–50, 2008

Grant JE, Kim SW: Demographic and clinical features of 131 adult pathological gamblers. J Clin Psychiatry 62:957–962, 2001

Grant JE, Kim SW: Gender differences in pathological gamblers seeking medication treatment. Compr Psychiatry 43:56–62, 2002

Grant JE, Potenza MN, Hollander E, et al: Multi-center investigation of the opioid antagonist nalmefene in the treatment of pathological gambling. Am J Psychiatry 163:303–312, 2006

Hollander E: Obsessive-Compulsive Related Disorders. Washington, DC, American Psychiatric Press, 1993

Hollander E, Decaria CM, Mari E, et al: Short-term single-blind fluvoxamine treatment of pathological gambling. Am J Psychiatry 155:1781–1783, 1998

Hollander E, DeCaria CM, Finkell JN, et al: A randomized double-blind fluvoxamine/placebo crossover trial in pathologic gambling. Biol Psychiatry 47:813–817, 2000

Ibáñez A, Blanco C, Donahue E, et al: Psychiatric comorbidity in pathological gamblers seeking treatment. Am J Psychiatry 158(10):1733–1735, 2001

Kausch O: Suicide attempts among veterans seeking treatment for pathological gambling. J Clin Psychiatry 64:1031–1038, 2003

Kessler RC, Hwang I, LaBrie R, et al: DSM-IV pathological gambling in the National Comorbidity Survey Replication. Psychol Med 38:1351–1360, 2008

Ladd GT, Petry NM: A comparison of pathological gamblers with and without substance abuse treatment histories. Exp Clin Psychopharmacol 11:202–209, 2003

LaPlante DA, Nelson SE, LaBrie RA, Shaffer HJ: Stability and progression of disordered gambling: lessons from longitudinal studies. Can J Psychiatry 53:52–60, 2008

Ledgerwood DM, Petry NM: Gambling and suicidality in treatment-seeking pathological gamblers. J Nerv Ment Dis 192(10):711–714, 2004

Ledgerwood D, Petry NM: Pathological experience of gambling and subtypes of pathological gamblers. Psychiatr Res 144:17–27, 2006

Lesieur HR: The compulsive gambler's spiral of options and involvement. Psychiatry 42(1):79–87, 1979

Lesieur HR, Blume SE: The South Oaks Gambling Screen (SOGS): a new instrument for identification of pathological gamblers. Am J Psychiatry 144:1184–1188, 1987

Lesieur HR, Blume SB: Characteristics of pathological gamblers identified among patients on a psychiatric admissions service. Hosp Community Psychiatry 41:1009–1012, 1990

Lesieur HR, Rosenthal RJ: Pathological gambling: a review of the literature. J Gambl Stud 7:5–39, 1991

Lesieur HR, Blume SB, Zoppa RM: Alcoholism, drug abuse, and gambling. Alcohol Clin Exp Res 10:33–38, 1986

Linden RD, Pope HG Jr, Jonas JM: Pathological gambling and major affective disorder: preliminary findings. J Clin Psychiatry 47:201–203, 1986

McCormick RA, Russo AM, Ramirez LF, Taber JI: Affective disorders among pathological gamblers seeking treatment. Am J Psychiatry 141:215–218, 1984

Meyer G, Stadler MA: Criminal behavior associated with pathological gambling. J Gambl Stud 15:29–43, 1999

Moody G: Quit Compulsive Gambling: The Action Plan for Gamblers and Their Families. Wellingborough, UK, Thorsons, 1990

Moran E: Varieties of pathological gambling. Br J Psychiatry 116:593–597, 1970

National Opinion Research Center: Gambling Impact and Behavior Study: Report to the National Gambling Impact Study Commission. Chicago, IL, National Opinion Research Center at the University of Chicago, April 1, 1999. Available at: www.norc.org/PDFs/publications/GIBSFinalReportApril1999.pdf. Accessed December 13, 2003.

Nower L, Martins SS, Lin KH, Blanco C: Subtypes of disordered gamblers: results from the National Epidemiologic Survey of Alcohol and Related Conditions. Addiction 108:789–798, 2012

Odlaug BL, Schreiber LRN, Grant JE: Personality disorder and dimensions in pathological gambling. J Person Disord 26:381–392, 2012

Park S, Cho MJ, Jeon HJ, et al: Prevalence, clinical correlations, comorbidities, and suicidal tendencies in pathological Korean gamblers: results from the Korean Epidemiologic Catchment Area Study. Soc Psychiatr Epidemiol 45:621–629, 2010

Pelletier O, Ladaceur R: Personality disorders and pathological gambling: comorbidity and treatment dropout predictors. Int Gambl Stud 8:299–313, 2008

Petry NM, Stinson FS, Grant BF: Comorbidity of DSM-IV pathological gambling and other psychiatric disorders: results from the National Epidemiologic Survey on Alcohol and Related Conditions. J Clin Psychiatry 66:564–574, 2005

Pietrzak, RH, Petry, NM: Antisocial personality disorder is associated with increased severity of gambling, medical, drug, and psychiatric problems among treatment-seeking pathological gamblers. Addiction 100:1183–1193, 2005

Potenza MN, Steinberg MA, McLaughlin SD, et al: Illegal behaviors in problem gambling: analysis of data from a gambling helpline. J Am Acad Psychiatry Law 28:389–403, 2000

Rosenthal RJ: Pathological gambling. Psychiatr Ann 22:72–78, 1992

Rosenthal RJ, Lorenz VC: The pathological gambler as criminal offender. Comments on evaluation and treatment. Psychiatr Clin North Am 15:647–660, 1992

Rugle L, Melamed L: Neuropsychological assessment of attention problems in pathological gamblers. J Nerv Ment Dis 181:107–112, 1993

Russo AM, Taber JI, McCormick RA, Ramirez LF: An outcome study of an inpatient treatment program for pathological gamblers. Hosp Community Psychiatry 35(8):823–827, 1984

Sartor CE, Scherrer JF, Shah KR, et al: Course of pathological gambling symptoms and reliability of the Lifetime Gambling History measure. Psychiatry Res 152:55–61, 2007

Shaffer HJ, Hall MN: The natural history of gambling and drinking problems among casino workers. J Soc Psychol 142:405–424, 2002

Shaw M, Forbush K, Schlinder J, et al: The effect of pathological gambling on families, marriages, and children. CNS Spectr 12:615–622, 2007

Slutske W: Natural recovery and treatment-seeking in pathological gambling: results of two national surveys. Am J Psychiatry 163:297–302, 2006

Slutske WS, True WR, Goldberg J, et al: A twin study of the association between pathological gambling and antisocial personality disorder. J Abnorm Psychol 110:297–308, 2001

Slutske W, Jackson KM, Sher KJ: The natural history of problem gambling from age 18 to 29. J Abnorm Psychol 112:263–274, 2003

Specker SM, Carlson GA, Christenson GA, Marcotte M: Impulse control disorders and attention deficit disorder in pathological gamblers. Ann Clin Psychiatry 7:175–179, 1995

Specker SM, Carlson GA, Edmonson KM, et al: Psychopathology in pathological gamblers seeking treatment. J Gambl Stud 12:67–81, 1996

Spunt B, Dupont I, Lesieur H, Liberty HJ: Pathological gambling and substance abuse: a review of the literature. Subst Use Misuse 33:2535–2560, 1998

Steel Z, Blaszczynski A: The factorial structure of pathological gambling. J Gambl Stud 12:3–20, 1996

Stinchfield RD, Winters KC: Outcome of Minnesota's gambling treatment programs. J Gambl Stud 17:217–245, 2001

Taber JI, McCormick RA, Russo AM, et al: Follow-up of pathological gamblers after treatment. Am J Psychiatry 144:757–761, 1987

Tavares H, Zilberman ML, Beites FJ, Gentil V: Gender differences in gambling progression. J Gambl Stud 17:151–159, 2001

Templer DI, Kaiser G, Siscoe K: Correlates of pathological gambling propensity in prison inmates. Compr Psychiatry 34:347–351, 1993

Vaddiparti K, Cottler LB: Personality disorders and pathological gambling. Curr Opin Psychiatry 30:45–49, 2017

Welte J, Barnes G, Wieczorek W, et al: Alcohol and gambling pathology among U.S. adults: prevalence, demographic patterns and comorbidity. J Stud Alcohol 62:706–712, 2001

Winters KC, Stinchfield RD, Botzet A, Anderon N: A prospective study of youth gambling behaviors. Psychol Addict Behav 16:3–9, 2002

Zimmerman M, Breen RB, Posternak MA: An open-label study of citalopram in the treatment of pathological gambling. J Clin Psychiatry 63:44–48, 2002

Zimmerman M, Chelminski I, Young D: Prevalence and diagnostic correlates of DSM-IV pathological gambling in psychiatric outpatients. J Gambl Stud 22:255–262, 2006

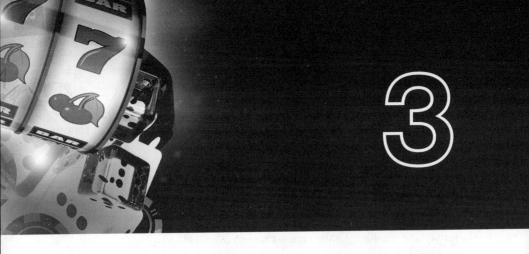

Older Adults

Georgina M. Gross, Ph.D.

Rani A. Hoff, M.P.H., Ph.D.

Adults older than 65 years represent a large and growing demographic of the U.S. population and arguably a key target market for the gambling industry. However, compared with younger age groups, much less is known about the effects of gambling on older adults. We begin this chapter with a review of what is known about the prevalence of and risk factors for problem gambling and gambling disorder among older adults. Next, we describe data on the health effects of gambling on older adults. Finally, we explore treatment issues that may differ between older and younger adults (or that may be unique to older adults).

Problem Gambling and Gambling Disorder

Prevalence Estimates

In general, prevalence rates for disordered gambling decrease as age increases (Kessler et al. 2008). However, disordered gambling is a significant problem associated with deleterious consequences among older adults. In a recent international review, Subramaniam et al. (2015) reported prevalence rates of lifetime gambling disorder for older adults ranging from 0.01% to 10.6% across studies.

Prevalence was higher among the younger age groups (of older adults) and among men compared with women. Population-based prevalence for current pathological gambling ranged from 0% (adults 61 years and older in the United States) to 1.2% (older adults in Manitoba, Canada), whereas rates from a combination of community and gambling venue samples ranged from 1% (adults age 65 years and older, Hamilton, New Zealand) to 11% (adults age 65 years and older, United States). Population-based prevalence for lifetime pathological gambling ranged from 0.29% (adults 60 years and older, United States) to 10.4% (adults age 60 years and older, Detroit, Michigan), whereas rates from a combination of community and gambling venue samples ranged from 3.8% to 4.7%.

Phenomenology

Problem gambling and gambling disorder involve many of the same symptoms as other addictive disorders: tolerance (the need to gamble more for the same effect), symptoms of withdrawal (restlessness or irritability when attempting to cut down or stop gambling), and loss of control over the addictive behavior. This pattern has been demonstrated among gamblers of all ages.

> Bill and Sue were a retired couple living on Long Island, with their one surviving child living in upstate New York and few surviving friends in their neighborhood. They worked several jobs each throughout most of their lives, and they found retirement to be boring. These feelings were exacerbated by the fact that Sue used a wheelchair and had both circulatory and cardiovascular conditions, making it difficult to find leisure activities that were both accessible and enjoyable for both of them.
>
> An acquaintance suggested they join a group going to Atlantic City, and the couple decided to go. They spent an enjoyable weekend, winning more than $500 between them, and decided to make such a trip a more regular part of their routine. Within a few months, they were going nearly once a week and had added daily lotto play to their gambling routines.
>
> Within a year, they were gambling almost continuously. They were rarely at home and spent most of their time on the road, traveling up and down the eastern seaboard to various casinos from Connecticut to Florida. Their conversations with family were almost exclusively centered on recent wins and "near wins," the prizes they had won from casinos for being such good customers, and their wish to own a mobile home so that they would not have to pay for hotel rooms.
>
> A "crisis" ensued when Sue had to be hospitalized for surgery and remained in the hospital to recover. After a few days, both Bill and Sue became very restless, talked of nothing else except going to the casino, bought large numbers of daily lotto tickets, and spent hours strategizing their lottery number picks. After a week, Sue left the hospital, and despite doctor recommendations to rest at home, they immediately embarked on another casino trip.
>
> During this time, the couple had neglected their home and their home insurance. When an electrical fire resulted in the destruction of their home, they were unable to recoup losses. Sue died a few days later of an apparent heart attack,

possibly related to the stress of losing their home. With no home and virtually no financial assets, Bill subsequently moved to Georgia to live with his brother. He continues to gamble occasionally, although he says that the "fun is gone out of it." He spends most of his time helping his brother in a contracting business and playing in a country-western band.

Traditional frameworks for addictive disorders suggested that the development of gambling disorder follows a chronic course, with early wins progressing to more pathological gambling behaviors until treatment or extreme adverse events force a change in gambling behavior (Custer 1984). However, more recent work has presented a more nuanced view, in which the course of gambling disorder (without treatment) is a dynamic process, with some people worsening, some people naturally improving or remitting, and some people moving in and out of pathological gambling behavior over time (Hodgins and Peden 2005; LaPlante et al. 2008). Little is known about the course of gambling disorder in older adults, though evidence has not suggested differences from younger adults. For example, Black et al. (2017) reported that week-by-week gambling trends showed significant downward trends over a 2.5-year time period for both older and younger adults.

However, manifestations of gambling difficulties are likely different for different people, depending on factors such as sources of income, spending behaviors, borrowing behaviors, and engagement in criminal behavior. The financial repercussions of problem gambling for older adults make them an extremely vulnerable group. Older adults are more likely to be retired and thus to be surviving on annuity income (e.g., Social Security, pensions, savings, and investment income). Older gamblers are less likely to have employment income, a fact that may either change patterns of spending on gambling or change the impact of that spending. Older adults have more difficulty recovering from financial losses and may be more likely than younger gamblers to exhaust savings, cash in investments, and spend annuity income (Subramaniam et al. 2015). The amount of money spent by a younger, working individual may have less overall impact than the same amount spent by a retired gambler with limited ability to recover from a loss.

Although the effects of financial losses may be more pronounced among older adults, the effects of gambling on work and family relationships may appear less pronounced. Gambling's impact on work and family relationships, represented in DSM-5 by the criterion "has jeopardized or lost a significant relationship, job, or educational or career opportunity because of gambling," may be less relevant particularly for older adults who are retired or widowed. For example, retired gamblers are less likely to commit work-related white-collar crimes (e.g., embezzlement) to obtain gambling money. Similarly, they may have fewer family members than younger gamblers from whom to borrow money to continue gambling. Because there may be less opportunity to engage in certain behaviors that constitute symptoms of gambling disorder, the impact of gambling on these aspects of life for older adults may be underestimated.

Unique Triggers and Risk Factors for Gambling Disorder

Several risk factors for the onset of problem gambling and gambling disorder have been identified, and some of these risk factors may be stronger or entirely unique to older adults. These include social isolation and role changes, depression and anxiety, cognitive and biological changes, and sociodemographic subgroup membership associated with both older age and gambling behavior.

> Anna, a 67-year-old woman, was in excellent health until the death of her husband of 40 years. After her husband's death, she became depressed and withdrawn. Having never held a full-time job outside of the home, she had difficulty filling her time now that she no longer was cooking and cleaning for her husband. In addition, she had very little understanding of her financial assets. After several falls, she moved to a supportive-care housing unit, paid for by life insurance and other savings set aside by her husband.
>
> Anna's mood improved after the move, partially because she had a network of friends and a regular schedule of social activities, including bingo games. She and a small group of friends played bingo several times a week, traveling to various sites for games on different nights. Although she never spent very much at any one time, Anna's financial assets were quite small and were taxed by the costs of her housing. She began to respond to mail solicitations for credit cards, taking cash advances to finance her gambling that she was unable to pay back. She also regularly asked her children for cash sums to gamble, saying that she needed money for medications or unexpected expenses.
>
> Becoming suspicious of these increasingly frequent requests, her son investigated and found that his mother was losing about $100 a week playing bingo. Because this was a substantial portion of her disposable income and because she was in a substantial amount of debt because of her cash advances, her son became very concerned. When confronted, Anna angrily objected to being treated like a child, and she accused her son of wanting to get her money. Initially refusing to seek treatment, Anna cut off contact with her son. After her lease at the supported housing community was terminated because of her inability to pay the rent, she agreed to attend Gamblers Anonymous meetings. She subsequently received treatment for both her gambling problem and her depression, allowed her son to manage her money, reduced and eventually eliminated her credit card debt with the help of a debt counselor, and rebuilt a network of social ties around activities other than gambling.

As adults age, they often experience the loss of traditional social roles associated with being parents, having employment, and even being in a marriage. These changes can lead to feelings of social isolation, boredom, loss of a sense of meaning or purpose, and even depression and anxiety. Recreational gambling may help to alleviate these negative feelings by providing entertainment, a chance to socialize, and a chance to escape from everyday problems. However, these feelings may in turn place older adults at increased risk for developing gambling problems (Guillou Landreat et al. 2019). For example, one study reported that compared with married older adults, unpartnered older adults were less likely to gamble with family or friends, were more likely to gamble because of loneliness, and had higher rates of problem gambling (Elton-Marshall et al. 2018). Another reported that loneliness predicted problem gambling for unmarried older men (Botterill et al. 2016). Overall, late-life problem gambling may develop as older adults gamble to escape anxiety and depression caused by deteriorating physical well-being and social support (Parke et al. 2018).

Another risk factor relatively unique to older adults is the cognitive decline associated with normal aging and age-related conditions such as Parkinson's disease and dementia. In late adulthood, the total volume and weight of the brain shrink gradually, including atrophy in the prefrontal cortex, which is responsible for executive functioning. Declining executive functioning, including impaired self-control, has been linked to increased risk for problem gambling. In one study, older adults recruited from gambling venues endorsed more gambling problems if they also experienced deficits in executive functioning (von Hippel et al. 2009). Likewise, evidence suggests that impaired executive functioning places older adults at risk for impaired decision-making while gambling (Rogalsky et al. 2012). Gambling may also enhance dopaminergic function in adults and may thus be more strongly reinforced in older adults, who have naturally diminishing dopamine levels. In addition, compulsive behavior, including pathological gambling, is associated with initiation of dopamine agonist therapies for adults with Parkinson's disease (Singh et al. 2007). Finally, case reports have suggested that early forms of dementia may place older adults at greater risk for pathological gambling (Cimminella et al. 2015). Although this is not likely to be an extremely important risk factor in the population, it nevertheless requires further study.

Sociodemographic subgroups of older adults likely have differential risk for the development of gambling disorder and associated health consequences. Women make up a majority of older adults because of their longer life expectancies, and their proportion will likely continue to increase as the population ages. Older women may be at even greater risk for the effects of problem gambling than older men because of even lower sources of income, a higher likelihood of being widowed and thus socially isolated, and a higher likelihood of living with chronic diseases such as diabetes and hypertension. Older women may be more likely to gamble as an escape from problems or anxiety than men and may be more vulnerable to gambling market strategies (e.g., bus tours) and electronic gaming machines (EGMs) (McKay 2005). Much more research on gambling among older women is needed, given that the majority of extant research has focused on men despite evidence that men and women may actually gamble at somewhat equal rates (McCarthy et al. 2018).

Lower socioeconomic status is associated with more frequent gambling and gambling disorder for adults in general (e.g., Welte et al. 2011), and specifically among older adults. Older adults with an income of less than $20,000 annually are more likely to exhibit problem gambling behavior than those making more than $20,000 (Zaranek and Lichtenberg 2008). Older adults with a small, fixed income are more likely to develop problem gambling, thus possibly worsening their financial difficulties. Finally, racial minority groups in the United States, such as Black and Native American groups, are at increased risk for gambling disorder (Alegria et al. 2009), though almost no research has focused on these groups among older adults. One study of Black older Americans reported gambling rates comparable to those in the general population, despite having much lower incomes (only 26.9% reported a yearly income greater than $10,000; Christensen and Patsdaughter 2004). Older adults who fall into one or more of these gender, socioeconomic, and racial subcategories are likely at the highest risk for negative gambling-related consequences; however, they remain among the least frequently studied groups.

Access to Games of Chance

Adults older than 65 years constituted 16% of the United States population in the 2018 census (U.S. Census Bureau 2019), and this segment is expected to continue growing as the population ages and life expectancies increase. Research has consistently shown that opportunity plays an important role in the prevalence of gambling, and by extension the prevalence of problem gambling and gambling disorder. Although older adulthood is associated with restrictions in the accessibility of certain types of activities (e.g., caused by physical or mental decline), barriers to older adult participation in gambling have been dramatically, and intentionally, reduced. Rates of gambling are consistently lower among older compared with younger adults; however, studies have shown that gambling rates for older adults rose dramatically between the 1970s and 2000 and continue to be on the rise (Tse et al. 2012). As gambling venues multiply, Americans, including older adults, have increasing and more convenient access to various types of gambling. Gaming corporations have adapted their facilities to be easily accessible for older adults, including through the provision of scooters and wheelchairs, as well as oxygen and diabetic needle disposal options (Surface 2009).

Many forms of gambling, such as slot machines and EGMs, are relatively passive forms of entertainment requiring little cognitive ability. These are the preferred gambling method for older adults and have been linked to a particularly fast progression to addiction. For example, one study reported that frequent gambling at slots or EGMs was associated with an odds ratio of 8.57 for problem gambling among older adults (Van der Maas et al. 2017). States that have high numbers of retired citizens (e.g., Florida, Arizona) have seen increases in the availability of gambling activities, and many such venues have incentive programs specifically targeting older adults (e.g., free bus rides, discounted meals). Finally, many extended-care facilities offer gambling activities (e.g., bingo games for money or casino day trips) as a means of social interaction and activity. This increased opportunity to gamble may place older people at greater risk for development of gambling-related problems. Overall, the participation in gambling among older Americans will likely continue to increase as younger gamblers age, access to gambling continues to increase (e.g., online gambling from home), and there is more widespread social acceptance of gambling as a recreational activity.

Patterns of Gambling Behavior

The limited research on older adults and problem gambling indicates that people older than 65 years differ from younger adults in their reasons for gambling, preferred games, and frequency of gambling.

Reasons for Gambling

Both older and younger adults engage in gambling for a wide variety of reasons. The motivational pathways framework conceptualizes motivation as the product of various internal or external forces that trigger and lead to the persistence of gambling behaviors (e.g., socialization, amusement, avoidance, excitement, and monetary motives) (Lee et al. 2007). Retirement from employment, declining social networks, and decreased purpose in life motivate some older adults to gamble as a replacement for diminished social interaction and occupational fulfillment (Tira et al. 2014). Given age-related deterioration of physical functioning, gambling may represent one of few leisure activities that are both exciting and accessible. Some research also suggests, however, that older adults may be less motivated by excitement and monetary or other incentives (Martin et al. 2010) and more motivated by the desire to decrease or escape negative affect. As discussed, older adults often use gambling to modulate negative mood states, such as depression and anxiety, that are associated with physical decline and social isolation (Black et al. 2017; Parke et al. 2018). Furthermore, evidence suggests that when older adults gamble to reduce negative affect (as opposed to other motivations), the probability of experiencing negative consequences from gambling is significantly increased (Van der Maas et al. 2017).

Types of Games Preferred

Additional evidence for differing motivations for gambling over age groups may be reflected in preferred games. Evidence suggests that younger adults tend to prefer competitive action games, such as sports betting, whereas older adults prefer less competitive games, such as lottery, slots, bingo, and EGMs (Ariyabuddhiphongs 2012). It has been hypothesized that older adults are attracted to less competitive games because they gamble more for the entertainment value than to make money or to beat opponents. In one comparison study, whereas 74% of young adults preferred "action" games (cards, sports betting, video games, and horse or dog tracks), 66% of older adults preferred slots (19% of older adults preferred "other games," i.e., not slots or action) (Black et al. 2017).

About 39% to 45% of all casino users are older than 65 years old, which is concerning given casino gambling is associated with risk for problem gambling. In a study of urban older adults, of those who responded "yes" to any casino visitation, 18.2% reported problem gambling behaviors (Zaranek and Lichtenberg 2008). Casino use may replace other leisure activities: another study of older adults in Detroit reported that those who frequented casinos participated in fewer other, nongambling activities and had poorer mental health, lower incomes, and less social support than those who visited infrequently or not at all (Zaranek and Chapleski 2005). Among older adults, few studies have examined whether game type preference (e.g., pure chance games or those involving skill) varies between recreational and problem gambling. One study of older adults in Singapore reported that problem gamblers age 55 years or older were more likely to play continuous games without money limits, such as slots or online games, whereas recreational gamblers preferred time-limited and inexpensive games such as lotteries (Tse et al. 2013). It should be noted that there has been no longitudinal research on gambling patterns over a lifetime, and the cross-sectional data presented here could be heavily confounded by time-related effects such as recency of gambling onset. Future research should explore how patterns of gambling change in individuals over a lifetime.

Frequency of Gambling

Evidence indicates that among those who gamble, the frequency of gambling may be higher among older compared with younger adults, though the evidence is mixed. Data from the Gambling Impact and Behavior Study indicated that older gamblers were three times more likely than younger gamblers to gamble daily and were two times more likely to gamble one to three times a week (Desai et al. 2004). Other work has suggested that those who started to gamble at a younger age (as opposed to examining current age) were more frequent gamblers (Hodgins et al. 2012). Thus, older adults who have been gambling for a significant portion of their lives are likely to constitute a particularly high-risk group for the development of problem gambling behaviors. In a national U.S. survey, 75% of adults ages 61–70 years reported gambling in the past year, and 24% had gambled 52 times or more, compared with 62% and 18% for adults 71 years and older (Welte et al. 2011). This suggests there may be age-related within-group differences for older adults. Gambling frequency of older adult gambling patrons is higher, with studies reporting at least once a week.

High gambling frequency among older adults is likely explained by two factors: a marked increased amount of leisure time and the reduction in financial responsibilities (e.g., the support of children) later in life, which may result in relatively higher proportions of disposable income. No matter the reason, though, such high frequencies are a cause for concern, because gambling frequency is consistently linked to the development of gambling disorder.

Health Correlates of Gambling

The impact of gambling, whether recreational or pathological, on health is also relatively unexamined among older adults. The majority of older adults who gamble do so recreationally, which is associated with few negative consequences. In fact, recreational gambling may confer benefits such as increased socialization and health, as well as cognitive and sensory benefits (Alberghetti and Collins 2015). Recreational gambling affords the opportunity for new social networks and has been associated with reduced stress and anxiety and increased overall health among older adults (Zaranek and Chapleski 2005). In addition, bingo, for example, has been associated with benefits for cognitive functioning such as improved concentration, memory, and attention.

However, the link between gambling disorder and poorer physical and psychological health is well established. Furthermore, older adults show higher levels of psychological and physical comorbidity than younger age groups. Among older adults, problem gambling is associated with self-reported reduced general health and social functioning (Erickson et al. 2005); increased risk for arteriosclerosis and any heart condition (Pilver and Potenza 2013); elevated rates of comorbid psychiatric disorders, including mood, anxiety, and personality disorders (Kerber et al. 2008); increased severity of family, social, medical, psychiatric, and alcohol problems (Pietrzak et al. 2005); a greater number of stressful life events; a greater number of obsessive-compulsive symptoms; and a perceived lower level of control over their future health status (Bazargan et al. 2001). Evidence consistently suggests dramatically heightened risk for suicidal ideation and suicide mortality associated with gambling disorder (e.g., Petry and Kiluk 2002); however, studies have not examined this among older adults. In one study of problem gamblers who elected to participate in a casino self-exclusion program, older adults were more likely than younger and middle-age groups to endorse "suicide prevention" as their motivation for self-exclusion (Nower and Blaszczynski 2008). This highlights a critical need for future research.

Some health effects of gambling may be unique to older adults, particularly those who engage in casino gambling. First, poor health effects may be associated with sitting for long periods of time, often in smoke-filled environments, eating less frequently than normal, and participating in games that increase heart rates and excitement levels. Although none of these factors would be a particularly immediate concern for younger gamblers, they may be of greater concern for older adults, who may have diabetes, heart disease, or otherwise poor circulation.

Second, health consequences of large financial losses may be greater among older adults, who have limited abilities to recoup those losses through work. Large financial losses may be associated with depression and anxiety, poor medication management because of the inability to purchase medications, loss of independence because of the inability to live on diminished means, or increased social isolation resulting from borrowing money or strained family relations resulting from gambling. However, further empirical examination of these processes among older adults is needed. Furthermore, the temporality of the association between gambling and physical and mental health warrants future study. For example, are older adults with physical limitations drawn to sedentary activities, such as gambling; does the sedentary nature of gambling bring on physical limitations; or is a combination of the two involved?

Screening, Assessment, Prevention, and Treatment of Gambling Disorder

Despite the need for gambling disorder treatment research specific to older adults having been highlighted in the literature for well over a decade, this remains a starkly understudied area. Older patients with gambling disorder may be less likely than younger patients to be identified clinically for several reasons. To begin with, most people with gambling disorder, regardless of age, do not present for treatment, and older adults are even less likely to do so. This is likely attributable to several factors. Older adults are more likely to have transportation limitations; thus, barriers to accessing care (e.g., in rural areas) are likely pronounced among older adults. Furthermore, older adults are not socialized to share or seek help for their problems and often do not believe their problems are serious enough to warrant treatment. Even when asked directly, older patients may attach more stigma to gambling disorder and thus may minimize their experience of symptoms (Bjelde et al. 2008). Finally, an exaggerated sense of independence or the need to retain the limited independence that remains may prompt greater resistance to recognizing certain symptoms such as financial strain or disruption of family relations.

Given this reduced likelihood of treatment seeking and reporting of symptoms, the inclusion of gambling disorder in universal screening for addictive behaviors and mental health more broadly is needed (Pietrzak et al. 2007; Skinner et al. 2018). Older adults are more likely to present to primary care than mental health, and primary care clinicians may be less proficient at identifying psychiatric and substance abuse disorders, particularly those with relatively low prevalence. Thus, education and training of providers are also needed (Lucke and Wallace 2006). For adults who screen at the mild to moderate level, brief interventions in primary care or in the community will likely be sufficient. Older adults who screen at the moderate or severe level of gambling disorder should be referred to a specialized mental health setting for a comprehensive assessment. In these instances, providers should stay in contact with the patient during the care transition to promote treatment engagement and follow up (Skinner et al. 2018).

Assessment should include factors that may be uniquely salient for older adults. Of critical importance is initial and ongoing assessment of imminent risk for suicidal behavior or self-directed violence, given that both older adulthood and gambling disorder confer markedly increased risk. In addition, assessment should include any declines in cognitive functioning; depression and anxiety; the effects of prolonged gambling over many years; loss of peers, spouse, and social support; assumptions or biases regarding mental health and mental health care; and access to social and economic resources that promote mental and physical health (Skinner et al. 2018).

Several preventive measures would likely reduce risk for gambling problems among older adults (Matheson et al. 2018). Eucational incentives are needed. They should be culturally sensitive and tailored to issues relevant for older adults, for example, comorbidities and stigma regarding seeking help. Social marketing campaigns to create awareness should be designed to appeal to older adults and should include information on negative consequences such as health and financial effects. Education on prevention for primary care providers is needed and should include risk factors specific to older adults and resources for treatment or referral. Training of family members, medical providers, gambling venue staff, and staff at senior residences is needed and should prompt them to monitor the frequency of gambling venue patronage as a risk factor for problems developing (Matheson et al. 2018).[1]

Several modalities and types of treatment have been successfully implemented for gambling disorder. In general, treatment recommendations typically involve psychosocial interventions (e.g., cognitive-behavioral therapies, mindfulness, motivational interviewing, exercise, social support, and group and online treatment), possibly in combination with pharmacological intervention. No treatments for pathological gambling have been developed specifically for older adult patients. Furthermore, almost no research has examined treatment for gambling disorder among older adults (Matheson et al. 2018); therefore, little is known about which treatment modalities are likely to be most effective for older adults.

Furthermore, some of the current best practices for treatment of gambling disorder may be more difficult to implement with older patients (Matheson et al. 2018). Multimorbidity is common among older adults, and older adults are more likely to be prescribed several medications. Thus, pharmacological interventions may be ruled out or require more careful management. Evidence suggests that treatment outcomes tend to be improved by family involvement. Thus, family and friends should be included whenever possible, though this may not be an option for many older adults. Support groups such as Gamblers Anonymous offer the component of social connectedness, which may be especially beneficial for older adults without social networks (Kerber et al. 2011).

Providing or promoting leisure activities with a social component may foster healthier substitutes for gambling. Treatment engagement may be more challenging for those with cognitive or physical limitations; clinicians should consider this when selecting the appropriate intervention (e.g., cognitive-behavioral therapy may not be feasible for some). Self-directed online interventions may be helpful for those who experience shame about seeking help. Finally, expanding treatment

---

[1]For more information, see the article by Turner et al. (2018), who provide an extensive best-practices guide for prevention of problem gambling among older adults. Both Matheson et al. (2018) and Turner et al. (2018) note that their recommendations were heavily informed by research on gambling disorder among adults more broadly, given that little older adult–specific literature is available.

for gambling disorder beyond mental health should increase access, because older adults tend to be high health care users (Matheson et al. 2018).[2] Outside of the health care system, casino self-exclusion programs have shown promise for harm reduction among older adults (Nower and Blaszczynski 2008). Toll-free help lines may provide another source of support, assuming older adults are aware of and willing to use them (Alberghetti and Collins 2015).

Conclusion

Gambling among older adults has increased dramatically over the past few decades, and older adults represent a major target market for the gambling industry. This combination puts them at potentially increased risk for the development of problem gambling and gambling disorder. Although prevalence rates of gambling-related disorders generally decrease with age, these differences may be diminishing over time. In fact, as gambling becomes more socially acceptable and widely available, rates of problem gambling among older adults are likely to continue increasing substantially. Older gamblers also have different patterns of gambling than younger adults, and these differences may have implications for the health and well-being of older gamblers. Although the condition is less prevalent than in younger patients, older adults with gambling disorder may have unique treatment challenges as a result of their age, comorbid medical conditions, and attitudes about mental health treatment.

References

Alberghetti A, Collins PA: A passion for gambling: a generation-specific conceptual analysis and review of gambling among older adults in Canada. J Gambl Stud 31:343–358, 2015

Alegria AA, Petry NM, Hasin DS, et al: Disordered gambling among racial and ethnic groups in the US: results from the national epidemiologic survey on alcohol and related conditions. CNS Spectr 14:132–143, 2009

Ariyabuddhiphongs V: Older adults and gambling: a review. Int J Ment Health Addict 10:297–308, 2012

Bazargan M, Bazargan SH, Akanda M: Gambling habits among aged African Americans. Clin Gerontol 22:51–62, 2001

Bjelde K, Chromy B, Pankow D: Casino gambling among older adults in North Dakota: a policy analysis. J Gambl Stud 24:423–440, 2008

Black DW, Coryell W, McCormick B, et al: A prospective follow-up study of younger and older subjects with pathological gambling. Psychiatry Res 256:162–168, 2017

---

[2]For more information, see the comprehensive report by Skinner et al. (2018) on best practices for treatment of older adults with gambling disorder.

Botterill E, Gill PR, McLaren S, Gomez R: Marital status and problem gambling among Australian older adults: the mediating role of loneliness. J Gambl Stud 32:1027–1038, 2016

Christensen MH, Patsdaughter CA: Gambling behaviors in Black older adults: perceived effects on health. J Gerontol Nurs 30:34–39, 2004

Cimminella F, Ambra FI, Vitaliano S, et al: Early onset frontotemporal dementia presenting with pathological gambling. Acta Neurol Belg 115:759–761, 2015

Custer RL: Profile of the pathological gambler. J Clin Psychiatry 45:35–38, 1984

Desai RA, Maciejewski PK, Dausey DJ, et al: Health correlates of recreational gambling in older adults. Am J Psychiatry 161:1672–1679, 2004

Elton-Marshall T, Wijesingha R, Sendzik T, et al: Marital status and problem gambling among older adults: an examination of social context and social motivations. Can J Aging 37:318–322, 2018

Erickson L, Molina CA, Ladd GT, et al: Problem and pathological gambling are associated with poorer mental and physical health in older adults. Int J Geriatr Psychiatry 20:754–759, 2005

Guillou Landreat M, Cholet J, Grall Bronnec M, et al: Determinants of gambling disorders in elderly people—a systematic review. Front Psychiatry 10:837, 2019

Hodgins DC, Peden N: Natural course of gambling disorders: forty-month follow-up. Journal of Gambling Issues 14:117–131, 2005

Hodgins DC, Schopflocher DP, Martin CR, et al: Disordered gambling among higher-frequency gamblers: who is at risk? Psychol Med 42:2433–2444, 2012

Kerber CS, Black DW, Buckwalter K: Comorbid psychiatric disorders among older adult recovering pathological gamblers. Issues Ment Health Nurs 29:1018–1028, 2008

Kerber CS, Schlenker E, Hickey K: Does your older adult client have a gambling problem? J Psychosoc Nurs Ment Health Serv 49:38–43, 2011

Kessler RC, Hwang I, LaBrie R, et al: DSM-IV pathological gambling in the National Comorbidity Survey Replication. Psychol Med 38:1351–1360, 2008

LaPlante DA, Nelson SE, LaBrie RA, Shaffer HJ: Stability and progression of disordered gambling: lessons from longitudinal studies. Can J Psychiatry 53:52–60, 2008

Lee H, Chae PK, Lee H, Kim Y: The five-factor gambling motivation model. Psychiatry Res 150:21–32, 2007

Lucke S, Wallace M: Assessment and management of pathological and problem gambling among older adults. Geriatr Nurs 27:51–57, 2006

Martin F, Lichtenberg PA, Templin TN: A longitudinal study: casino gambling attitudes, motivations, and gambling patterns among urban elders. J Gambl Stud 27:287–297, 2010

Matheson FI, Sztainert T, Lakman Y, et al: Prevention and treatment of problem gambling among older adults: a scoping review. Journal of Gambling Issues 39:6–66, 2018

McCarthy S, Thomas SL, Randle M, et al: Women's gambling behaviour, product preferences, and perceptions of product harm: differences by age and gambling risk status. Harm Reduct J 15(1):22, 2018

McKay C: Double jeopardy: older women and problem gambling. Int J Ment Health Addict 3:35–53, 2005

Nower L, Blaszczynski A: Characteristics of problem gamblers 56 years of age or older: a statewide study of casino self-excluders. Psychol Aging 23:577–584, 2008

Parke A, Griffiths MD, Pattinson J, Keatley D: Age-related physical and psychological vulnerability as pathways to problem gambling in older adults. J Behav Addict 7:137–145, 2018

Petry NM, Kiluk BD: Suicidal ideation and suicide attempts in treatment-seeking pathological gamblers. J Nerv Ment Dis 190:462–469, 2002

Pietrzak RH, Molina CA, Ladd GT, et al: Health and psychosocial correlates of disordered gambling in older adults. Am J Geriatr Psychiatry 13:510–519, 2005

Pietrzak RH, Morasco BJ, Blanco C, et al: Gambling level and psychiatric and medical disorders in older adults: results from the National Epidemiologic Survey on Alcohol and Related Conditions. Am J Geriatr Psychiatry 15:301–313, 2007

Pilver CE, Potenza MN: Increased incidence of cardiovascular conditions among older adults with pathological gambling features in a prospective study. J Addict Med 7:387–393, 2013

Rogalsky C, Vidal C, Li X, Damasio H: Risky decision-making in older adults without cognitive deficits: an fMRI study of VMPFC using the Iowa Gambling Task. Soc Neurosci 7:178–190, 2012

Singh A, Kandimala G, Dewey RB Jr, O'Suilleabhain P: Risk factors for pathologic gambling and other compulsions among Parkinson's disease patients taking dopamine agonists. J Clin Neurosci 14:1178–1181, 2007

Skinner WJW, Littman-Sharp N, Leslie J, et al: Best practices for the treatment of older adult problem gamblers. Journal of Gambling Issues 39:166–203, 2018

Subramaniam M, Wang P, Soh P, et al: Prevalence and determinants of gambling disorder among older adults: a systematic review. Addict Behav 41:199–209, 2015

Surface D: High risk recreation—problem gambling in older adults. Social Work Today 9:18–23, 2009

Tira C, Jackson AC, Tomnay JE: Pathways to late-life problematic gambling in seniors: a grounded theory approach. Gerontologist 54:1035–1048, 2014

Tse S, Hong SI, Wang CW, Cunningham-Williams RM: Gambling behavior and problems among older adults: a systemic review of empirical studies. J Gerontol B Psychol Sci Soc Sci 67:639–652, 2012

Tse S, Hong S, Ng K: Estimating the prevalence of problem gambling among older adults in Singapore. Psychiatry Res 210:607–611, 2013

Turner NE, Wiebe J, Ferentzy P, et al: Developing a best practices guide for the prevention of problem gambling among older adults. Journal of Gambling Issues 39:112–165, 2018

U.S. Census Bureau: 2018 Population Estimates by Age, Sex, Race and Hispanic Origin. April 1, 2010 to July 1, 2018. Washington, DC, U.S. Census Bureau, 2019. Available at: https://data.census.gov/cedsci/all?q=age%20and%20sexandhidePreview=false-andtid=ACSST1Y2018.S0101andt=Age%20and%20Sexandvintage=2018. Accessed April 23, 2020.

Van der Maas M, Mann RE, McCready J, et al: Problem gambling in a sample of older adult casino gamblers: associations with gambling participation and motivations. J Geriatr Psychiatry Neurol 30:3–10, 2017

von Hippel W, Ng L, Abbot L, et al: Executive functioning and gambling: performance on the trail making test is associated with gambling problems in older adult gamblers. Aging Neuropsychol Cogn 6:654–670, 2009

Welte JW, Barnes GM, Tidwell MO, Hoffman JH: Gambling and problem gambling across the lifespan. J Gambl Stud 27:49–61, 2011

Zaranek RR, Chapleski EE: Casino gambling among urban elders: just another social activity? J Gerontol B Psychol Sci Soc Sci 60:S74–S81, 2005

Zaranek RR, Lichtenberg PA: Urban elders and casino gambling: are they at risk of a gambling problem? J Aging Stud 22(1):13–23, 2008

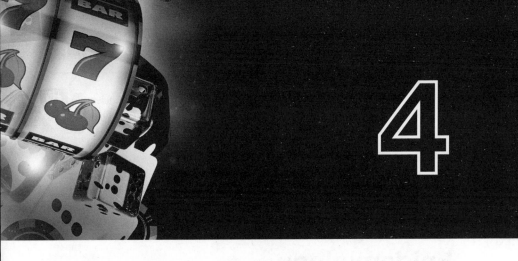

Gender Differences

Jon E. Grant, M.D., M.P.H., J.D.

Samuel R. Chamberlain, M.B./B.Chir., Ph.D., MRCPsych

The notion of meaningful differences between men and women in various aspects of gambling disorder is a topic that has received increasing attention over the past 20 years. Although gambling disorder is considered to be primarily a male problem, the recent focus on gambling disorder in women has brought attention to important gender differences in epidemiology, phenomenology, psychiatric comorbidity, and biology. These differences have important treatment implications. In this chapter, we review findings concerning gender differences within a clinical context.

Case Vignette

Rochelle did not start gambling until she was 48 years old. Rochelle remembers the first time she went to a casino. Friends asked her to join them for dinner and entertainment. She and her friends began to go to the casino twice a month. Rochelle began playing nickel slot machines. Because winning at the nickel machines gradually lost its excitement, over the next 2 years, Rochelle found that only dollar slot machines produced a "thrill."

Within 2 years of starting casino gambling, Rochelle felt she had a problem. She no longer wanted to go to the casino with her friends. She found her friends too distracting and reported that they did not take gambling seriously. Instead, Rochelle started going by herself. This also allowed her to go to the casino more frequently and to stay for longer periods of time. Even though Rochelle recognized on some level that her gambling might be a problem, she tended to feel she could "keep control" and was also reluctant to seek help because she felt guilty about the extent of her gambling and how she had concealed it from others.

Rochelle reported that her interest in gambling was often prompted by her mood. If she was feeling anxious because of work or feeling sad or lonely because of problems within her marriage, Rochelle would choose to go to the casino. In fact, when stress at work was at its highest, Rochelle often chose to leave work early. Because of her frequent absences, she eventually lost her job. Rochelle avoided telling her husband about her problem until it got out of hand, and their marriage eventually ended in divorce.

Epidemiology

Community Populations

The lifetime prevalence of gambling disorder ranges from 0.4% to 2.0% in North America, and a recent epidemiological study found that men were more likely to report current problems with gambling that reflected some degree of psychopathology (rates of problem or pathological gambling of 0.7% in men and 0.4% in women) (Desai and Potenza 2008). Similarly, a meta-analysis of gambling problems among non-treatment-seeking older adults (age 60 years or older) found that problem gambling was more common among men (Subramaniam et al. 2015). This is in keeping with previous research (Pietrzak et al. 2007) but seems to differ from some previous reports (Afifi et al. 2010). Although men may be more likely to have gambling disorder, there are clinically important differences to consider between men and women with gambling disorder in terms of age at onset, gambling attitudes, time course, motivation to gamble, types of gambling preferred, and treatment outcome.

Clinical Populations

The gender ratio in many clinical populations suggests a higher percentage of women seeking treatment for gambling disorder than has been found in community samples. Nonetheless, and although reasons have not been rigorously examined, there has long been a suggestion that women are underrepresented in treatment programs (Mark and Lesieur 1992). In part, this finding may reflect female gamblers' decreased tendency to seek treatment for gambling problems (Grant and Kim 2002; Ladd and Petry 2002; Ronzitti et al. 2016). Alcohol treatment literature suggests that women experience gender-specific barriers to treatment such as lack of funding, childcare and custody issues, and difficulty obtaining transportation (Brady and Randall 1999). Whether similar barriers exist for female gamblers seeking treatment is currently unknown. Another explanation drawn from the alcohol treatment literature is that whereas women may seek treatment after a severe episode of gambling, men seek treatment after a more chronic period (Kim et al. 2016; Ladd and Petry 2002). Whether some women have not sought treatment because they simply have not yet "hit bottom" is unclear, but this difference in motivation for treatment may offer clues to the gender ratios found in clinical samples.

The gender ratio of subjects in clinical samples, however, may be influenced by age. Two studies of older pathological gamblers have found that a high percentage of women in older-age cohorts seek treatment (Grant et al. 2001; Petry 2002). Women tend to start gambling at a later age, so the age of the sample may influence the gender ratio. Thus, in clinical settings, women, particularly of middle to older age, should be screened for gambling disorder because it may be more common than was previously estimated.

Phenomenology

Course of Illness

Perhaps the most replicated finding in studies has been that the course of illness seems to be different for women. Men tend to start gambling earlier in life (Lahti et al. 2013). The interval between the age of initially gambling for money and the age of recognizing problems because of gambling seems to be shorter for women (Grant et al. 2012b; Ibáñez et al. 2003; Jiménez-Murcia et al. 2016; Ladd and Petry 2002; Martins et al. 2002; Potenza et al. 2001; Tavares et al. 2001; but see Slutske et al. 2015). This accelerated development of addiction in women, the so-called telescoping effect (Grant et al. 2012a; 2012b), has been documented in other addictive disorders such as alcohol use disorder and opiate dependence (Brady and Randall 1999; Randall et al. 1999).

Triggers to Gambling

Whereas women with gambling disorder are also more likely to report that they gamble as a means of escaping from stressful or unsatisfying life situations or from states of depression, men often report urges to gamble that are unrelated to their emotional state (Grant and Kim 2002; Ladd and Petry 2002; Potenza et al. 2001; Sacco et al. 2011; Trevorrow and Moore 1998). Although some studies have found that female gamblers have high rates of mood disorders that might explain the triggers for gambling (Ibáñez et al. 2003), similar rates of mood disorders have been found among samples of predominantly male gamblers (Black and Moyer 1998). A recent study helped to explain the directionality of these variables and found that having experienced anxiety or depression before gambling onset constituted a risk for developing problem gambling for the women but not for the men (Sundqvist and Rosendahl 2019). Furthermore, women initiated gambling after their first period of anxiety, depression, and problems with substances, and problem gambling was the last condition to evolve. Men, on the other hand, initiated gambling before any mood or addiction symptoms developed, and depression and suicidal events emerged after problem gambling onset (Sundqvist and Rosendahl 2019).

Social situations may also explain why affective state is a more prominent trigger for disordered gambling in women. Ladd and Petry (2002) suggested that the home environment may be more unstable, stressful, and unsupportive for female pathological gamblers. More recent research suggests, however, that cultural factors may also influence the triggers and other clinical aspects of gender (Medeiros et al. 2016).

The emotional state that women with gambling disorder report as the trigger to gambling appears to correlate with the type of gambling women prefer. Although choice of gambling activity depends on availability, women tend to prefer and to develop problems with nonstrategic forms of gambling such as bingo or slot machines (Grant and Kim 2002; Potenza et al. 2001; Tavares et al. 2001). Nonstrategic forms of gambling may be more escape oriented, while men's choice of strategic gambling may be more action oriented (e.g., sports gambling or blackjack) (Potenza et al. 2001). Furthermore, action-oriented gambling may also reflect a higher level of sensation seeking among male gamblers (Blaszczynski et al. 1997; Bonnaire et al. 2017; Vitaro et al. 1997).

Although women often report pronounced mood symptoms as the prompt for their gambling behavior, many do not meet diagnostic criteria for a mood disorder. These women, however, may have subclinical mood symptoms that predispose them to gambling. Therefore, it is clinically important to inquire not only about possible depression and anxiety but also about the emotional context in which the woman finds herself when gambling. The alcohol treatment literature advises that women may require more assistance in finding alternatives to drinking to cope with negative affect (Rubin et al. 1996). Having patients maintain a diary of their mood and gambling behavior may be helpful in demonstrating a possible link between these factors and identifying high-risk times for gambling. If the emotional cues for gambling are not identified, treatment may not focus on the cause of the disordered gambling.

Comorbidity

Studies have consistently reported that subjects with gambling disorder experience high rates of lifetime mood, anxiety, substance use, and personality disorders, as well as ADHD (Karlsson and Håkansson 2018; Petry et al. 2005; Ronzitti et al. 2018; Waluk et al. 2016). In terms of gender differences in comorbidity, some studies have found that whereas men with gambling disorder were more likely to have a current alcohol use disorder, women were more likely to have a comorbid mood disorder (Ibáñez et al. 2001; Ronzitti et al. 2016). The higher rates of comorbid mood disorders among women with gambling disorder may also explain the higher reported rates of attempted suicide among women with these disorders (Potenza et al. 2001). In fact, several reports have concluded that female sex may be a risk factor of suicidality or suicide attempts in patients with gambling disorder (Bischof et al. 2015; Husky et al. 2015; Komoto 2014; Manning et al. 2015).

Potenza and colleagues (2001) found that men with gambling disorder were more likely to report problems with drug use. Consistent with these findings, Ladd and Petry (2002) found that male gamblers were more likely to have had prior treatment for substance abuse than were female gamblers. Other research disputes these findings, however, suggesting that associations between alcohol dependence and any drug use disorder and gambling disorder may be stronger among women than men (Petry et al. 2005). Evidence further suggests that female gamblers may be more likely to have compulsive buying problems (another putative behavior addiction) than male gamblers (Granero et al. 2016).

Other aspects of comorbidity have been found less consistently in the literature. For example, one study found that women with gambling disorder were more likely to report anxiety because of their gambling (Potenza et al. 2001). Differences in scores on the Hamilton Anxiety Scale, however, have not been found to differ between genders (Grant and Kim 2002). Also, there is no clear evidence that women compared with men with gambling disorder experience higher rates of categorical anxiety disorders (Ibáñez et al. 2003). Rates of personality disorders also do not appear to generally differ between genders, although there is some indication that antisocial traits may be higher among male pathological gamblers (Ibáñez et al. 2003).

In critically reviewing the area of gender differences in comorbidity with gambling disorder, physicians must keep in mind the gender differences in psychiatric disorders in the general population. Epidemiological surveys indicate that in the general population, affective disorders are more common in women (Kessler et al. 1994), but alcohol use disorder is more common in men (Helzer et al. 1991). Thus, it is possible that the gender differences in comorbidity in gambling disorder reflect the gender differences for these psychiatric disorders found in the general population.

Problems Due to Gambling

Problems arising from gambling behavior may differ on the basis of gender. Although legal problems tend to be fairly common in patients with gambling disorder (Adolphe et al. 2019), recent studies have examined illegal behavior in gambling subjects and have reported inconsistent findings. For example, some research suggests that men with gambling disorder have more gambling-related illegal activities (Ladd and Petry 2002; Svensson et al. 2013). A separate study, however, found similar rates of acknowledgment of gambling-related illegal activities reported by male and female problem gamblers (21.4% of women and 22.3% of men) (Potenza et al. 2000). Two other studies also found no differences in illegal behavior based on gender (Grant and Kim 2001; Ibáñez et al. 2003). Finally, two studies have found that male gamblers are more likely to report illegal behaviors resulting in arrest than are female gamblers (Ladd and Petry 2002; Potenza et al. 2001).

Some studies have found that female problem gamblers are more likely to have financial problems due to gambling (Potenza et al. 2001), high rates of financial problems have been found in both genders (Grant and Kim 2001; Ibáñez et al. 2003; Potenza et al. 2001). In particular, the majority of both men and women with gambling disorder report credit card problems secondary to gambling (Grant and Kim 2001; Potenza et al. 2001), and approximately one-fourth of both groups have filed for bankruptcy because of gambling debt (Grant and Kim 2001). In addition, Ibáñez et al. (2003) found that men were more likely to have marital consequences from their gambling than were women.

Personality Differences

Although the number of categorical personality disorders does not appear to differ between male and female pathological gamblers (Ibáñez et al. 2003), gender may still influence personality characteristics of those with gambling disorder. The extent to which male and female gamblers differ with respect to personality traits, however, remains unclear. One study found that those with gambling disorder reported significantly more novelty seeking and impulsiveness than control subjects, and these traits did not distinguish male and female gamblers (Kim and Grant 2001). Another study, using a different scale to assess personality traits, found that male compared with female gamblers were more sensation seeking (Ibáñez et al. 2003). Of course, these personality traits may be moderated by other variables. For example, one study found that men with gambling disorder and co-occurring ADHD report higher negative emotionality and lower positive emotionality (Cairncross et al. 2019). With so few studies having been conducted using different scales, meaningful comments concerning personality differences in men and women with gambling disorder require data from further investigations.

Patterns of Heredity

Behavioral genetic studies can provide estimates of the extent of genetic versus environmental contributions to specific behaviors and conditions by contrasting the concordance of these behaviors and conditions between monozygotic and dizygotic twin pairs. In one study of male twins, familial factors (both genetic and environmental) explained 56%–62% of the occurrence of gambling disorder. The lifetime prevalence rates of gambling disorder were 22.6% for monozygotic twins and 9.8% for dizygotic twins (Eisen et al. 1998).

A second twin study, again including only men with gambling disorder, specifically examined the association between gambling disorder and alcohol use disorder (Slutske et al. 2000). In that study, 12%–20% of the genetic variation in risk for gambling disorder was held in common by both gambling and alcohol use disorders. In addition, genetic factors accounted for 64% of the overlap between these two disorders. The study also found that 3%–8% of the nonshared environmental variation was common for both conditions. In the same cohort, it was also found that the co-occurrence of gambling disorder and antisocial behavior disorders was greater than that due to chance and that the co-occurrence was at least partially due to a common genetic vulnerability (Slutske et al. 2001).

Because these studies involved only male gamblers, it remains unclear how these findings may apply to women with gambling disorder. However, one study produced a hint about differences in genetic influences with the finding that rates of first-degree relatives with alcohol use disorder were equally high among both male and female probands with gambling disorder (Grant and Kim 2001).

Other genetic differences have also been examined. One study found a possible significant association between gambling in females and a dopamine D_4 receptor gene (*DRD4*) polymorphism that leads to less efficient functioning of this particular dopamine receptor (Perez de Castro et al. 1997). In addition, serotonergic functioning has been implicated in gambling, and a possible association has been discovered between DNA polymorphisms in monoamine oxidase A genes and a subgroup of men with severe gambling disorder (Ibáñez et al. 2000). Another finding related to serotonergic function is that male gamblers may more frequently have a less functional variant of a polymorphism of the serotonin transporter gene (Perez de Castro et al. 1999). These findings suggest a contribution of genetic factors in the pathophysiology of gambling and suggest that these genetic factors may differ based on gender.

In one study that examined the genetics of personality traits that underpin gambling disorder, the authors found that genetic influences contributing to individual differences in normal-range personality traits explained more than 40% of the genetic risk for gambling disorder, with the largest and most robust contributions from the higher-order personality dimension of negative emotionality and its two lower-order dimensions of alienation and aggression. The higher-order dimension of constraint (i.e., low self-control) was associated with the genetic risk for gambling disorder only among women (Slutske et al. 2013). Risk taking or sensation seeking did not explain genetic risk for gambling disorder in either sex.

Neurocognitive and Neurobiological Underpinnings

Previous research has shown that women may be more prone to gamble as an escapist motivation. In a study by Ledgerwood and Petry (2006) involving treatment-seeking problem gamblers, it was found that a principal motivator for women to gamble was to escape negative emotions (Ledgerwood and Petry 2006). There has also been some suggestion that gender may moderate neural correlates in decision-making during gambling (Clark 2010). A recent meta-analysis of cognition in gambling disorder, however, found that gambling disorder was associated with significant impairments in motor and attentional inhibition, discounting, and decision-making tasks (Ioannidis et al. 2019). Importantly, moderation analyses did not indicate a significant effect of gender (Ioannidis et al. 2019).

Women and men in the general community have been shown to differ in self-report assessments of gambling-related cognitions (Raylu and Oei 2004). Cognitions relating to gambling expectancies or desired outcomes may be moderated by gender (Balodis et al. 2014; Bonnaire et al. 2009; Raylu and Oei 2004). One recent study found that men reported statistically significantly stronger levels of gambling-related urge and interpretive bias relative to women (Smith et al. 2015).

Very little neuroimaging research has attempted to understand gender differences in gambling disorder. One functional magnetic resonance imaging study ($n=28$ gamblers [8 women]) found that in the region encompassing the posterior putamen and insula, women with gambling disorder (but not men) exhibited increased activity in response to gambling videos. This finding suggests that women with gambling disorder may have a different sensory and motivational response in these regions when encountering gambling-related stimuli (Kober et al. 2016).

Access and Responsiveness to Treatment

In terms of seeking treatment, a recent study found that men and women with gambling disorder both felt shame associated with gambling-related financial difficulties and that it prevented them from seeking help. Specifically, whereas for men, the addictive qualities of and emotional responses to gambling were perceived as stigma-related barriers to help seeking, for women, their denial of their addiction and shame from being perceived as dishonest were seen as barriers to help seeking (Baxter et al. 2016). Finally, whereas women more typically report abstinence, men often report moderation as their end goal (Kim et al. 2016).

Little systematic research on gender-specific treatment response has been conducted. A recent meta-analysis showed that male gender was one of the most consistent predictors of successful psychotherapy treatment outcomes across multiple time points (Merkouris et al. 2016). A more recent study, however, found some slight evidence that men may be less likely than women to respond to internet-based cognitive-behavioral therapy (Rozental et al. 2019). Furthermore, another study of psychotherapy treatment found that whereas men rated treatment components to be more helpful, women found specific gambling-related treatment interventions (e.g., identification of high-risk situations, gambling beliefs and attitudes) to be less helpful (Toneatto and Wang 2009).

In terms of pharmacological treatment of individuals with gambling disorder, there appears to be little difference in response to treatment based on gender. A study of opioid antagonist medications found that gender was not associated with a differential response to medication (Grant et al. 2008). Recent research also shows that men and women with gambling disorder are equally likely to respond to placebo (Grant and Chamberlain 2017).

Moving forward, stress and posttraumatic regulation in women might be helpful as a preventive measure before treatment, given the particularly strong links between trauma and gambling problems in women and female-predominant tendencies to gamble as an escape from negative emotions (Dion et al. 2010; Petry and Steinberg 2005).

Conclusion

Gambling disorder is commonplace and undertreated. A number of important gender differences in gambling disorder are highly relevant to understanding this condition, including how it may present and how it can be optimally treated.

We have seen that men and women differ in terms of gambling trajectories over time, aspects of comorbidity, the nature of gambling-related cognitions (but not overall cognitive function), perceived barriers to treatment, and even—potentially—response to particular psychological interventions. Some of these gender differences are exemplified in the case vignette of Rochelle, who had a relatively rapid progression from recreational to pathological gambling, tended to gamble because of mood and anxiety triggers, and did not seek treatment because of treatment barriers such as feeling guilty. Although there are "average" differences between men and women with gambling disorder, it is important to consider patients on a case-by-case basis. Additionally, more research on gender differences in gambling disorder is needed, including studies of how existing treatments can be adapted to help maximize treatment outcomes for all gamblers.

References

Adolphe A, Khatib L, van Golde C, et al: Crime and gambling disorders: a systematic review. J Gambl Stud 35(2):395–414, 2019

Afifi TO, Cox BJ, Martens PJ, et al: Demographic and social variables associated with problem gambling among men and women in Canada. Psychiatry Res 178:395–400, 2010

Balodis S, Thomas A, Moore S: Sensitivity to reward and punishment: horse race and EGM gamblers compared. Pers Individ Dif 56:29–33, 2014

Baxter A, Salmon C, Dufresne K, et al: Gender differences in felt stigma and barriers to help-seeking for problem gambling. Addict Behav Rep 3:1–8, 2016

Bischof A, Meyer C, Bischof G, et al: Suicidal events among pathological gamblers: the role of comorbidity of axis I and axis II disorders. Psychiatry Res 225(3):413–419, 2015

Black DW, Moyer T: Clinical features and psychiatric comorbidity of subjects with pathological gambling behavior. Psychiatr Serv 49(11):1434–1439, 1998

Blaszczynski A, Steel Z, McConaghy N: Impulsivity in pathological gambling: the antisocial impulsivist. Addiction 92(1):75–87, 1997

Bonnaire C, Bungener C, Varescon I: Subtypes of french pathological gamblers: comparison of sensation seeking, alexithymia and depression scores. J Gambl Stud 25(4):455–471, 2009

Bonnaire C, Bungener C, Varescon I: Sensation seeking in a community sample of French gamblers: comparison between strategic and non-strategic gamblers. Psychiatry Res 250:1–9, 2017

Brady KT, Randall CL: Gender differences in substance use disorders. Psychiatr Clin North Am 22:241–252, 1999

Cairncross M, Milosevic A, Struble CA, et al: Clinical and personality characteristics of problem and pathological gamblers with and without symptoms of adult ADHD. J Nerv Ment Dis 207(4):246–254, 2019

Clark L: Decision-making during gambling: an integration of cognitive and psychobiological approaches. Phil Trans R Soc B: Biol Sci 365(1538):319–330, 2010

Desai RA, Potenza MN: Gender differences in the associations between past-year gambling problems and psychiatric disorders. Soc Psychiatry Psychiatr Epidemiol 43(3):173–183, 2008

Dion J, Collin-Vézina D, De La Sablonnière M, et al: An exploration of the connection between child sexual abuse and gambling in aboriginal communities. Int J Mental Health Addict 8:174–189, 2010

Eisen SA, Lin N, Lyons MJ, et al: Familial influences on gambling behavior: an analysis of 3359 twin pairs. Addiction 93:1375–1384, 1998

Granero R, Fernández-Aranda F, Steward T, et al: Compulsive buying behavior: characteristics of comorbidity with gambling disorder. Front Psychol 7:625, 2016

Grant JE, Chamberlain SR: The placebo effect and its clinical associations in gambling disorder. Ann Clin Psychiatry 29(3):167–172, 2017

Grant JE, Kim SW: Demographic and clinical features of 131 adult pathological gamblers. J Clin Psychiatry 62:957–962, 2001

Grant JE, Kim SW: Gender differences in pathological gamblers seeking medication treatment. Compr Psychiatry 43:56–62, 2002

Grant JE, Kim SW, Brown E: Characteristics of geriatric patients seeking medication treatment for pathologic gambling disorder. J Geriatr Psychiatry Neurol 14:125–129, 2001

Grant JE, Kim SW, Hollander E, Potenza MN: Predicting response to opiate antagonists and placebo in the treatment of pathological gambling. Psychopharmacology (Berl) 200(4):521–527, 2008

Grant JE, Chamberlain SR, Schreiber L, Odlaug BL: Gender-related clinical and neurocognitive differences in individuals seeking treatment for pathological gambling. J Psychiatr Res 46, 1206–1211, 2012a

Grant JE, Odlaug BL, Mooney ME: Telescoping phenomenon in pathological gambling: association with gender and comorbidities. J Nerv Ment Dis 200:996–998, 2012b

Helzer JE, Burnam A, McEvoy LT: Alcohol abuse and dependence, in Psychiatric Disorders in America: The Epidemiologic Catchment Area Study. Edited by Robins LN, Regier DA. New York, Free Press, 1991, pp 81–115

Husky MM, Michel G, Richard JB, et al: Gender differences in the associations of gambling activities and suicidal behaviors with problem gambling in a nationally representative French sample. Addict Behav 45:45–50, 2015

Ibáñez A, de Castro IP, Fernandez-Piqueras J, et al: Pathological gambling and DNA polymorphic markers at MAO-A and MAO-B genes. Mol Psychiatry 5:105–109, 2000

Ibáñez A, Blanco C, Donahue E, et al: Psychiatric comorbidity in pathological gamblers seeking treatment. Am J Psychiatry 158:1733–1735, 2001

Ibáñez A, Blanco C, Moreyra P, Saiz-Ruiz J: Gender differences in pathological gambling. J Clin Psychiatry 64:295–301, 2003

Ioannidis K, Hook R, Wickham K, et al: Impulsivity in gambling disorder and problem gambling: a meta-analysis. Neuropsychopharmacology 44(8):1354–1361, 2019

Jiménez-Murcia S, Granero R, Tárrega S, et al: Mediational role of age of onset in gambling disorder: a path modeling analysis. J Gambl Stud 32(1):327–340, 2016

Karlsson A, Håkansson A: Gambling disorder, increased mortality, suicidality, and associated comorbidity: a longitudinal nationwide register study. J Behav Addict 7(4):1091–1099, 2018

Kessler RC, McGonagle KA, Zhao S, et al: Lifetime and 12-month prevalence of DSM-III-R psychiatric disorders in the United States: results from the National Comorbidity Survey. Arch Gen Psychiatry 51(1):8–19, 1994

Kim HS, Hodgins DC, Bellringer M, Abbott M: Gender differences among helpline callers: prospective study of gambling and psychosocial outcomes. J Gambl Stud 32:605–623, 2016

Kim SW, Grant JE: Personality dimensions in pathological gambling disorder and obsessive-compulsive disorder. Psychiatry Res 104:205–212, 2001

Kober H, Lacadie CM, Wexler BE, et al: Brain activity during cocaine craving and gambling urges: an fMRI study. Neuropsychopharmacology 41(2):628–637, 2016

Komoto Y: Factors associated with suicide and bankruptcy in Japanese pathological gamblers. Int J Ment Health Addict 12(5):600–606, 2014

Ladd GT, Petry NM: Gender differences among pathological gamblers seeking treatment. Exp Clin Psychopharmacol 10:302–309, 2002

Lahti T, Halme J, Pankakoski M, et al: Characteristics of treatment seeking Finnish pathological gamblers: baseline data from a treatment study. Int J Ment Health Addict 11(3):307–314, 2013

Ledgerwood DM, Petry NNM: Psychological experience of gambling and subtypes of pathological gamblers. Psychiatry Res 144(1):17–27, 2006

Manning V, Koh PK, Yang Y, et al: Suicidal ideation and lifetime attempts in substance and gambling disorders. Psychiatry Res 225(3):706–709, 2015

Mark ME, Lesieur HR: A feminist critique of problem gambling research. Br J Addiction 87:549–565, 1992

Martins SS, Lobo DS, Tavares H, Gentil V: Pathological gambling in women: a review. Rev Hosp Clin Fac Med Sao Paulo 57:235–242, 2002

Medeiros GC, Leppink EW, Redden SA, et al: A cross-cultural study of gambling disorder: a comparison between women from Brazil and the United States. Braz J Psychiatry 38(1):53–57, 2016

Merkouris SS, Thomas SA, Browning CJ, Dowling NA: Predictors of outcomes of psychological treatments for disordered gambling: a systematic review. Clin Psychol Rev 48:7–31, 2016

Perez de Castro I, Ibáñez A, Torres P, Fernandez-Piqueras J: Genetic association study between pathological gambling and a functional DNA polymorphism at the D4 receptor gene. Pharmacogenetics 7:345–348, 1997

Perez de Castro I, Ibáñez A, Saiz-Ruiz J, Fernandez-Piqueras J: Genetic contribution to pathological gambling: possible association between a functional DNA polymorphism at the serotonin transporter gene (5-HTT) and affected men. Pharmacogenetics 9:397–400, 1999

Petry NM: A comparison of young, middle-aged, and older adult treatment-seeking gamblers. Gerontologist 42:92–99, 2002

Petry NM, Steinberg KL: Childhood maltreatment in male and female treatment-seeking pathological gamblers. Psychol Addict Behav 19:226–229, 2005

Petry NM, Stinson FS, Grant BF: Comorbidity of DSM-IV pathological gambling and other psychiatric disorders: results from the National Epidemiologic Survey on Alcohol and Related Conditions. J Clin Psychiatry 66(5):564–574, 2005

Pietrzak RH, Morasco BJ, Blanco C, et al: Gambling level and psychiatric and medical disorders in older adults: results from the National Epidemiologic Survey on Alcohol and Related Conditions. Am J Geriatr Psychiatry 15:301–313, 2007

Potenza MN, Steinberg MA, McLaughlin SD, et al: Illegal behaviors in problem gambling: analysis of data from a gambling helpline. J Am Acad Psychiatry Law 28:389–403, 2000

Potenza MN, Steinberg MA, McLaughlin SD, et al: Gender-related differences in the characteristics of problem gamblers using a gambling helpline. Am J Psychiatry 158:1500–1505, 2001

Randall CL, Roberts JS, Del Boca FK, et al: Telescoping of landmark events associated with drinking: a gender comparison. J Stud Alcohol 60:252–260, 1999

Raylu N, Oei T: The Gambling Related Cognitions Scale (GRCS): development, confirmatory factor validation and psychometric properties. Addiction 99(6): 757–769, 2004

Ronzitti S, Lutri V, Smith N, et al: Gender differences in treatment-seeking British pathological gamblers. J Behav Addict 5(2):231–238, 2016

Ronzitti S, Kraus SW, Hoff RA, et al: Problem-gambling severity, suicidality and DSM-IV Axis II personality disorders. Addict Behav 82:142–150, 2018

Rozental A, Andersson G, Carlbring P: In the absence of effects: an individual patient data meta-analysis of non-response and its predictors in internet-based cognitive behavior therapy. Front Psychol 10:589, 2019

Rubin A, Stout RL, Longabaugh R: Gender differences in relapse situations. Addiction 91(suppl):111–120, 1996

Sacco P, Torres LR, Cunningham-Williams RM, et al: Differential item functioning of pathological gambling criteria: an examination of gender, race/ethnicity, and age. J Gambl Stud 27(2):317–330, 2011

Slutske WS, Eisen S, True WR, et al: Common genetic vulnerability for pathological gambling and alcohol dependence in men. Arch Gen Psychiatry 57:666–673, 2000

Slutske WS, Eisen S, Xian H, et al: A twin study of the association between pathological gambling and antisocial personality disorder. J Abnorm Psychol 110:297–308, 2001

Slutske WS, Cho SB, Piasecki TM, Martin NG: Genetic overlap between personality and risk for disordered gambling: evidence from a national community-based Australian twin study. J Abnorm Psychol 122(1):250–255, 2013

Slutske WS, Piasecki TM, Deutsch AR, et al: Telescoping and gender differences in the time course of disordered gambling: evidence from a general population sample. Addiction 110(1):144–151, 2015

Smith D, Battersby M, Harvey P: Does gender moderate the subjective measurement and structural paths in behavioural and cognitive aspects of gambling disorder in treatment-seeking adults? Addict Behav 48:12–18, 2015

Subramaniam M, Wang P, Soh P, et al: Prevalence and determinants of gambling disorder among older adults: a systematic review. Addict Behav 41:199–209, 2015

Sundqvist K, Rosendahl I: Problem gambling and psychiatric comorbidity—risk and temporal sequencing among women and men: results from the Swelogs Case-Control Study. J Gambl Stud 35(3):757–771, 2019

Svensson J, Romild U, Shepherdson E: The concerned significant others of people with gambling problems in a national representative sample in Sweden—a 1 year follow-up study. BMC Public Health 13:1087, 2013

Tavares H, Zilberman ML, Beites FJ, Gentil V: Gender differences in gambling progression. J Gambl Stud 17:151–159, 2001

Toneatto T, Wang JJ: Community treatment for problem gambling: sex differences in outcome and process. Community Ment Health J 45(6):468–475, 2009

Trevorrow K, Moore S: The association between loneliness, social isolation, and women's electronic gaming machine gambling. J Gambl Stud 14:263–284, 1998

Vitaro F, Arseneault L, Trenblay RE: Dispositional predictors of problem gambling in male adolescents. Am J Psychiatry 154:1769–1770, 1997

Waluk OR, Youssef GJ, Dowling NA: The relationship between problem gambling and attention deficit hyperactivity disorder. J Gambl Stud 32(2):591–604, 2016

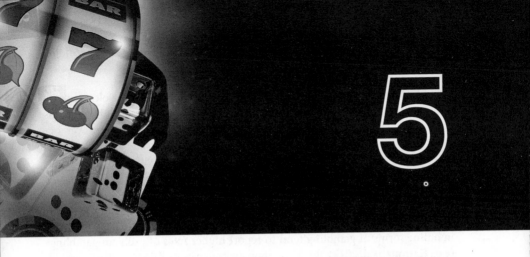

Online Gambling and Gambling-Gaming Convergence

Daniel L. King, Ph.D.

Sally M. Gainsbury, Ph.D.

Paul H. Delfabbro, Ph.D.

Advances in digital technology, including the growth of interactive platforms, have given rise to many innovations in gambling products. There are now more ways to access gambling products, new player experiences and reward structures, greater tailoring of products to individual players, and increasing integration of gambling with other popular online activities such as gaming and social media (Delfabbro et al. 2020; King and Delfabbro 2020). Research suggests that many of these products are capturing new gambling cohorts, including people who would not otherwise be gambling. Instead of growth being principally confined to land-based activities such as casinos and slot machine venues, there are now a myriad of online wagering and gaming products from which prospective gamblers can choose.

Public health approaches to gambling advocate for delayed or older age at first gambling experiences and for experiences to involve responsible parental supervision (Dickson-Gillespie et al. 2008). These principles may, however, be more difficult to satisfy as gambling becomes more accessible and promoted within widely accessible, "everyday" technology-based activities (e.g., browsing the internet, using social media, visiting sports websites). The relative risks of technology-driven gambling activities to users have been difficult to assess and track over time, particularly in studies that fail to differentiate types of users and activities. Although some early research has reported that gamblers who engage in online forms of gambling tend to report higher rates of problem gambling (e.g., Kairouz et al. 2012), this association may often be explained by demographic or other characteristics of these users or their involvement in a wide range of activities (including land-based gambling) rather than as a consequence of aspects of the technology itself (Blaszczynski et al. 2016).

In this chapter, we highlight some of the major intersection points between gambling and technology and consider research that has examined online and digital gambling and gambling-like activities in relation to problem gambling. It will be evident that the intersection of gambling and technology has sometimes enabled major changes in gambling behavior and created some regulatory challenges, including difficulties in determining when an activity is legally considered gambling. We describe some of the major forms of online and digital gambling and gambling-like activities and present research evidence on their potential impact on users, and then highlight regulatory challenges associated with these technologies.

Internet Gambling

The internet gambling industry has grown rapidly since its inception and is expected to continue to thrive and expand its market. Wood and Williams (2007) reported that although accurate revenue figures were difficult to obtain, the global online gambling market was worth an estimated $12 billion in 2005 and $15.2 billion in 2006. This continued growth trajectory is evident in more recent data. In 2019, it was estimated that the global online gambling market was valued at $46 billion and projected to more than double, to reach $94 billion, by 2024 (Lock 2019). Although this prediction was made prior to the current (mid-2020) context of the coronavirus pandemic and thus does not account for associated economic uncertainties, the accessibility of online gambling has not been affected by the closures and restrictions that have affected land-based gambling venues, although sporting events have been largely canceled, impacting online wagering companies.

Internet gambling, or "interactive gambling" as it is known in Australia, is a broad term used to refer to any gambling activity that is primarily facilitated online. In this sense, internet gambling technically refers to a mode of access (e.g., computer, laptop, mobile, and similar devices) rather than a type of gambling per se. Its most popular forms include online versions of conventional betting or wagering options (including betting on sports and racing), lottery products, and online or virtual casinos (e.g., poker, roulette, blackjack). Reviews of internet gambling have referred to its distinguishing characteristics (Gainsbury 2015; Lawn et al. 2020). These include 24-hour accessibility, ease of use and convenience, the wide array of options, and the capacity for continuous and simultaneous play. All of these features are thought to contribute to the popularity and higher frequency of involvement in these activities (Chagas and Gomes 2017; Gainsbury 2015).

Many jurisdictions globally, including the United States, have taken steps in the past decade to legalize and regulate internet gambling. This has typically followed the recognition of the practical difficulties of enforcing prohibition, overseas competition including unregulated marketplaces, and the benefits of a local regulated market, including taxation revenue and harm minimization measures to enhance consumer protection (Laffey et al. 2016; Procter et al. 2019; Wood and Williams 2007). Moves to legalize a local online market have been desirable or necessary in some regions to combat the illegal, predatory, or questionable tactics used by some overseas operators to lure customers.

There have been debate and conjecture on the public health risks and harms associated with internet gambling (LaPlante et al. 2019). Varying terminology and ways of differentiating types of online gambling activities have sometimes complicated this discussion. For example, there has been critical discussion of the nature of the internet as an object of addiction versus a virtual environment for existing gambling activities (Griffiths 2003; Shaffer et al. 2000). There have been studies that have differentiated online and land-based forms of problem gambling to evaluate whether online gambling may be distinct from land-based gambling (Blaszczynski et al. 2016; Lawn et al. 2020). The latest revision of the *International Classification of Diseases* (ICD-11) has reinforced this view with its inclusion of specifiers for "predominantly online" and "predominantly offline" (which is consistent with "gaming disorder" in the same category of addictive disorders) to differentiate these broad types of gambling behaviors.

Internet vs. Land-Based Gambling Participation

Research on online gambling has attempted to identify some typical profiles of users and determine how they may differ from land-based gamblers (Gainsbury et al. 2019; Höllén et al. 2020; Lopez-Gonzalez et al. 2019). This research has sometimes assumed that online and offline gamblers may represent mutually exclusive groups or activities. However, studies have shown that exclusively online gambling is relatively rare and that online gambling tends to overlap with land-based gambling activities (Blaszczynski et al. 2016). This includes participation in the same basic gambling activity (i.e., online and offline poker) and in different activities (e.g., buying lottery tickets and playing online poker). Although internet gamblers are not a homogenous group (Khazaal et al. 2017), studies have reported that online gamblers tend to report certain characteristics more often than their land-based counterparts. It bears noting that internet gambling has changed significantly over time and that studies conducted in the 2000s and early 2010s are unlikely to be representative of current gamblers and activities, operators, and their regulation. There is a need to replicate some of the earlier studies, particularly those that inform the basis of current policies.

Wood and Williams (2011) presented data from 1,954 internet gamblers and 5,967 non-internet gamblers, reporting that internet gamblers were more likely to be male (78% vs 58%) and younger (45 vs. 51 years of age), have higher incomes, and have more past-month substance use (i.e., tobacco, alcohol, and other drugs). They reported that internet gamblers had higher yearly and weekly involvement in almost every kind of gambling and reported higher levels of sports betting, betting on horse or dog races, and betting on games of skill, such as poker. Another large study by Wardle et al. (2011) presented findings from the 2010 British Gambling Prevalence Survey. This was a large-scale random probability survey of adults ($n=7,756$) that examined how people gamble and the extent to which online and offline gambling may be integrated into overall gambling participation. Only 2% of participants were exclusively online gamblers, compared with about 10% who were "mixed-mode" gamblers who gambled in-person and online on the same activity. They found that online gamblers typically had higher levels of education and higher incomes than their land-based-only counterparts. Furthermore, it was the mixed-mode group of gamblers who were the most frequent gamblers compared with the other gambling groups.

More recently, Blaszczynski et al.'s (2016) study of 4,594 respondents evaluated different groups of exclusively online, land-based, and mixed-mode gamblers. Participants were surveyed on participation in all forms of gambling; use of alcohol, tobacco, and drugs; help seeking; and personal problems experienced because of gambling, as well as problem gambling and psychological distress. The exclusively online gamblers were the smallest group in the study (13% of the total number) and were less psychologically complex than land-based and mixed-mode gamblers. These findings were consistent with those of Wardle et al. (2011), who reported that mixed-mode gamblers reported more frequent gambling involvement and greater psychological distress and alcohol consumption while gambling than exclusively online gamblers. Land-based gamblers experienced more psychological distress, self-acknowledged need for treatment, and help-seeking behavior. The authors suggested that several factors may contribute to lower levels of gambling and associated problems among internet gamblers, including their lower alcohol consumption rates during gambling, lower general psychological distress, and possible use of responsible gambling features when online to minimize the extent of their losses.

Gainsbury et al. (2019) investigated the associations between specific gambling activities and modalities (internet and venue or land based) and problem gambling and psychological distress. The authors surveyed 998 Australian adults who had gambled online in the previous 30 days. They observed that those who engaged in an online version of a gambling activity were likely to have also engaged in the offline activity. When controlling for overall gambling frequency, the authors found that problem gambling was significantly positively associated with the frequency of online gambling and land-based gambling using electronic gaming machines (EGMs) and sports betting. Psychological distress was uniquely associated with higher frequency of venue gambling using EGMs, sports betting, and casino card or table games. Although higher overall gambling engagement was an important predictor of gambling-related harms, the authors noted that participation in venue-based EGMs, sports betting, and casinos among internet gamblers was uniquely positively associated with distress.

Internet Gambling and Problem Gambling

With its greater convenience and accessibility, online gambling has been proposed to give rise to more frequent patterns of gambling, which in turn may contribute to higher rates of problem gambling (Effertz et al. 2018). At face value, this appears to make sense because the internet can be accessed almost anywhere and could be engaged in for long periods while in psychological states that impair decision-making (e.g., depression, intoxication) with no responsible oversight. However, one counterargument to this is that many forms of land-based gambling are also highly accessible, including EGM gambling in venues where there may be more incentives (e.g., amenities, free drinks or food, comfort) to visit and stay in the venue than an online casino. Research evidence suggests that internet gambling may not be inherently more harmful than land-based gambling activities that enable similar continuous forms of gambling (e.g., EGMs). Instead, any harms that appear to be associated with internet gambling (e.g., financial) could arise from the cumulative involvement in a range of activities.

In support of this, Wardle et al.'s (2011) study in the United Kingdom found no problem gamblers in a subsample of online-only gamblers classified on the basis of DSM-IV pathological gambling criteria. By contrast, prevalence rates were 0.9% for land-based-only gamblers, 2.4% for mixed-mode same activity gamblers, and 4.3% for mixed-mode different activity gamblers. In their study of 9,910 French adolescents (age 17 years), Baggio et al. (2017) reported that 10.5% of participants were internet gamblers (i.e., they had gambled online at least one time during the previous 12 months). Internet gamblers had significantly higher levels of problem gambling, spent more money gambling, spent more time gambling, and reported a wider range of gambling activities than land-based gamblers. However, these relationships weakened and became nonsignificant when participation in other gambling forms and time spent gambling were controlled for separately. The authors concluded that time spent gambling and the diversity of gambling formats, rather than internet gambling, were the best predictors of problem gambling.

Further work has examined how problem online gamblers may differ from nonproblem online gamblers. Gainsbury et al.'s (2016) study examined different groups of Australian gamblers (N=4,482) according to preferred modes for accessing online gambling as well as personal and behavioral factors. Gamblers who preferred to gamble online on computers had lower rates of gambling problems compared with those using mobile and supplementary devices. Problem gamblers were younger, gambled on more activities, had more irrational beliefs about gambling, and were more likely to use drugs while gambling than nonproblem and at-risk gamblers. However, consistent with previous studies, a significant proportion of these respondents also had problems related to land-based gambling. These findings suggested that gambling-related problems often arose from engagement in many gambling activities rather than from principally internet gambling.

Khazaal et al. (2017) investigated the psychosocial profiles of 584 internet gamblers recruited online through gambling websites and forums. The study examined their gambling motives and cognitions, mood differences, and impulsivity in addition to "social" variables of indebtedness (owing money to others), loneliness, and in-game behaviors. Using cluster analysis, the authors identified three main types of gamblers: 1) lonely, indebted gamblers (6.5%); 2) nonlonely, non-indebted gamblers (75.4%), and 3) nonlonely, indebted gamblers (18%). Groups 1 and 3 were at higher risk of problem gambling than those in group 2. Furthermore, the three groups differed on most assessed variables, including problem gambling scores, general mood, and impulsivity scores. These results showed that online gamblers are not a homogenous group in terms of psychosocial variables and risk of problem gambling.

As highlighted previously, Gainsbury et al.'s (2019) study enabled comparisons of different types of gambling in relation to gambling-related problems among 998 Australian adult online gamblers. They reported that frequency of participation in EGM gambling online and in venues uniquely predicted greater problem gambling severity scores even when controlling for the frequency of gambling on other activities. The authors suggested that there may be features of EGMs that are inherently problematic (i.e., in both venues and online forms), for example, the short interval between bets and outcomes enabling rapid, continuous periods of betting. Similarly, research suggests there may be unique features of online gambling activities that contribute to greater gambling frequency and harms. Lopez-Gonzalez et al. (2019) surveyed 659 online sports gamblers to examine online betting characteristics in relation to problem gambling. Measurement of these characteristics included coverage of 1) live in-play betting, 2) cash-out feature use, 3) fantasy sports gaming, 4) location of betting, and 5) device or platform used to make bets. They reported that participants who scored higher on gambling problems engaged more often with these structural characteristics than low-risk and nonproblem gamblers and that this difference was not fully accounted for by their higher overall gambling activity.

Together, these findings suggest that there are a minority of exclusively online gamblers who report gambling-related problems. This group tends to be much smaller than other groups of gamblers, including those who engage in a mixture of online and land-based gambling. Studies suggest that problem gambling is predicted by the level of involvement in multiple forms of gambling activities (Blaszczynski et al. 2016) and by some specific features and activities, including EGMs (Gainsbury et al. 2019). Internet gambling offers another means of accessing gambling activities for vulnerable gamblers, and this may contribute to further harms in addition to their involvement in other activities.

Gambling-Gaming Convergence

Another growing area of study of gambling and technology has been the overlap or "convergence" of gambling and gaming activities (Gainsbury 2019; King and Delfabbro 2018a). Since the 1990s, there has been interest in whether there might be a connection between video gaming and gambling (Griffiths 1991; Ladouceur and Dube 1995). Such speculation, as Griffiths (1991) argued, is not unsurprising given that the two activities share much in common at a structural level (Griffiths and Wood 2000). Recent technological developments have led to some video games resembling, promoting, or intersecting with gambling products or facilitating continuous in-game purchasing to obtain random rewards (King et al. 2019b, 2019b).

Some examples of this convergence include video games that realistically simulate gambling without money being directly involved (aside from being used to purchase virtual currency), such as social casino games; video games that include options to acquire monetized items (e.g., skins) that enable unregulated gambling on external platforms; gambling operators promoting gambling using video games on social media; and the presence of gambling within competitive gaming events and online broadcasts (King and Delfabbro 2016b). In terms of product availability, a scoping study suggested that about 54% of games on Facebook include gambling themes (Jacques et al. 2016). A 2018 review of 22 popular video games available in Australia found that 5 retail games met the conventional criteria for gambling, including the option to cash out winnings (Drummond and Sauer 2018).

Some studies have examined the broad overlap of involvement in video gaming and gambling participation to identify whether gaming might be a risk factor for gambling (Kim et al. 2017). This literature has generally referred to the similarities between gaming and electronic gambling machines, such as variable-ratio reinforcement (Delfabbro et al. 2009; Griffiths 2005). A study by McBride and Derevensky (2016), using a student sample of both adolescents and young adults, reported that 94% of gamblers played video games, compared with 86% of nongamblers, and that 55% of video game players gambled, compared with 31% of non–video game players. Sanders and Williams (2019) surveyed a panel of 3,942 adults and found that 79% of video gamers gambled and that 70% of gamblers played video games (a reversal of the pattern observed by McBride and Derevensky [2016]). Other relevant findings include those of Kristiansen and Severin (2020), who reported that 55% of Danish adolescents (nearly all of whom played video games) had engaged in some form of gambling, and Brooks and Clark (2019), who reported that 53% of 144 recruited video gamers gambled.

Taken together, these results suggest that nearly all young people (a focus of these studies) play video games and that around 50%–60% are gamblers, a figure generally consistent with international reviews (King et al. 2020b; Volberg et al. 2010). However, engagement in one activity appears to modestly increase the likelihood of participation in the other. These associations do not imply causation, nor do they indicate whether the relationship might still occur after one has controlled for factors that might predict engagement in both activities. In addition to age, studies would need to control for gender (because both video gaming and gambling are more likely to be reported by males [Delfabbro et al. 2009]), impulsivity (Sanders and Williams 2019), and a range of other variables that might relate to risk-taking propensity (Biegun et al. 2020; Walther et al. 2012).

Loot Boxes

The "loot box" is a feature within monetized games that has received growing regulatory and research attention for its resemblance to gambling (Delfabbro and King 2020; Drummond et al. 2020; Griffiths 2018; King and Delfabbro 2019a, 2019b). A loot box refers to an in-game reward system that can be purchased with real money (but sometimes only with virtual credits), usually repeatedly, to obtain a random selection of virtual items. In some implementations, these virtual items can be purchased from or sold to other users via trading applications outside of the game in which they are located. In some jurisdictions, there have been recommendations that loot boxes should be considered an illegal form of gambling when they operate in an "open economy" (i.e., loot-boxed rewards have monetary value outside the source game) (BBC News 2018).

Some virtual items, called "skins," that are purchased or won from loot boxes in games can also be externally traded and therefore used as a form of virtual currency for betting purposes on some third-party gambling sites. This development has essentially led to an unregulated online gambling market, with some researchers noting that the popularity of gaming among younger people may lead them to experiment with skin gambling opportunities. There is some research evidence indicating that people, including underage users, are familiar with and engage in the activity (Li et al. 2019). A large-scale study by the UK Gambling Commission (2017) investigated young people's awareness of and participation in "skin betting" as part of its broader survey of gambling in this population. Overall, 45% of 11- to 16-year-old participants were aware of the options to bet with in-game items when playing computer games or app-based games. Almost 6 in 10 boys (59%) knew about this activity, compared with less than one third of girls (31%). In terms of actual participation, 11% of 11- to 16-year-old participants claimed to have personally bet with in-game items, with this being much more prevalent among boys (20%) than girls (3%).

Some limited research has examined cross-sectional relationships between loot-box spending and problematic gambling symptoms (Li et al. 2019). A study by Zendle and Cairns (2018), involving a large-scale cross-sectional survey of 7,422 online gamers using the Problem Gambling Severity Index (PGSI), measured loot-box spending and other microtransaction spending. The authors reported that higher PGSI scores were positively associated with loot-box spending (with a small to medium effect). Zendle and Cairns (2018) noted that the association between the PGSI and loot-box spending was comparable to many other risk factors in the gambling literature, but also acknowledged that causality could not be inferred from their data. As Delfabbro and King (2020) have pointed out, it is probably more likely that people who have a preexisting interest in gambling tend to migrate toward loot-box playing because of its gambling-like content. For loot boxes to be considered a possible "gateway" product for gambling, one would need to be able to show that there was a direct link between external gambling activities and loot-box use. Examples of more persuasive evidence might include reports that people were betting with the skins obtained in loot boxes on third-party gambling sites.

Other research teams have examined loot-box spending and its association with gambling-related indicators. A study by Brooks and Clark (2019) surveyed a population of adults (through MTurk) ($n=144$) and an undergraduate student population ($n=113$). Gaming and loot-box-related variables included estimated time spent gaming and monthly expenditure, measures of problematic gambling and gaming, and perceptions and behaviors related to loot boxes. Most participants reported that they believed that loot boxes were a form of gambling (68.1% and 86.2% for MTurk and undergraduate samples, respectively). The authors identified a subset of survey items that were then used to create a Risky Loot-box Index (RLI). Consistent with Zendle and Cairns' (2018) studies, participants' RLI scores were significantly associated with their PGSI scores. In addition, RLI scores were associated with problematic gaming and all subscales on the Gambling Related Cognitions Scale (small to medium effects).

Recent calls for regulation and consumer protection measures (e.g., by the House of Lords Gambling Committee in the United Kingdom) for monetized games across jurisdictions have encountered issues related to the lack of clarity regarding the legal status and associated risks of certain types of in-game purchases (Drummond et al. 2020; King et al. 2020a). The available research on loot boxes and gambling is complicated by the diversity of structural features of in-game monetization (e.g., random elements, cosmetic versus competitive options, closed vs. open economies) and suggests that there is a need for researchers to consider games on a case-by-case basis (King et al. 2019a, 2019b). Proposed regulatory measures have included age-appropriate marketing, greater transparency and consumer advice on odds for random in-game rewards, and limit-setting and parental controls (Drummond and Sauer 2018; King and Delfabbro 2018b; Király et al. 2018). Assuming the policy objective is to reduce the addictive potential of monetized gaming activities, it may not be necessary to implement wide-reaching restrictive policies that encompass all types of microtransactions, which may have some unforeseen consequences.

Social Casino Games

Social casino games (SCGs) occupy a unique place in the digital entertainment marketplace. SCGs are casino-style games that are accessed via social media or apps and usually played on mobile (phone or tablet) devices. SCGs offer close structural approximations to gambling, featuring comparable and sometimes identical audiovisual and game play design to casino games, and enable players to invest real money in exchange for virtual credits that can be won or lost. These activities, therefore, blur the line between gaming and gambling but evade legal definition as a gambling activity because of the absence of monetary return to the player (Dayanim 2014; Gainsbury et al. 2014; Rose 2014).

Social casino gaming is becoming more recognized in the academic literature, and attempts have been made to examine potential links between SCGs and engagement in formal gambling activities (Abarbanel and Rahman 2015; King and Delfabbro 2016a; King et al. 2016; Macey and Kinnunen 2020). Studies of SCGs (Gainsbury et al. 2016; Kim et al. 2015) have examined the association between SCG play and problem gambling symptoms (Gainsbury et al. 2016; Kim et al. 2015). Research evidence suggests that social games are popular among young adults (i.e., worldwide prevalence of 6% in the 18- to 21-year age range [Parke et al. 2013]), and a small proportion of adolescents are familiar with or have engaged in SCGs (King et al. 2014). This is borne out in data that show that the small number of young people ages 13–17 who spend money on SCGs spend, on average, $3.96 per day on credits (Harvest Strategy 2014).

However, there is limited evidence to support the notion that SCGs contribute to changes in the incidence and prevalence of gambling and potential problems associated with gambling (Gainsbury et al. 2015b; Kim et al. 2015; King et al. 2014). Qualitative studies of SCG users have reported that some users migrate to gambling, motivated by a desire to achieve monetary rewards (Dussault et al. 2017; Gainsbury et al. 2015b; Kim et al. 2016). However, these studies also suggest that some gamblers may turn to SCGs as a less financially risky option when attempting to limit or quit involvement in EGMs.

Fantasy Sports

Fantasy sports (including its faster-paced subtype, "daily fantasy sports" [DFS]) refers to an online-facilitated structured competition involving both chance and skill in which participants compete by assembling a virtual team of players of a professional sports league. Each player's team competes in imagined or theoretical rounds of play in which the outcomes are determined by the statistical performance of each player's team members, which corresponds to their real-world individual performances. In contrast to traditional fantasy sports leagues, which are generally played in real time over the corresponding sports season, DFS is more fast-paced, being conducted over a single game or one round of competition.

Fantasy sports involve money usually expressed in the form of a "cost-of-entry" fee by requiring players to deposit money into a pot or pool that is subsequently awarded to the winner. DFS players are required to pay entry fees that can range from 25 cents to $5,000, depending on the league's rules and requirements (Pickering et al. 2016). The main aspect of interactivity involves making decisions in relation to which virtual players select, trade, or delist from a player's team, and this is where players more familiar with or knowledgeable of the scoring systems at play or the status of the professional competition and its players have a marked competitive advantage over other participants in the fantasy sports league. Although fantasy sports has a considerable chance element (e.g., real-world players may get injured or unfit), a large proportion of the winnings tends to be awarded to the more highly skilled or knowledgeable players.

Fantasy sports have not been classified consistently across jurisdictions, such as the United States, where there have been many legal deliberations on their status as a potential form of gambling because of differences in the degree to which legislators believe the activity is a game of skill or luck (Pickering et al. 2016). In Australia, where in 2016 there were reportedly 1.65 million DFS players (Swinson 2016), DFS have generally been classified as gambling when money became involved. The DFS market in Australia is projected to continue to grow with DraftKings, a major DFS operator popular in the United States and Europe, joining several other large operators in this region.

Some limited research has been conducted on DFS in relation to gambling and other correlates. A study by Nower et al. (2018) surveyed 3,634 U.S. residents on gambling and leisure activities. Their sample included 299 past-year DFS players. Their results showed that more frequent and diverse involvement in gambling, male gender, and reports of suicidal thoughts in the past year were most predictive of DFS players. Being Hispanic (vs. white) or single (vs. married or living with a partner) doubled the likelihood of DFS play.

Esports Betting

Esports are organized video game competitions between highly skilled video game players or teams that audiences view either online or in a venue (Greer et al. 2019; Seo and Jung 2014). These sports cover a wide range of games but generally fall into game types in which players or teams of players compete against each other, such as shooters (e.g., first-person shooter games such as Counter-Strike: Global Offensive, Call of Duty), real-time strategy (e.g., StarCraft), multiplayer online battle arena (e.g., League of Legends, Defense of the Ancients), fighting (e.g., Mortal Kombat, Street Fighter, Super Smash Bros.), sports (e.g., FIFA, Madden NFL, Rocket League), survival (e.g., PlayerUnknown's Battlegrounds, Fortnite Battle Royale), and other popular games (e.g., the collectible card game Hearthstone). The rising popularity of esports has attracted the provision of esports gambling services offered by established sports wagering operators across the globe, as well as newer esports-exclusive betting operators (Macey and Hamari 2018). Many regulated sports wagering operators across the globe now offer esports cash betting. Esports betting is also increasingly available via online operators who offer esports betting exclusively (e.g., Unikrn, EGB.com, arcanebet). Some operators allow esports betting with cryptocurrencies, such as Bitcoin or Ethereum, which allow gamblers greater anonymity.

The estimated global combined esports cash and skin betting revenue was $56 billion in 2016 (Grove 2016). However, these estimates appear to have decreased in subsequent years because of game developer actions that affected the unregulated skin marketplace, with the 85% of the 2016 estimated revenue (cash and skins) attributable to skin betting ($4.9 billion) dropping to around 10% for 2019 ($670 million). Reliable data on the prevalence, characteristics, and gambling behaviors of esports bettors are hard to obtain (Gainsbury et al. 2017a, 2017b). Gainsbury et al.'s (2017a) study of esports bettors and sports bettors reported that both were predominantly male, but esports bettors were more likely to be younger, be more educated, report higher income, and be more ethnically diverse than sports bettors.

Regulatory Challenges

The dynamic and rapidly evolving nature of emerging gambling products creates numerous difficulties for regulators and policy makers (Harris and Griffiths 2017). Attempts at using evidence as a basis for regulatory decision-making is hindered by the lack of evidence on most new forms of gambling or products that may be considered by gambling regulators. Industry innovation and consumer adoption are much more rapid than the typical research cycle required to produce credible, reliable, and robust research to guide policy. When research does exist, it often uses small, nonrepresentative samples; has been conducted in just one jurisdiction; and may focus on a product already outdated.

Attempts to regulate industry may be limited because of jurisdictional reach, such as when an industry is based or owned in a particular place, or has a physical location that may be different from where it is targeting customers. This has repeatedly been noted by regulators in relation to internet gambling sites, leaving relatively little recourse against companies operating in breach of jurisdictional regulation. There are several products, including those discussed in this chapter, that may not be within the remit of a gambling regulator despite the impact that the product may have on gambling and gambling-related harms. There are few specific consumer regulations for gaming companies, particularly compared with the highly regulated gambling industry. The gaming industry is relatively unwilling to engage in discussions with various stakeholders, including researchers, about topics including research and consumer protection and corporate social responsibility.

A final challenge is a lack of consensus between regulators and jurisdictions in terms of best practices that is related to the lack of evidence of the impact of various policies on newly emerging gambling products. Ongoing dialogue between stakeholders across the gambling field, including researchers, industry, policy makers and regulators, treatment providers, and consumers, would be highly beneficial in guiding policies to minimize harms related to emerging gambling technologies.

Conclusion

New technologies have enabled many innovations and changes to gambling opportunities. The past 15 years has seen the expansion and sophistication of gambling products on the internet and the emergence of new forms of unregulated gambling with virtual currencies in addition to nongambling online content such as loot boxes and SCGs and gambling promotions on social media. The research literature in this diverse area is growing rapidly in response to the academic and regulatory interest in these activities, particularly in relation to younger users, who routinely use the underlying technologies. Many of these activities appear to expand and evolve at a rate that outpaces the research. Further research is needed to examine the potential impacts of digital gambling technologies and gambling hybrid products, including the identification of people who are more vulnerable to overinvolvement in these activities, and to develop regulatory and public health responses to address problem gambling and gambling-related harm.

References

Abarbanel B, Rahman A: eCommerce market convergence in action: social casinos and real money gambling. UNLV Gaming Research Review Journal 19:51–62, 2015

Baggio S, Dupuis M, Berchtold A, et al: Is gambling involvement a confounding variable for the relationship between Internet gambling and gambling problem severity? Comput Hum Behav 71:148–152, 2017

BBC News: Video game loot boxes declared illegal under Belgium gambling laws. April 26, 2018. Available at: http://www.bbc.com/news/technology-43906306. Accessed December 30, 2018.

Biegun J, Edgerton JD, Roberts LW: Measuring problem online video gaming and its association with problem gambling and suspected motivational, mental health, and behavioural risk factors in a sample of university students. Games Culture, January 2, 2020 (Epub ahead of print)

Blaszczynski A, Russell A, Gainsbury S, Hing N: Mental health and online, land-based and mixed gamblers. J Gambl Stud 32:261–275, 2016

Brooks GA, Clark L: Associations between loot box use, problematic gaming and gambling, and gambling-related cognitions. Addict Behav 96:26–34, 2019

Chagas BT, Gomes JF: Internet gambling: a critical review of behavioural tracking research. Journal of Gambling Issues 36:1–27, 2017

Dayanim B: Social casino gaming: an evolving legal landscape. Gam Law Rev Econ 18:30–36, 2014

Delfabbro PH, King DL: Gaming-gambling convergence: evaluating evidence for the "gateway" hypothesis. Int Gambl Stud 20(3):380–392, 2020

Delfabbro PH, King DL, Lambos C, Puglies S: Is video-game playing a risk factor for pathological gambling in Australian adolescents? J Gambl Stud 25:391–405, 2009

Delfabbro PH, King DL, Gainsbury SM: Understanding gambling and gaming skill and its implications for convergence of gaming with electronic gaming machines. Int Gambl Stud 20:171–183, 2020

Dickson-Gillespie L, Rugle L, Rosenthal R, Fong T: Preventing the incidence and harm of gambling problems. J Prim Prev 29:37–55, 2008

Drummond A, Sauer JD: Video game loot boxes are psychologically akin to gambling. Nat Hum Behav 2:530–532, 2018

Drummond A, Sauer JD, Hall LC, et al: Why loot boxes could be regulated as gambling. Nat Hum Behav 4:986–988, 2020

Dussault F, Kalke J, Meyer G, et al: Transition from playing with simulated gambling games to gambling with real money: a longitudinal study in adolescence. Int Gambl Stud 17:386–400, 2017

Effertz T, Bischof A, Rumpf HJ, et al: The effect of online gambling on gambling problems and resulting economic health costs in Germany. Eur J Health Econ 19:967–978, 2018

Gainsbury SM: Online gambling addiction: the relationship between internet gambling and disordered gambling. Curr Addict Rep 2:185–193, 2015

Gainsbury SM: Gaming-gambling convergence: research, regulation, and reactions. Gaming Law Review 23:80–83, 2019

Gainsbury SM, Hing N, Delfabbro PH, King DL: A taxonomy of gambling and casino games via social media and online technologies. Int Gambl Stud 14:196–213, 2014

Gainsbury SM, Russell A, Wood R, et al: How risky is Internet gambling? A comparison of subgroups of Internet gamblers based on problem gambling status. New Med Soc 17:861–879, 2015a

Gainsbury SM, Hing N, Delfabbro P, et al: An exploratory study of interrelationships between social casino gaming, gambling, and problem gambling. Int J Ment Health Addict 13:136–153, 2015b

Gainsbury SM, Russell AM, King DL, et al: Migration from social casino games to gambling: motivations and characteristics of gamers who gamble. Comput Hum Behav 63:59–67, 2016

Gainsbury SM, Abarbanel B, Blaszczynski A: Game on: comparison of demographic profiles, consumption behaviors, and gambling site selection criteria of esports and sports bettors. Gaming Law Review 21:575–587, 2017a

Gainsbury SM, Abarbanel B, Blaszczynski A: Intensity and gambling harms: exploring breadth of gambling involvement among esports bettors. Gaming Law Review 21:610–615, 2017b

Gainsbury SM, Angus DJ, Blaszczynski A: Isolating the impact of specific gambling activities and modes on problem gambling and psychological distress in internet gamblers. BMC Public Health 19:1372, 2019

Greer N, Rockloff M, Browne M, et al: Esports betting and skin gambling: a brief history. J Gambl Issues 43:128–146, 2019

Griffiths MD: Amusement machine playing in childhood and adolescence: a comparative analysis of video games and fruit machines. J Adolesc 14:53–73, 1991

Griffiths M: Internet gambling: issues, concerns, and recommendations. CyberPsychology & Behavior 6:557–568, 2003

Griffiths MD: Relationship between gambling and video-game playing: a response to Johansson and Gotestam. Psychol Rep 96:644–646, 2005

Griffiths MD: Is the buying of loot boxes in video games a form of gambling or gaming? Gaming Law Review 22:52–54, 2018

Griffiths MD, Wood RTA: Risk factors in adolescence: the case of gambling, videogame playing, and the Internet. J Gambl Stud 16:199–225, 2000

Grove C: Esports and Gambling: Where's the Action? Irvine, CA, Eilers and Krejcik Gaming, 2016. Available at: www.thelines.com/wp-content/uploads/2018/03/Esports-and-Gambling.pdf. Accessed January 7, 2020.

Harris A, Griffiths MD: A critical review of the harm-minimisation tools available for electronic gambling. J Gambl Stud 33:187–221, 2017

Harvest Strategy: A snapshot of youth in the digital playground: Digsogames and Digsinos. London, International Social Games Association, 2014. Available at: http://blogs.dlapiper.com/all-in/files/2014/11/ISGA-Research-A-Snapshot-of-Youth-in-the-Digital-Playground.pdf. Accessed January 7, 2020.

Hollén L, Dörner R, Griffiths MD, Emond A: Gambling in young adults aged 17–24 years: a population-based study. J Gambl Stud 36(3):747–766, 2020

Jacques C, Fortin-Guichard D, Bergeron PY, et al: Gambling content in Facebook games: a common phenomenon? Comput Hum Behav 57:48–53, 2016

Kairouz S, Paradis C, Nadeau L: Are online gamblers more at risk than offline gamblers? Cyberpsychol Behav Soc Netw 15:175–180, 2012

Khazaal Y, Chatton A, Achab S, et al: Internet gamblers differ on social variables: a latent class analysis. J Gambl Stud 33:881–897, 2017

Kim HS, Wohl MJ, Salmon MM, et al: Do social casino gamers migrate to online gambling? An assessment of migration rate and potential predictors. J Gambl Stud 31:1819–1831, 2015

Kim HS, Wohl MJ, Gupta R, Derevensky J: From the mouths of social media users: a focus group study exploring the social casino gaming–online gambling link. J Behav Addict 5:115–121, 2016

Kim HS, Hollingshead S, Wohl MJ: Who spends money to play for free? Identifying who makes micro-transactions on social casino games (and why). J Gambl Stud 33(2):525–538, 2017

King DL, Delfabbro PH: Adolescents' perceptions of parental influences on commercial and simulated gambling activities. Int Gambl Stud 16:424–441, 2016a

King DL, Delfabbro PH: Early exposure to digital simulated gambling: a review and conceptual model. Comput Hum Behav 55:198–206, 2016b

King DL, Delfabbro PH: Internet Gaming Disorder: Theory, Assessment, Treatment, and Prevention. London, Academic Press, 2018a

King DL, Delfabbro PH: Predatory monetization features in video games (e.g., "loot boxes") and Internet gaming disorder. Addiction 113:1967–1969, 2018b

King DL, Delfabbro PH: Loot box limit-setting is not sufficient on its own to prevent players from overspending: a reply to Drummond, Sauer, and Hall. Addiction 114:1324–1325, 2019a

King DL, Delfabbro PH: Video game monetization (e.g., "loot boxes"): a blueprint for practical social responsibility measures. Int J Ment Health Addict 17:166–179, 2019b

King DL, Delfabbro PH: The convergence of gambling and monetised gaming. Curr Opin Behav Sci 31:32–36, 2020

King DL, Delfabbro PH, Kaptsis D, Zwaans T: Adolescent simulated gambling via digital and social media: an emerging problem. Comput Hum Behav 31(2):305–313, 2014

King DL, Russell A, Gainsbury S, et al: The cost of virtual wins: an examination of gambling-related risks in youth who spend money on social casino games. J Behav Addict 5:401–409, 2016

King DL, Delfabbro PH, Gainsbury SM, et al: Unfair play? Video games as exploitative monetized services: an examination of game patents from a consumer protection perspective. Comput Hum Behav 101:131–143, 2019a

King DL, Koster E, Billieux J: Study what makes games addictive. Nature 573:346, 2019b

King DL, Russell AR, Delfabbro PH, Polisena D: Fortnite microtransaction spending was associated with peers' spending behaviors but not gaming disorder symptoms. Addict Behav 104:106311, 2020a

King DL, Russell A, Hing N: Adolescent land-based and online gambling: Australian and international prevalence rates and measurement issues. Curr Addict Rep 7:137–148, 2020b

Király O, Griffiths MD, King DL, et al: Policy responses to problematic video game use: a systematic review of current measures and future possibilities. J Behav Addict 7:503–517, 2018

Kristiansen S, Severin MC: Loot box engagement and problem gambling among adolescent gamers: findings from a national survey. Addict Behav 103:106254, 2020

Ladouceur R, Dube D: Prevalence of pathological gambling and associated problems in individuals who visit non-gambling video arcades. J Gambl Stud 11:361–365, 1995

Laffey D, Della Sala V, Laffey K: Patriot games: the regulation of online gambling in the European Union. J Eur Public Policy 23:1425–1441, 2016

LaPlante DA, Gray HM, Williams PM, Nelson SE: An empirical review of gambling expansion and gambling-related harm. Sucht 64:295–306, 2019

Lawn S, Oster C, Riley B, et al: A literature review and gap analysis of emerging technologies and new trends in gambling. Int J Enviro Res Publ Heal 17:744, 2020

Li W, Mills D, Nower L: The relationship of loot box purchases to problem video gaming and problem gambling. Addict Behav 97:27–34, 2019

Lock S: Market value of online gambling worldwide 2017 and 2024. Statista, 2019. Available at: www.statista.com/statistics/270728/market-volume-of-online-gaming-worldwide. Accessed January 7, 2020.

Lopez-Gonzalez H, Estévez A, Griffiths MD: Internet-based structural characteristics of sports betting and problem gambling severity: is there a relationship? Int J Ment Health Addict 17:1360–1373, 2019

Macey J, Hamari J: Investigating relationships between video gaming, spectating esports, and gambling. Comput Hum Behav 80:344–353, 2018

Macey J, Kinnunen J: The convergence of play: interrelations of social casino gaming, gambling, and digital gaming in Finland. Int Gambl Stud 20(3):414–435, 2020

McBride J, Derevensky J: Gambling and video game playing among youth. Journal of Gambling Issues 34:156–178, 2016

Nower L, Caler KR, Pickering D, Blaszczynski A: Daily fantasy sports players: gambling, addiction, and mental health problems. J Gambl Stud 34:727–737, 2018

Parke J, Wardle H, Rigbye J, Parke A: Exploring social gambling: scoping, classification and evidence review. London, Gambling Commission, 2013. Available at: www.gamblingcommission.gov.uk/Gambling-data-analysis/Social-media/Exploring-social-gambling.aspx. Accessed January 7, 2020.

Pickering D, Blaszczynski A, Hartmann M, Keen B: Fantasy sports: skill, gambling, or are these irrelevant issues? Curr Addict Rep 3:307–313, 2016

Procter L, Angus DJ, Blaszczynski A, Gainsbury SM: Understanding use of consumer protection tools among Internet gambling customers: utility of the Theory of Planned Behavior and Theory of Reasoned Action. Addict Behav 99:106050, 2019

Rose IN: Should social casino games be regulated? Gam Law Rev Econ 18:134–137, 2014

Sanders J, Williams R: The relationship between video gaming, gambling, and problematic levels of video gaming and gambling. J Gambl Stud 35:559–569, 2019

Seo Y, Jung SU: Beyond solitary play in computer games: the social practices of eSports. Journal of Consumer Culture 16(3):635–655, 2014

Shaffer HJ, Hall MN, Bilt JV: "Computer addiction": a critical consideration. Am J Orthopsychiatr 70:162–168, 2000

Swinson M: Living in a fantasy (sports) world. Melbourne, Australia, King and Wood Mallesons, 2016. Available at: www.kwm.com/en/au/knowledge/insights/living-in-fantasy-sports-world-regulation-virtual-team-20160601. Accessed January 7, 2020.

UK Gambling Commission: Young people and gambling: a study among 11–16 year olds in Great Britain. Birmingham, UK, UK Gambling Commission, 2017

Volberg R, Gupta R, Griffiths MD, et al: An international perspective on youth gambling prevalence studies. Int J Adolesc Med Health 22:3–38, 2010

Walther B, Morgenstern M, Hanewinkel R: Co-occurrence of addictive behaviours: personality factors related to substance use, gambling and computer gaming. Eur Addict Res 18:167–174, 2012

Wardle H, Moody A, Griffiths M, et al: Defining the online gambler and patterns of behaviour integration: evidence from the British Gambling Prevalence Survey 2010. Int Gambl Stud 11:339–356, 2011

Wood RT, Williams RJ: Problem gambling on the Internet: implications for Internet gambling policy in North America. New Media & Society 9:520–542, 2007

Wood RT, Williams RJ: A comparative profile of the Internet gambler: demographic characteristics, game-play patterns, and problem gambling status. New Media & Society 13:1123–1141, 2011

Zendle D, Cairns P: Video game loot boxes are linked to problem gambling: results of a large-scale survey. PloS One 13:e0206767, 2018

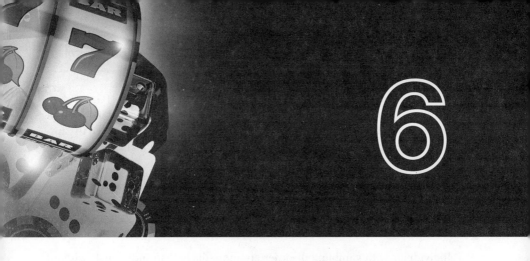

Legal and
Forensic Aspects

Austin W. Blum, M.D., J.D.
Jon E. Grant, M.D., M.P.H., J.D.

Robert, a 26-year-old college graduate,
began working as a bank teller approximately 3 years ago. He has been a model
employee and gets along well with coworkers. He started gambling at a local casino about 2 years ago, playing blackjack on Friday evenings. At first, he relished
the challenge of trying to beat the house. During the past 6 months, however, he
has been going to the casino more frequently and enjoying it less. Instead of feeling like he is having fun, he has become obsessed with gambling, thinking all
day about strategies to enhance his chances of winning. Unfortunately, he has
been losing more as well. Not particularly good at managing finances, Robert finds
himself with considerable debt, unable to pay rent or even his minimum credit
card payments each month. In a desperate move, he impulsively "borrows"
money from the bank by stealing from his register. He claims he intended to re-
pay the money the next day after winning at the casino. He loses $500 that night,
however, and his theft is discovered. He is fired for embezzlement and reported
to the authorities for legal action.

Patients like Robert are not rare. The social and economic costs of disordered gambling are high: disturbed marital and family functioning (Black et al.
2012; Dowling et al. 2009), loss of employment (Gerstein et al. 1999), and signif-

icant financial difficulties, including insolvency and bankruptcy (Grant et al. 2010). In many cases, individuals with gambling disorder become involved in the criminal justice system. In this chapter, we summarize issues related to gambling disorder and the law that are relevant to practicing clinicians.

Clinical Aspects of Gambling and Crime

Individuals with gambling disorder are more likely than individuals without gambling disorder to report engaging in criminal behavior. Illegal activities of problem gamblers commonly include embezzlement, theft, writing bad checks, and other forms of fraud. The precise relationship between disordered gambling and crime, however, has resisted easy explanation.

A previous edition of the *Diagnostic and Statistical Manual of Mental Disorders* (DSM-IV-TR) included among the diagnostic criteria for pathological gambling (now gambling disorder) a history of "illegal acts such as forgery, fraud, theft, or embezzlement to finance gambling" (American Psychiatric Association 2000). Subsequent research found that the "illegal acts" criterion had little diagnostic value because individuals who engage in gambling-related crime are likely to meet criteria for disordered gambling based on other symptoms. Although the "illegal acts" criterion was subsequently removed in the fifth edition (DSM-5; American Psychiatric Association 2013), the presence of such behaviors should be considered an important marker of gambling severity (Granero et al. 2014; Jiménez-Murcia et al. 2009; Petry et al. 2013). In fact, several studies of clinical samples have found that individuals with gambling disorder who have a history of illegal behavior tend to have more severe gambling symptoms (Mestre-Bach et al. 2018; Strong and Kahler 2007).

Gambling has long been associated with criminal behavior (Rosenthal and Lorenz 1992), often in a bidirectional way, with people engaging in crimes either to obtain money for gambling or conversely to solve financial problems stemming from gambling (Laursen et al. 2016; May-Chahal et al. 2017; Petry and O'Brien 2013). It is estimated that between 25% and 43% of individuals with disordered gambling have engaged in criminal acts to support their gambling (Turner et al. 2016). In one study, Ledgerwood and colleagues (2007) interviewed 231 people with gambling problems and found that 27.3% reported engaging in gambling-related illegal behavior over the previous year. Only 5 of these 63 participants had been arrested for their illegal behavior (Ledgerwood et al. 2007). In a study of callers to a gambling helpline, those who reported gambling-related illegal behaviors were more likely to have a severe gambling problem, owe debts to acquaintances, and have a substance use disorder (Potenza et al. 2000).

Whether there is in fact a causal relationship between illegal behavior and gambling, however, remains unclear (for a review, see Adolphe et al. 2019). Some of the many factors that may mediate the relationship between gambling and criminal activity include personality disorders or features such as impulsivity and risk acceptance, as well as co-occurring substance use disorders (Adolphe et al. 2019; Gorsane et al. 2017; Pastwa-Wojciechowska 2011; Turner et al. 2009).

Researchers have identified three putative links between problem gambling and crime: a direct or "instrumental" connection (e.g., theft to pay off gambling debts); a "co-symptomatic" relationship in which a mediating factor (e.g., poor impulse control) increases the risk of both gambling and criminal offending; and, finally, a "coincidental" connection in which the offending bears no relationship to a gambling problem (Perrone et al. 2013). Although most gamblers in self-report studies attribute their criminal activity to financial need (Blaszczynski and McConaghy 1994; Blaszczynski et al. 1989; Meyer and Stadler 1999; Turner et al. 2009), the overall evidence is mixed. Some gamblers, to be sure, seem to turn to crime only when legal means of obtaining gambling funds have been exhausted (Binde 2016; Lesieur 1984). For many other gamblers, however, criminal behaviors are motivated by more than simple financial considerations. A growing number of studies suggest that problem gamblers commit assault and other violent crimes at a higher-than-expected rate—not only income-generating crimes (Dowling et al. 2016; McCorkle 2002; Roberts et al. 2016; Smith et al. 2003; Suomi et al. 2013). These violent offenders may represent a particularly impaired subset of gamblers (Rudd and Thomas 2016). In short, the relationship between problem gambling and criminal offending is complex and multifactorial.

Some researchers have considered whether gamblers with a history of illegal acts may represent a distinct pathological gambling phenotype—for example, a group characterized by higher levels of impulsivity. In one recent study, gamblers who engaged in illegal activity were more likely than gamblers without such a history to report experiencing high levels of urgency (i.e., a tendency to act rashly when experiencing heightened emotional states) and increased lack of premeditation (Mestre-Bach et al. 2018). As such, impulsivity (or other related constructs) may represent an important and clinically relevant construct for better understanding the complex relationship between problem gambling and crime.

Relationship of Gambling Disorder to Antisocial Personality Disorder

For some gamblers—especially those with a long history of criminal activities (Abbott et al. 2005)—illegal behaviors may be better explained by a third factor: antisocial personality disorder (ASPD), characterized by a pervasive pattern of poor social conformity, deceitfulness, impulsivity, and lack of remorse. Although ASPD is relatively rare in the general population, with approximately 3.6% of people meeting criteria (Grant et al. 2005), it is estimated that between 13% and 15% of individuals with disordered gambling have co-occurring ASPD (Black and Moyer 1998; Slutske et al. 2001). Compared with gamblers without ASPD, gamblers with ASPD are younger and more likely to be male, to be divorced, and to have fewer years of education (Pietrzak and Petry 2005). They are also more likely to report earlier onset of gambling behavior, greater severity of gambling and substance use problems, and more severe psychopathology (on measures of paranoid ideation, somatization, and phobic anxiety) than problem gamblers without ASPD (Pietrzak and Petry 2005). In a forensic setting, clinicians can recognize gamblers with ASPD by their pattern of illegal behavior, the underlying motivation of the offender, and the presence of other antisocial behaviors.

Gambling Disorder and Domestic Abuse

Although we tend to think of the crimes committed by problem gamblers as being largely financial, clinicians should be aware of an association that has received relatively less attention: that between gambling disorder and intimate partner or family violence (IPV) (Dowling et al. 2016). One study found that women whose partners had a gambling problem were 10.5 times more likely to be a victim of IPV than women whose partners did not gamble (Muelleman et al. 2002). When the gambling partner had a co-occurring alcohol use disorder, the odds increased to 50.4 times as likely. Thus, if Robert (from the opening vignette) were in a relationship, screening for evidence of abuse or other serious dysfunction within the family unit would be warranted. Finally, although empirical data on this topic are still limited, problem gambling appears to increase one's likelihood not only of perpetrating IPV (Brasfield et al. 2012) but of being victimized as well (Afifi et al. 2010; Korman et al. 2008).

Gambling and the Legal System

Compulsive gambling has raised challenging forensic issues in both criminal and civil legal contexts. How should the courts think about the rights and obligations of a compulsive gambler such as Robert in the case vignette?

Gamblers as Criminal Defendants

In a criminal justice setting, putative behavioral addictions (e.g., gambling disorder) have raised thorny questions about criminal responsibility. In and of itself, carrying a psychiatric diagnosis such as gambling disorder does not mitigate or excuse criminal responsibility (Wills and Gold 2014). Rather, according to a standard devised by the American Law Institute (ALI) currently used in 20 states (Scott 2018), a defendant is free from criminal liability if he or she "lacks substantial capacity either to appreciate the wrongfulness of his conduct or to conform his conduct to the requirements of law" (Model Penal Code § 401; American Law Institute 1985). The ALI's rule is an example of an *insanity defense*. Even if a defendant does not meet insanity criteria, his or her mental illness may still be taken into account at sentencing (e.g., as a mitigating factor) (Felthous 2016).

For the purpose of federal criminal law, the Federal Insanity Defense Reform Act holds that a defendant may be found not guilty by reason of insanity only if he or she "was unable to appreciate the nature and quality or the wrongfulness of his acts" (Insanity Defense Reform Act 1984). Under the federal statute, therefore, simply having lost control over one's behavior is not enough. One's very rationality must be impaired. The Federal Sentencing Guidelines, however, authorize downward departure at sentencing on the basis of "a significantly impaired ability to (A) understand the wrongfulness of the behavior comprising the offense or to exercise the power of reason; or (B) control behavior that the defendant knows is wrongful" (U.S. Sentencing Commission 2018). Therefore, a reduction in federal sentencing may be available to defendants who were unable to control their behavior—even if they knew their actions were wrong at the time. That distinction played a key role in the sentencing of former Wall Street executive Andrew W. W. Caspersen.

In *United States v. Caspersen* (2016), Andrew Caspersen pleaded guilty to federal securities and wire fraud charges and admitted to defrauding investors of $38.5 million. In a Ponzi-like scheme, Mr. Caspersen solicited investors for a deal he claimed would earn a 15%–20% annual return. However, instead of investing the funds as promised, Mr. Caspersen misdirected them to his personal bank account. He then used the money to make a series of highly speculative options trades based on the performance of Standard & Poor's 500 stock index (S&P 500). In one transaction, Mr. Caspersen made what amounted to a $17 million bet that the S&P 500 would increase in value; when the market moved in the opposite direction, he lost $14.6 million. In the end, Mr. Caspersen was left with only $40,000 in his trading account. When one investor asked Mr. Caspersen to return their original $25 million investment, the fraud was quickly discovered. At sentencing, defense attorneys asked for leniency, arguing that Mr. Caspersen was impaired by a gambling addiction. According to the defense, Mr. Caspersen had also lost all of his $20 million personal fortune over the previous decade because of compulsive gambling. U.S. District Judge Jed S. Rakoff, also a founding member of the MacArthur Foundation Project on Law and Neuroscience, accepted the defense argument and concluded that a downward departure from the plea agreement was warranted. Accordingly, Mr. Caspersen was sentenced to a lesser term of 4 years in prison.

Before *Caspersen*, sentencing reductions based on disordered gambling were rare. In *United States v. Grillo* (2004), a compulsive gambler who was found guilty of mail theft and fraud raised gambling addiction as a means of reducing his sentence. The court noted that as long as the defendant had funds to support his gambling habit, he did not steal; he stole only when he ran out of money. In other words, compulsive gambling merely provided a motive for the defendant's criminal behavior. And, the court noted, all crimes have a motive of some sort—including those motivated by behavior that might be described as addictive or compulsive.

The *Grillo* court was concerned about setting a precedent that might be abused. It if had granted a downward departure in that case, then defendants charged with many other crimes would be able to seek a lesser sentence as well. As an example, the court referred to the possibility of a compulsive shopper seeking a reduced sentence because he or she started to steal after running out of money. In addition, the court aligned itself with the U.S. Court of Appeals for the Seventh Circuit, which has held that the defendant's capacity to control his or her conduct must have been significantly impaired at the time of the offense (*United States v. Roach* 2002).

In summary, the law tends to hold individuals with disordered gambling responsible for their criminal conduct. Whether *Caspersen* will lead other courts to show leniency toward defendants with gambling disorder remains to be seen.

Civil Context:
Gamblers as Plaintiffs

In civil litigation, individuals with disordered gambling have brought suit against casinos based on a theory of negligence. Does the casino owe Robert (or other compulsive gamblers) protection from the harm caused by his addiction? Although courts in the United States have not been receptive to such claims, they have met with some success in Canada.

One significant U.S. case is *Stevens v. MTR Gaming Group, Inc.* (2016). Scott Stevens went to Mountaineer Casino (in West Virginia) and began to gamble on his favorite slot machine. After losing $10,000, he completed suicide by gunshot wound. Mr. Stevens' spouse, Stacy Stevens, filed a lawsuit against both Mountaineer Casino and International Game Technology, the slot machine manufacturer. In her suit, Ms. Stevens argued that Mountaineer Casino "had a duty to protect Scott Stevens from *itself* . . . yet no attempts were made to intervene." Mr. Stevens had gambled regularly at Mountaineer Casino in the 5 years before his death and been offered various inducements, including complimentary meals, drinks, hotel rooms, and access to lines of credit ("markers"). The West Virginia Supreme Court of Appeals rejected Ms. Stevens' argument, holding that "no duty of care under West Virginia law exists on the part of manufacturers of video lottery terminals, or the casinos in which the terminals are located, to protect users from compulsively gambling." Specifically, the Court noted that the state of West Virginia had adopted a "self-exclusion" program, which provided an alternative avenue for compulsive gamblers to seek help. Thus, the casino itself had no legally recognized duty to protect its patrons from their own behavior.

However, even problem gamblers who have availed themselves of state self-exclusion programs have few rights under the law. In *Merrill v. Trump Indiana,*

Inc. (2003), a compulsive gambler brought suit in federal court seeking $6 million in damages from Trump Indiana, Inc., the operator of a riverboat casino. Mr. Merrill had been treated for problem gambling and asked to be placed on the casino's "eviction list." Two years later, Mr. Merrill returned to the casino and lost heavily. Applying Indiana law, the U.S. Court of Appeals for the Seventh Circuit determined that a casino operator does not have a duty to protect problem gamblers from their own gambling addiction. At most, the Court held, "the rules impose upon [casinos] a duty to the state through the gaming commission"—not to the individual gambler. Other American courts have also held that compulsive gamblers do not have a cause of action against casinos that have failed to exclude them (see *Taveras v. Resorts International Hotel, Inc.* 2008; *Williams v. Aztar Indiana Gaming Corp.* 2003).

By contrast, in Canada, litigation by compulsive gamblers has sometimes led to settlement. In one case, Lisa Dickert was allowed to return to a casino just 6 weeks after signing a self-exclusion form. After gambling for 52 hours straight, Ms. Dickert drove home and was subsequently involved in a motor vehicle accident. Ms. Dickert filed a $1 million lawsuit against the Ontario Lottery and Gaming Corporation (OLG)—the government agency that runs Ontario's casinos—for failing to enforce the exclusion order. The case was subsequently resolved pursuant to a confidential settlement. Several years later, the OLG had settled all 10 problem gambling–related lawsuits filed against it. More recently, the Ontario Court of Appeal appears to have opened the door to possible claims by third parties defrauded by problem gamblers (see *Paton Estate v. Ontario Lottery and Gaming Corporation* 2016).

In addition to these legal interactions involving gamblers and gaming operators, plaintiffs have also brought suit against pharmaceutical manufacturers based on reports of serious medication side effects, one of which has been the claim of causing a gambling addiction. These cases began to surface in the medical literature in 2000 with reports of dopaminergic drugs (e.g., Parkinson's disease drugs and the antipsychotic medication aripiprazole) resulting in gambling behavior, as well as other impulsive behaviors. In hundreds of separate lawsuits, patients have alleged that their use of these drugs caused them to engage in compulsive gambling. These cases have all reached undisclosed settlements and have resulted in warnings by regulatory agencies in many countries. In the wake of this litigation, the authors of DSM-5 specified that patients whose gambling had taken place only while they were using a dopaminergic agent should not receive a diagnosis of gambling disorder.

Implications for Treatment

For many clinicians, the prospect of being involved in the care of a patient like Robert could be intimidating or even daunting. As previously mentioned, gamblers who commit crimes tend to have more severe levels of psychopathology than their non–legally involved counterparts. Indeed, the presence of illegal behaviors has been linked by Ledgerwood and colleagues to worse treatment outcomes, implying that different (or more intensive) therapies may be indicated (Ledgerwood et al. 2007). In a commentary following the work by Ledgerwood et al., Grant and Potenza (2007) proposed that the complex relationship between illegal behavior and disordered gambling should be studied in large clinical samples. If it became apparent, for example, that illegal acts and disordered gambling are rooted in the same underlying pathology (e.g., impulsivity or sociopathy), then treatments could be targeted accordingly. At the time of this writing, however, there are no published studies, to our knowledge, examining whether individuals with disordered gambling with a propensity for illegal behavior respond preferentially to particular pharmacological or psychosocial treatments.

Conclusion

Problem gambling and illegal activity may be linked by multiple pathways. Depending on the context, illegal acts may be motivated by the need for money, part of a larger pattern of risk-seeking behavior, or simply secondary to antisocial personality. Thus, gamblers who commit crime are a heterogeneous population with different psychiatric comorbidities, underlying risk factors (e.g., impulsive traits), and potentially different treatment needs. Patients with a history of gambling-related crime should therefore be carefully assessed and managed on a case-by-case basis.

Returning to the case vignette, the clinical assessment of Robert should include an inquiry into other impulsive behaviors (including antisocial behaviors and drug and alcohol use), prescribed medications, and any salient family history. The clinician should consider a detailed examination of both the gambling behavior and the criminal behavior, including motivations beforehand and feelings about these acts in retrospect (such as regret). The assessment could also include a full screening for ASPD, consisting of a structured diagnostic interview and a discussion of conduct problems during adolescence. Based on this evaluation, the clinician should be able to determine whether Robert's behavior is attributable to gambling disorder or better explained by more chronic personality pathology. In addition, the clinician could consider screening Robert using a self-report measure for impulsivity, such as the Barratt Impulsiveness Scale, as well as for specific impulsive behaviors, including those related to ADHD and sexual impulsivity. The clinician should ask Robert about his sexual relationships and make every reasonable effort to ascertain whether intimate partner violence is present.

On the basis of a detailed assessment, a treatment plan for Robert can be initiated. Preliminary treatment options include the use of therapy (especially cognitive and behavioral therapies), pharmacological treatments, or both (see Chapter 11, "Psychosocial Treatments," and Chapter 12, "Pharmacological Treatments," in this volume for evidence-based treatment approaches to gambling disorder). Because of his criminal behavior, Robert may have a more serious gambling disorder than other patients. With that in mind, the clinician may consider using cognitive-behavioral therapy (CBT), but perhaps for a longer period of time than the evidence might suggest for gamblers without criminal histories. If ASPD is noted in the assessment, CBT augmented with insight-oriented therapy and therapy focusing on otherness may be beneficial. Referral to Gamblers Anonymous should also be part of the treatment plan.

The clinician should also consider referring Robert for legal counseling. Assuming that Robert is charged with a crime, it is not exactly clear what the outcome would (or should) be. For the most part, courts have treated individuals with disordered gambling like other offenders—as possessing a sufficient degree of understanding and self-control to be held responsible for their actions. However, after conviction, evidence of disordered gambling has led to a reduced sentence in some cases. Will other jurisdictions follow the lead of the *Caspersen* court in granting leniency to these defendants? And as scientific experts continue to bring neuroscientific evidence (e.g., neuroimaging and genetics data) into the courtroom at an ever-growing pace, will the law adapt to take advantage of emerging biological insights?

References

Abbott MW, McKenna BG, Giles LC: Gambling and problem gambling among recently sentenced male prisoners in four New Zealand prisons. J Gambl Stud 21(4):537–558, 2005

Adolphe A, Khatib L, van Golde C, et al: Crime and gambling disorders: a systematic review. J Gambl Stud 35(2):395–414, 2019

Afifi TO, Brownridge DA, MacMillan H, Sareen J: The relationship of gambling to intimate partner violence and child maltreatment in a nationally representative sample. J Psychiatr Res 44(5):331–337, 2010

American Law Institute: Model Penal Code, §4.01, 1962

American Law Institute: Model Penal Code and Commentaries. Philadelphia, PA, American Law Institute, 1985

American Psychiatric Association: Diagnostic and Statistical Manual of Mental Disorders, 4th Edition, Text Revision. Washington, DC, American Psychiatric Association, 2000

American Psychiatric Association: Diagnostic and Statistical Manual of Mental Disorders, 5th Edition. Arlington, VA, American Psychiatric Association, 2013

Binde P: Gambling-related embezzlement in the workplace: a qualitative study. Int Gambl Stud 16(3):391–407, 2016

Black DW, Moyer T: Clinical features and psychiatric comorbidity of subjects with pathological gambling behavior. Psychiatr Serv 49(11):1434–1439, 1998

Black DW, Shaw MC, McCormick BA, Allen J: Marital status, childhood maltreatment, and family dysfunction: a controlled study of pathological gambling. J Clin Psychiatry 73(10):1293–1297, 2012

Blaszczynski AP, McConaghy N: Antisocial personality disorder and pathological gambling. J Gambl Stud 10(2):129–145, 1994

Blaszczynski A, McConaghy N, Frankova A: Crime, antisocial personality and pathological gambling. J Gambl Behav 5(2):137–152, 1989

Brasfield H, Febres J, Shorey R, et al: Male batterers' alcohol use and gambling behavior. J Gambl Stud 28(1):77–88, 2012

Dowling N, Smith D, Thomas T: The family functioning of female pathological gamblers. Int J Ment Health Addict 7(1):29–44, 2009

Dowling N, Suomi A, Jackson A, et al: Problem gambling and intimate partner violence: a systematic review and meta-analysis. Trauma Violence Abuse 17(1):43–61, 2016

Felthous AR: Criminal responsibility, in Principles and Practice of Forensic Psychiatry, 3rd Edition. Edited by Rosner R, Scott CL. Boca Raton, FL, CRC Press, 2016, pp 267–275

Gerstein D, Hoffman J, Larison C, et al: Gambling impact and behavior study: report to the National Gambling Impact Study Commission. Chicago, National Opinion Research Center at the University of Chicago, 1999

Gorsane MA, Reynaud M, Vénisse JL, et al: Gambling disorder-related illegal acts: regression model of associated factors. J Behav Addict 6(1):64–73, 2017

Granero R, Penelo E, Stinchfield R, et al: Contribution of illegal acts to pathological gambling diagnosis: DSM-5 implications. J Addict Dis 33(1):41–52, 2014

Grant JE, Potenza MN: Commentary: illegal behavior and pathological gambling. J Am Acad Psychiatry Law 35(3):302–305, 2007

Grant BF, Hasin DS, Stinson FS, et al: Co-occurrence of 12-month mood and anxiety disorders and personality disorders in the US: results from the national epidemiologic survey on alcohol and related conditions. J Psychiatr Res 39(1):1–9, 2005

Grant JE, Schreiber L, Odlaug BL, Kim SW: Pathologic gambling and bankruptcy. Compr Psychiatry 51(2):115–120, 2010

Insanity Defense Reform Act: Pub. L. No. 98–473, 98 Stat. 2057, 1984

Jiménez-Murcia S, Stinchfield R, Alvarez-Moya E, et al: Reliability, validity, and classification accuracy of a Spanish translation of a measure of DSM-IV diagnostic criteria for pathological gambling. J Gambl Stud 25(1):93–104, 2009

Korman LM, Collins J, Dutton D, et al: Problem gambling and intimate partner violence. J Gambl Stud 24(1):13–23, 2008

Laursen B, Plauborg R, Ekholm O, et al: Problem gambling associated with violent and criminal behaviour: a Danish population-based survey and register study. J Gambl Stud 32(1):25–34, 2016

Ledgerwood DM, Weinstock J, Morasco BJ, Petry NM: Clinical features and treatment prognosis of pathological gamblers with and without recent gambling-related illegal behavior. J Am Acad Psychiatry Law 35(3):294–301, 2007

Lesieur HR: The Chase: Career of the Compulsive Gambler. Rochester, VT, Schenkman Publishing Company, 1984

May-Chahal C, Humphreys L, Clifton A, et al: Gambling harm and crime careers. J Gambl Stud 33(1):65–84, 2017

McCorkle R: Pathological gambling in arrestee populations. Final report prepared for National Institute of Justice. Las Vegas, NV, Department of Criminal Justice, 2002

Merrill v Trump Indiana, Inc., 320 F3d 729, 7th Cir (2003)

Mestre-Bach G, Steward T, Granero R, et al: Gambling and impulsivity traits: a recipe for criminal behavior? Front Psychiatry 9:6, 2018

Meyer G, Stadler MA: Criminal behavior associated with pathological gambling. J Gambl Stud 15(1):29–43, 1999

Muelleman RL, DenOtter T, Wadman MC, et al: Problem gambling in the partner of the emergency department patient as a risk factor for intimate partner violence. J Emerg Med 23(3):307–312, 2002

Pastwa-Wojciechowska B: The relationship of pathological gambling to criminality behavior in a sample of Polish male offenders. Med Sci Monit 17(11):CR669–CR675, 2011

Paton Estate v Ontario Lottery and Gaming Corporation (Fallsview Casino Resort and OLG Casino Brantford), 2016 ONCA 458, Ontario, CA (2016)

Perrone S, Jansons D, Morrison L: Problem Gambling and the Criminal Justice System. Melbourne, Australia, Victorian Responsible Gambling Foundation, 2013

Petry NM, O'Brien CP: Internet gaming disorder and the DSM-5. Addiction 108(7):1186–1187, 2013

Petry NM, Blanco C, Stinchfield R, Volberg R: An empirical evaluation of proposed changes for gambling diagnosis in the DSM-5. Addiction 108(3):575–581, 2013

Pietrzak RH, Petry NM: Antisocial personality disorder is associated with increased severity of gambling, medical, drug and psychiatric problems among treatment-seeking pathological gamblers. Addiction 100(8):1183–1193, 2005

Potenza MN, Steinberg MA, McLaughlin SD, et al: Illegal behaviors in problem gambling: analysis of data from a gambling helpline. J Am Acad Psychiatry Law 28(4):389–403, 2000

Roberts A, Coid J, King R, et al: Gambling and violence in a nationally representative sample of UK men. Addiction 111(12):2196–2207, 2016

Rosenthal RJ, Lorenz VC: The pathological gambler as criminal offender: comments on evaluation and treatment. Psychiatr Clin North Am 15(3):647–660, 1992

Rudd C, Thomas SDM: The prevalence, mental health and criminal characteristics of potential problem gamblers in a substance using treatment seeking population. Int J Ment Health Addict 14(5):700–714, 2016

Scott CL: Evaluation of criminal responsibility, in The American Psychiatric Association Publishing Textbook of Forensic Psychiatry, 3rd Edition. Edited by Gold LH, Frierson RL. Arlington, VA, American Psychiatric Association, 2018, pp 281–296

Slutske WS, Eisen S, Xian H, et al: A twin study of the association between pathological gambling and antisocial personality disorder. J Abnorm Psychol 110(2):297–308, 2001

Smith GJ, Wynne HJ, Hartnagel T: Examining Police Records to Assess Gambling Impacts: A Study of Gambling-Related Crime in the City of Edmonton: A Study Prepared for The Alberta Gaming Research Institute. Edmonton, AB, Alberta Gaming Research Institute, 2003

Stevens v MTR Gaming Group, Inc., 237 W Va 531, 788 SE2d 59 (2016)

Strong DR, Kahler CW: Evaluation of the continuum of gambling problems using the DSM-IV. Addiction 102(5):713–721, 2007

Suomi A, Jackson A, Dowling NA, et al: Problem gambling and family violence: family member reports of prevalence, family impacts and family coping. Asian J Gambl Issues Public Health 3(1):13, 2013

Taveras v Resorts International Hotel, Inc., 2008 US Dist LEXIS 71670, DNJ (2008)

Turner NE, Preston DL, Saunders C, et al: The relationship of problem gambling to criminal behavior in a sample of Canadian male federal offenders. J Gambl Stud 25(2):153–169, 2009

Turner NE, Stinchfield R, McCready J, et al: Endorsement of criminal behavior amongst offenders: implications for DSM-5 gambling disorder. J Gambl Stud 32(1):35–45, 2016

United States v Caspersen, No 16-Cr-0414, SDNY, Dec 7, 2016

United States v Grillo, 111 Fed Appx 631; 2004 US App LEXIS 19087, 2nd Cir (2004)

United States v Roach, 296 F3d 565, 7th Cir (2002)

U.S. Sentencing Commission: Guidelines Manual. §5K2.13—Diminished Capacity, Commentary, Application Note 1. Washington, DC, U.S. Sentencing Commission, 2018

Williams v Aztar Indiana Gaming Corp, 351 F3d 290, 7th Cir (2003)

Wills CD, Gold LH: Introduction to the special section on DSM-5 and forensic psychiatry. J Am Acad Psychiatry Law 42(2):132–135, 2014

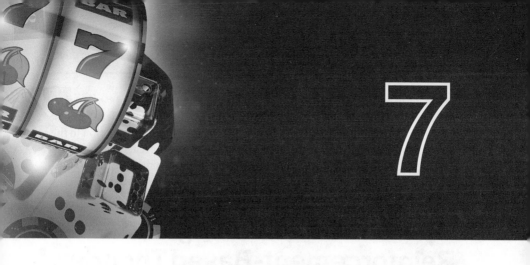

7

Cognitive and Behavioral Underpinnings

Elijah Otis, B.A.
Igor Yakovenko, Ph.D.
Sherry H. Stewart, Ph.D.

What makes a person gamble and continue to gamble even when faced with mounting losses? In this chapter, we attempt to answer this complex question by investigating the etiology of gambling behaviors from a wide variety of theoretical perspectives, with a special focus on factors that mark the transition from healthy to disordered gambling. Drawing from the behavioral (learning) perspective, we highlight the role of operant and classical conditioning processes relevant to gambling, including design features of gambling games that encourage excessive play. From the cognitive perspective, we provide an overview of the major cognitive biases relevant to gambling, as well as the current state of research on the impact of explicit and implicit cognitive pro-

Dr. Stewart is supported through a Canadian Institutes of Health Research Tier 1 Canada Research Chair in Addictions and Mental Health at Dalhousie University.

cesses on gambling outcomes. We also discuss the importance of certain personality traits and motives for gambling as important individual differences that may impact learning and cognitive biases. We finish with an introduction to the pathways model (Blaszczynski and Nower 2002) as a comprehensive model of disordered gambling that incorporates key findings from various theoretical orientations to identify how gambling behaviors can become pathological.

Operant Conditioning and Reinforcement-Based Theories of Gambling

The core tenets of operant conditioning theory posit that whereas behaviors that are consistently rewarded will increase in frequency or intensity over time, behaviors that are consistently punished will diminish over time, a process known as extinction (Ferster and Skinner 1957; Goddard 2012). Within this theory, rewards that follow a behavior can take the shape of positive reinforcers, in which the consequences of a behavior involve something pleasurable or of value, or negative reinforcers, which reward the behavior by removing something unpleasant from the individual's experience as a consequence of the behavior.

Applying the operant conditioning theoretical framework to gambling, money (or any item of value that can be won through a wager) can act as a powerful positive reinforcer. Yet most gambling games have a negative expected value in the long run for the average player (Hannum 2012). This means that over a long period of play, most gamblers lose more money than they win. Under the principles of operant conditioning, one would expect mounting losses from repeated play of games with negative expected value to act as a punishment. This should serve to discourage continued play, overcoming the positively reinforcing effect of occasionally winning money. However, there are several reasons why the discouraging effects of punishment from losses do not always overcome the encouraging effects of reinforcement for many gamblers. As we discuss in further detail later in the chapter, the prospect of winning money is not the only element of gambling that reinforces gambling behaviors. Other examples of positive reinforcers that motivate continued play include social factors (i.e., enjoyment derived from playing with and interacting with others), the excitement or arousal derived from the prospect of winning (Brown 1986), complimentary or "comped" items from the casino (e.g., free hotel rooms, free drinks), and elements of gambling games designed to stimulate the senses (e.g., flashing lights, interesting sounds from a slot machine) (Parke and Griffiths 2006). Moreover, research into gambling motivations has also found evidence that many gamblers use gambling as a means of relief or escape from boredom or other negative emotional states (i.e., anxiety, depression, shame), thus providing evidence that negative reinforcers contribute to gambling behavior as well (Stewart and Zack 2008).

Reinforcement Schedules

Based on operant conditioning theory, another important feature of gambling games that contributes to persistence is the presence of a random-ratio reinforcement schedule. A reinforcement schedule refers to how often a certain behavior is reinforced under the principles of operant conditioning. Underlying most gambling games is a random-ratio reinforcement schedule in which reinforcement is received randomly after a certain number of responses; how many responses are needed before the reward is delivered varies randomly. Under a random-ratio reinforcement schedule, every response has a constant probability of being rewarded (Madden et al. 2007). For example, a slot machine programmed with a random-ratio reinforcement schedule might have a 10% probability of paying out on any given spin, regardless of the results of all previous spins. This means that even if the last 10 consecutive spins were all unsuccessful (or all successful), the next spin still has a 10% chance of payout. Random-ratio reinforcement schedules involve a high degree of unpredictability with respect to when the next reward will arrive. This is what makes this schedule so powerful—gamblers never know when the next reward will come, so they keep playing because it could be on the next spin. In fact, animal model studies have demonstrated that random-ratio reinforcement schedules elicit more target behavioral responses than fixed-ratio schedules (in which rewards are predictable) for a number of rewards, including food pellets (Laskowski et al. 2019; Madden et al. 2005) and drugs of abuse such as cocaine (Lagorio and Winger 2014). A related psychological phenomenon is the partial reinforcement effect, in which behaviors that are reinforced intermittently (as is the case with the random-ratio reinforcement schedules typical of gambling) rather than consistently are demonstrably more resistant to extinction (Capaldi 1966). The presence of random-ratio schedules and intermittent reinforcement in most gambling games has been theorized as one of the risk factors in behavioral acquisition of gambling problems (Blaszczynski and Nower 2002).

Psychophysiology of Gambling and Arousal

To understand the role of arousal in the reinforcement of gambling behaviors, we must first briefly mention the role of the dopaminergic mesolimbic system in reward. This neural system is thought to contain both a consummatory element that controls the hedonic experience of liking a particular reward and an appetitive element that controls the degree to which individuals want to obtain a reward (Alcaro et al. 2007; Berridge 2007). One way that arousal may reinforce gambling behavior is by contributing to the hedonic enjoyment of gambling by producing a feeling of excitement. The expectancy that one might be rewarded by winning money has been demonstrated to be an important factor in producing physiological arousal while gambling (Ladouceur et al. 2003; Wulfert et al. 2005). Ladouceur et al. (2003) found that video lottery terminal players who played for money had a higher pulse rate while playing and rated their machines as subjectively more exciting than those who played for nonmonetary points. In a similar experimental study, Wulfert et al. (2005) found that participants who had wagered on a horse race experienced significantly higher heart rates while watching the race and reported greater subjective excitement than those who had not wagered. Other research has demonstrated that the effect of wins on physiological arousal is correlated with the magnitude of the win (Lole et al. 2012) but not for individuals with disordered gambling (Lole and Gonsalvez 2017). Individuals with disordered gambling have also been shown to experience lower overall physiological arousal than individuals without disordered gambling in response to wins during slot machine game play (Lole et al. 2014). This latter finding lends some support to the theory that individuals with disordered gambling are chronically underaroused, which may encourage excessive play to compensate (e.g., Jacobs 1986). It is also possible that through continued play, gamblers' hedonic enjoyment of gambling becomes dampened through habituation, thus resulting in a lower arousal response while gambling (Koob and Le Moal 2008).

Although feelings of excitement engendered by arousal may act as positive reinforcer for further gambling, there is some evidence that arousal can indicate frustration, rather than excitement, in certain scenarios. Heart rate deceleration in tandem with increases in skin conductance response (SCR) are physiological indicators of frustration (Clark et al. 2011; Lobbestael et al. 2008; Osumi and Ohira 2009). Certain gambling outcomes, such as a "near miss" (a loss that is almost a win, described in greater detail later in the chapter), have been shown to elicit these physiological frustration responses (Clark et al. 2011; Dixon et al. 2010). In a study conducted by Dixon et al. (2013), gamblers had their SCR monitored while playing a simulated slot machine. Additionally, the researchers tracked the length of participants' postreinforcement pauses (PRPs), a measure of time between receiving the outcome of a previous spin and the initiation of a subsequent spin. PRPs have been observed to be longer after winning trials than losing trials and to scale in duration with the quantity of the win (e.g., Delfabbro and Winefield 1999; Dixon et al. 2013). One possible explanation for this scaling is that PRPs represent the time during which a reward is being enjoyed, which inhibits the desire to continue gambling (Dixon et al. 2013). By comparing participants' SCRs and PRPs after losing, winning, and near-miss trials, Dixon et al. (2013) found that both wins and near misses elicited high arousal (large spikes in SCR). However, whereas wins were followed by longer PRPs than losses, near misses were followed by very short PRPs. The researchers suggested that this pattern of psychophysiological responses to near misses indicated that these experiences were frustrating but nonetheless motivational toward continued play. The finding that these frustrating, nonpleasurable outcomes can nonetheless be motivational toward continued gambling highlights the power of the appetitive or "wanting" component of the mesolimbic system in promoting behavioral reinforcement even in the absence of enjoying or "liking" the outcome of the behavior. This observation may help explain why individuals with disordered gambling continue gambling even when their gambling causes them more harm than good. Moreover, neurological studies have demonstrated that individuals differ in their sensitivity to the effects of reward and punishment (Gray and McNaughton 2000). Reward sensitivity has been implicated in greater bet size during gambling (Brunborg et al. 2011) and more symptoms of disordered gambling (MacLaren et al. 2012; Jiménez-Murcia et al. 2017; MacLaren et al. 2011). Such results suggest that certain people may be especially vulnerable to becoming behaviorally conditioned into disordered gambling.

Early Big Win Hypothesis

Winning large sums of money early on during one's exposure to gambling, or the "big win hypothesis," has also been suggested as a possible contributing factor to the development of future gambling problems (Custer 1984; Snyder 1978; Walker 1992). This hypothesis is consistent with reinforcement-based theories of disordered gambling, with winning a large sum early in one's gambling career acting as a powerful positive reinforcer for future gambling. However, several studies have failed to demonstrate this hypothesized association between early "big wins" and potentially problematic gambling behaviors (Kassinove and Schare 2001; Mentzoni et al. 2012; Weatherly et al. 2004). In fact, Weatherly et al. (2004) found evidence for an opposite effect, wherein research participants who played a slot machine programmed to yield a large payout at the beginning of their gambling session actually chose to stop gambling earlier than those who did not experience this big early win. It may be that early big wins only pose significant risks for a subset of gamblers who are especially sensitive to behavioral conditioning (e.g., Blaszczynski and Nower 2002; Turner 2012). Overall, however, the body of evidence does not seem to strongly support the "big win hypothesis" as a major risk factor in the acquisition of disordered gambling.

Classical Conditioning

Classical conditioning, also known as Pavlovian conditioning, is a type of behavioral learning facilitated through the pairing of a conditioned and an unconditioned stimulus. For classical conditioning to occur, the conditioned stimulus (which does not naturally elicit a response) is repeatedly paired with an unconditioned stimulus that does naturally elicit a particular response. In Pavlov's classic experiment demonstrating this learning mechanism in dogs, a bell was rung (conditioned stimulus) during the presentation of food (unconditioned stimulus), the smell of which caused the dogs to automatically salivate (Rehman et al. 2020). After repeated pairings of the bell and the food, the dogs eventually began to salivate when the bell was rung even if it was not followed by food, thus demonstrating that the unconditioned response (salivation in response to the smell of food) had become a conditioned response (salivation in response to the ringing of a bell). Despite the wealth of research implicating operant conditioning processes in the acquisition of gambling and gambling disorder, there has been far less research on the role of classical conditioning in gambling (Ramnerö et al. 2019). Theoretically, the audiovisual feedback that accompanies wins on a gambling machine could act as a conditioned stimulus that reinforces gambling behavior; Parke and Griffiths (2006) note that the constant noise of winning sounds from the multitude of machines being played by others in a casino may even increase the perceived odds of winning in the eyes of the individual gambler, thus encouraging them to gamble. Additionally, many electronic gaming machines (EGMs) include audiovisual effects from popular sources (e.g., TV show theme song, character voices, and video effects), which may condition gamblers to believe that playing these machines is socially acceptable and safe because of these associations with benign pop culture (Griffiths and Parke 2005). In a study comparing the physiological effects of gambling in a casino versus a laboratory setting, Anderson and Brown (1984) found that gamblers in a casino setting experienced more drastic changes in physiological arousal (heart rate) during play than those in the laboratory environment, an effect that may be attributable to the arousing effect of casino background music and sounds emitted by machines in the casino setting. The researchers noted that the repeated pairings of arousal (from arousing audiovisual stimuli in the casino environment) and gambling "is likely to have a powerful classical or Pavlovian conditioning effect on gambling behavior" (p. 406).

Another element of classical conditioning that seems relevant to disordered gambling is aversive conditioning. Aversive conditioning consists of pairing a neutral conditioned stimulus with an undesirable or unpleasant unconditioned stimulus, such as a painful electric shock. After repeated pairings of these stimuli, aversive conditioning posits that the presence of the neutral conditioned stimulus alone will lead to a conditioned response of fear or avoidance. Applying this framework to gambling, economic losses from gambling may act as aversive unconditioned stimuli when paired with gambling-related cues, leading to negative associations between gambling cues and economic loss that discourages future play via fear or avoidance. Theoretically, if some gamblers are less susceptible to these aversive conditioning processes, they may be less likely to stop gambling when faced by mounting economic losses. One study by Brunborg et al. (2010) found that gamblers who were less reactive to an aversive conditioning task also made more risky decisions on a gambling task. Another study by Brunborg et al. (2012) found that individuals with disordered gambling showed diminished conditioning compared with healthy control participants on an aversive conditioning task. Together, these studies suggest the presence of a relationship between aversive conditioning deficits and disordered gambling; however, more research is needed to replicate these findings and determine the directionality and causality of this relationship, as well as to further investigate the importance of traditional classical conditioning processes in gambling more generally.

Structural Features of Gambling Games

Beyond the universal aspects of nearly all gambling games that act to encourage future gambling, some specific gambling games have design features that can be manipulated to further promote gambling persistence. EGMs such as virtual slot machines and poker terminals offer game developers considerable freedom in manipulating features that affect the gamblers' gaming experience via the machine's programming. The manipulability of these features also presents a unique opportunity for conducting behavioral research. Two such features that are especially salient to disordered gambling are known as near misses and losses disguised as wins (LDWs). The presence of these design features may contribute to the fact that EGMs are thought to be one of the more potentially harmful forms of gambling (Binde 2011; MacLaren 2016).

Near Misses

A "near miss" occurs in a gambling context when a gambler "almost" wins a bet but does not. There are a myriad of ways in which a gambler might experience a near miss, but some examples include having a horse picked to win a race finish second, "busting" with a hand of 22 in blackjack, or getting two of three "7s" required for a jackpot on a slot machine line. Although the economic effect of a near miss is equivalent to that of a "full miss" in that the gambler fully loses his or her wager, near misses have a substantially different impact on a gambler's decision to continue play compared with full misses. Electronic slot machines programmed to yield near misses with moderate frequency have been consistently shown to increase persistence of play in gamblers (Cote et al. 2003; Daugherty and MacLin 2007; Kassinove and Schare 2001). Given that near misses are equivalent to full misses in that they result in an economic loss for the gambler, these results beg the question of why near misses seem to reinforce, rather than discourage, continued gambling. One proposed explanation of this effect is the skill-acquisition hypothesis, which posits that gamblers misattribute near misses as indicators that they are skilled at the game (Clark et al. 2013). There is some evidence supporting this hypothesis, particularly with respect to individuals with disordered gambling. Clark et al. (2013) found that a subgroup of their participants on a slot machine task responded to near misses with increased win expectancy for subsequent trials, which led to greater persistence. Moreover, a neuroimaging study conducted by Habib and Dixon (2010) examining both disordered and nondisordered gambling found that in the participants with nondisordered gambling, near misses on a slot machine task elicited a brain response that was similar to the response elicited by losses (full misses). In participants with disordered gambling, near misses elicited a response similar to the response elicited by wins. Together, these studies suggest near misses may trigger erroneous beliefs and thereby encourage excessive play in a subset of gamblers. We discuss the role of erroneous beliefs more fully later in this chapter.

Losses Disguised as Wins

Another manipulable design element that exists in certain gambling games is what are known as "losses disguised as wins," or LDWs. For an LDW to occur, a gambler must win some amount less than they wagered on a trial, resulting in a net loss. The most salient example of an LDW occurs in multiline slot machine play, in which a player can win one or more of their multiple played lines but still lose money overall because of losses on other lines played concurrently (Dixon et al. 2010). A key feature of LDWs is that despite an overall economic loss for the player, many slot machines will still react to LDWs by engaging the same audiovisual effects that normally accompany real wins, thus "disguising" a loss as a win through the use of these effects as an unconditioned stimulus (Dixon et al. 2010). By measuring the SCR of participants while they played a multiline slot machine, Dixon et al. (2010) found that the levels of arousal elicited by LDWs were similar to those elicited by real wins. Another study by Graydon et al. (2018) found that when given the choice between playing otherwise identical multiline slot machines with or without LDWs, participants consistently preferred playing the machines that included LDWs. Yet another study by Dixon et al. (2014) found that playing machines with reinforcing sounds that accompany both real wins and LDWs led participants to significantly overestimate their total winnings. Similarly, Jensen et al. (2012) found that participants misremembered LDWs as real wins on a slot machine task. Gambling machines that incorporate LDWs may encourage problematic gambling by effectively tricking gamblers into thinking they are winning even when they are losing.

Pace of Play

Gambling games vary considerably in their pace of play, or the speed at which successive bets and payouts occur. Whereas some gambling games have a relatively slow pace of play with a relatively long latency between wager and win or loss (e.g., lotteries), other games are very fast-paced (e.g., electronic slot machines), with minimal latency between betting and payoff allowing for a large number of wagers to be made in a single gambling session. Research into the effects of pace of play on gambling behaviors suggests that although most gamblers deem faster-paced games to be more exciting, individuals with disordered gambling have a particularly strong preference for these games; additionally, games with faster paces of play may encourage gamblers to place more bets and play for longer periods of time (see Harris and Griffiths 2018 for a review). Individuals with disordered gambling have also been shown to have greater difficulty ceasing play on machines with faster paces of play (Loba et al. 2001).

Additionally, games with faster paces of play such as electronic slot machines have been demonstrated to cause more gambling-related harms than slower-paced games, such as lotteries (Binde 2011).

Maximum Bet Size or Prize Level

Another important design element of gambling games is the maximum amount of money that can be wagered on an individual trial (e.g., a "spin" of a slot machine). Sharpe et al. (2005) conducted a study in which three design elements (pace of play, maximum bill denomination accepted, and maximum bet size) of otherwise identical electronic slot machines were manipulated and compared with control machines to assess the effect of these design characteristics on play habits in order to determine whether these modifications could be used to reduce gambling-related harms. Of these three modifications, only reducing the maximum bet size had a significant effect in reducing play time, total losses, and net losses. Although the researchers did find that problem gamblers preferred machines that allowed for higher-denomination bill deposits, this did not translate to more potentially harmful play. Similarly, in a study conducted by Crewe-Brown et al. (2014), the researchers investigated the effect of prize level (e.g., size of the "jackpot") on participants' willingness to play and bet large sums of money on EGMs. Participants were presented with a series of vignettes that asked about how much they would bet on hypothetical EGMs with identical payout ratios but varying maximum prize levels. As the prize level increased, participants indicated being both more willing to place a bet and willing to bet more money on these machines even though their overall rate of return was identical across all prize values.

Audiovisual Stimuli

A notable design element of most EGMs, both casino based and online, is the fact that play, as well as wins and losses, is generally accompanied by an array of appealing audiovisual stimuli. The average modern EGM is programmed with close to 400 distinct sounds related to gameplay (Rivlin 2004). Under classical conditioning theory, these sounds have been theorized to act as a conditioned stimulus toward the conditioning of gambling behavior when paired with monetary wins (Parke and Griffiths 2006). In a study testing the physiological effects of gameplay audio on slot machine players, Dixon et al. (2014) found that participants exhibited stronger arousal responses when playing with the sound on than with the sound off. This is notable given that arousal is theorized to be an independent positive reinforcer of gambling behavior (Brown 1986). Additionally, Dixon et al. (2014) found that participants preferred playing with the sound on and tended to overestimate their number of winning trials when the sound was on, ostensibly because of remembering more LDWs as real wins. In a follow-up study, Dixon et al. (2015) replicated this latter finding that "positive" or celebratory sounds increase the rate at which LDWs are misremembered as true wins. However, the researchers also observed that when "negative" sounds are paired with losses and LDWs, this effect is reversed, such that participants are more accurate in remembering LDWs as true losses. Although there has been less research into the effects of visual stimuli on gambling behavior, Spenwyn et al. (2010) found that exposure to red light concurrent with fast-tempo music led to faster play during an online roulette game. Additionally, there is some evidence that the presence of flashing lights, which are ubiquitous in many casino settings, increases an individual's willingness to gamble in a potentially harmful manner, perhaps as an effect of increased information load (Finlay et al. 2010).

Slot Machine Immersion

Another troubling feature of multiline slot machines that can contribute to the addictive potential of these machines is their immersive properties. Because of the presence of LDWs, multiline slot machines result in more frequent "win" experiences, shorter streaks without a win or LDW, and smaller payouts per win or LDW than single-line slot machines, all of which contribute to a "smoother" play experience (Dixon et al. 2018; Schüll 2005). Multiline slot machines can induce a quasi-dissociative state in players, characterized by narrow attention, dissociation, and dulled response to external stimuli (e.g., Diskin and Hodgins 1999, 2001; Schüll 2005). Contrary to the positive "flow state" described by Csikszentmihalyi (1992) in which an individual is fully engaged and immersed in an activity, Dixon et al. (2018) coined the term "dark flow" to refer to this more maladaptive immersive state brought on by slot machine play that can lead to negative gambling-related consequences. Experiences of dark flow in slot machine play are amplified by playing on multiple lines (Dixon et al. 2018; Murch and Clark 2019). The experience of dark flow during multiline slot machine play has been associated with disordered gambling (Dixon et al. 2014; Murch et al. 2017), as well as depression (Dixon et al. 2018, 2019), a condition commonly comorbid with disordered gambling (Petry et al. 2005). Taken together, these results suggest that the dark flow state elicited by multiline slot play may act as a powerful negative reinforcer for problem gamblers, particularly those with comorbid mood pathology.

Behavioral Markers of Disordered Gambling

Several behaviors have been identified as risk factors associated with disordered gambling. One of the defining behavioral characteristics of individuals with disordered gambling is a tendency to try to win back their money lost to gambling. This tendency is also known as "chasing losses." Because of the negative expected value of gambling for most gamblers, chasing losses can create a vicious cycle in which larger and larger bets are necessary to win back one's losses. Chasing losses is the most commonly endorsed symptom of disordered gambling (Toce-Gerstein et al. 2003). Other behavioral markers that have been identified as risk factors for disordered gambling include high betting frequency, high variability in the amount of money wagered, and steadily increasing bet sizes (Braverman and Shaffer 2012).

Another important behavioral phenomenon that relates to gambling is delay discounting. This refers to the natural tendency for people to prefer receiving smaller and more immediate rewards while "discounting" the value of larger rewards that they would receive in the more distant future (Ramnerö et al. 2019). Delay discounting has been demonstrated to be a relatively stable phenomenon in a variety of studies (see Reynolds 2006 for a review). On tasks in which participants choose between lesser immediate rewards and larger delayed rewards, individuals with disordered gambling tend to discount the value of delayed rewards more heavily than healthy control participants (Ledgerwood et al. 2009; MacKillop et al. 2006). Heavy delay discounting has similarly been associated with substance use disorders (see Yi et al. 2010 for a review), suggesting that severity of delay discounting may be broadly associated with addiction.

Related to delay discounting is the concept of probability discounting. This refers to the degree to which an individual discounts larger, less likely rewards in favor of smaller, more likely rewards. In a recent meta-analysis of 12 studies investigating the relationship between probability discounting and disordered gambling, Kyonka and Schute (2018) found consistent evidence across all studies for an association between shallow probability discounting (overvaluing unlikely larger rewards or undervaluing likely larger losses) and disordered gambling. Another study conducted by Ligneul et al. (2013) comparing individuals with disordered gambling with healthy control participants found that when presented with a choice between a lesser, certain reward and a greater probabilistic or "risky" reward, individuals with disordered gambling consistently chose the risky reward more often than did controls.

Cognitive Theories of Gambling Behavior

Cognitive Biases

Many cognitive theories of gambling focus on the influence of erroneous thought patterns, also known as cognitive distortions or cognitive biases, on gambling behavior. Ladouceur and Walker (1996) noted that although it is well documented that gambling activities generally have a negative expected monetary outcome, cognitive biases may influence gamblers' subjective expectations of gambling to a degree that they actually believe that they can "beat the odds" and profit.

Illusion of Control

One of the most important cognitive biases related to gambling is known as the illusion of control (IOC). With this cognitive bias, individuals erroneously believe that they have undue influence over outcomes that are largely or entirely determined by other factors, such as chance (Langer 1975). A classic experiment by Langer (1975) illustrated the IOC in a gambling context. In Langer's study, office workers were given the opportunity to pay $1 for a lottery ticket and were randomly assigned to either pick their ticket themselves or be given one by an experimenter. Later, when all participants were asked what price they would sell their lottery ticket for, the participants who picked their own ticket demanded an average of $8.67, more than eight times what they paid for their ticket and more than four times the value demanded by participants who did not pick their ticket. This suggests that the former group falsely believed that by choosing the ticket themselves, they had increased their chances of winning. As noted by Ladouceur and Walker (1996), superstitious beliefs and behaviors, such as the use of good-luck charms while gambling, are an example of the IOC. The IOC can be robust even after losing sessions because gamblers high in IOC have been shown to focus on their largest individual win during an overall losing session when determining their overall enjoyment derived from the session (Cowley et al. 2015). This is consistent with what Ladouceur and Walker (1996) refer to as a "biased evaluation of outcomes," in which gambling losses are attributed to external factors (i.e., bad luck) and wins are attributed to internal factors (i.e., skill).

The Gambler's Fallacy and Hot Hand Fallacy

Another cognitive bias commonly observed among gamblers is aptly named the "gambler's fallacy." This bias refers to the erroneous belief that the outcome of prior events influences the probability of a future outcome, when in fact each event is probabilistically independent. A common example of the gambler's fallacy in a gambling context is the observed tendency for roulette players to bet on the opposite color (e.g., red) after the ball falls on one color (e.g., black) several times in a row, even though the probability of the roulette ball landing on either color is the same for each spin regardless of prior results (Ayton and Fischer 2004; Studer et al. 2015). The gambler's fallacy has been conceptualized as an example of the representativeness heuristic, such that gamblers expect a normal distribution of probability outcomes that would be present in the long run to also be present in the short run, when there is much more room for variability (Kahneman and Tversky 1972). A similar concept is the "hot hand fallacy," wherein a gambler's confidence in future successful predictions (or bets) increases as a function of the length of their ongoing "run" of wins (Ayton and Fischer 2004).

Given that cognitive distortions can distort a gambler's subjective appraisal of the odds of winning, it stands to reason that individuals who endorse these distortions might be more susceptible to disordered gambling. Indeed, there is a wealth of evidence supporting this theorized association between cognitive distortions and disordered gambling (see Goodie and Fortune 2013 for a review). Moreover, in a longitudinal study conducted over 5 years, Yakovenko et al. (2016) found evidence that increases in gambling-related cognitive distortions preceded increases in gambling behavior and gambling problem severity, suggesting that emergence of these distortions may signal a transition from recreational gambling into more problematic gambling.

Gambling Expectancies

Just as actual positive outcomes of gambling episodes can reinforce potentially problematic gambling behaviors, so too can expectations of positive gambling outcomes. Several studies have found evidence supporting an association between positive gambling expectancies (i.e., beliefs that gambling behavior will result in desirable consequences) and gambling involvement using self-report measures (e.g., Grubbs and Rosansky 2020; St-Pierre et al. 2014). Moreover, several distinct types of positive expectancies may be relevant to different types of gamblers. For example, reward expectancies refer to an expectation that gambling will lead to a positive mood state (e.g., relaxation, excitement), and relief expectancies refer to the expectation that gambling will provide relief or distraction from a negative mood state (e.g., sadness, irritability) (Yi et al. 2015). Other, more specific positive (reward) gambling expectancies that have been identified include enjoyment or arousal, self-enhancement (positive social outcomes and increased feelings of independence), and monetary gain, and negative gambling expectancies include overinvolvement in gambling and experiencing a negative emotional impact from gambling (Gillespie et al. 2007).

Interestingly, St-Pierre et al. (2014) found that participants in their sample who endorsed more negative gambling expectancies also endorsed more symptoms of disordered gambling, a finding that may seem somewhat counterintuitive. It may be that although individuals with disordered gambling are able to learn that gambling will lead to negative consequences, this learning occurs later in the addictive process. By the time these negative expectancies have developed, other factors that encourage harmful play may be too entrenched for these expectancies to function as an effective deterrent. Investigating change in gambling expectancies over time using a longitudinal design could be a fruitful area for future research to further understand how disordered gambling is affected by explicit gambling expectancies.

The use of self-report measures taps into expectancies about gambling that participants are actively aware of. However, individuals may also have implicit expectancies about gambling of which they are not consciously aware or that occur relatively automatically. A study conducted by Stewart et al. (2015) investigated the relationship between implicit gambling expectancies and gambling behaviors or gambling problem severity through the use of an affective priming task. Participants were primed with either gambling-related or non-gambling-related images before the presentation of a word signifying either a negative or positive outcome of gambling (e.g., "anxiety" or "relaxation," respectively). Participants were then asked to quickly identify whether the word was negative or positive by clicking a corresponding key. In this task, implicit positive gambling expectancy was operationalized as faster response times in identifying positive gambling outcome words after a gambling cue, indicating strong memory associations between gambling and positive outcomes. The researchers found associations between implicit positive gambling expectancies on the affective priming task and gambling behavior intensity as well as problem gambling severity.

In a separate study conducted by Stiles et al. (2017), the researchers investigated implicit gambling expectancies using a word association task. In this task, participants were presented with a list of phrases denoting positive outcomes (e.g., "I feel relaxed") and asked to write down the first two behaviors that these phrases brought to mind. The researchers found that participants who were more involved in gambling and endorsed more symptoms of disordered gambling were more likely to indicate gambling behaviors in response to positive outcome phrases. These results suggest that positive gambling expectancies may contribute to disordered gambling even if individuals are not consciously aware of these expectancies. Recent work shows that implicit and explicit gambling expectancies are not redundant; each explains significant and unique variance in the prediction of gambling behavior involvement and problem gambling severity (Stewart et al. 2015).

Automatic Approach Bias

Another implicit cognitive process that is relevant to gambling is that of automatic approach bias. A wealth of research from the substance use literature has shown that individuals who misuse alcohol and drugs exhibit an automatic tendency to "approach" environmental cues related to their substance of choice (e.g., Braunstein et al. 2016; Zhou et al. 2012). This automatic approach tendency may increase the likelihood of engaging in impulsive and potentially harmful behaviors, such as heavy drug use or excessive gambling, before one has time to properly consider the consequences of engaging in said behavior (Stacy and Wiers 2010). Boffo et al. (2018) investigated the approach bias in gamblers using a computerized approach avoidance task in which gamblers were tasked with deciding whether to "push" or "pull" neutral and gambling-related images as fast as possible based on the rotation of the image. In this task, deciding to "pull" the image resulted in the image zooming in closer, thus simulating an approach behavior. By analyzing participant reaction times when deciding whether to "pull" or "push" these related images, the researchers found that individuals with disordered gambling were quicker to "pull" gambling-related images than neutral images relative to those with nondisordered gambling, thus demonstrating an approach bias toward gambling-related stimuli. The presence of these approach biases in individuals with disordered gambling may make it particularly difficult for these individuals to abstain from gambling.

Personality and Gambling

Do certain personality traits confer an increased risk for disordered gambling? There is a wealth of empirical evidence implicating impulsivity as one such trait. Impulsivity is a multifaceted personality trait that broadly refers to an enduring tendency toward behavior that is "poorly conceived, prematurely expressed, unduly risky, or inappropriate to the situation and that often result[s] in undesirable consequences" (Daruna and Barnes 1993, p. 23). A number of studies using self-report measures of impulsivity have found an association between high trait impulsivity and disordered gambling severity (e.g., Hodgins and Holub 2015; MacLaren et al. 2011, 2012; Myrseth et al. 2009; Otis et al. 2021). Additionally, a longitudinal cohort study followed up with participants 30 years after they were initially assessed as children. It showed that impulsive behaviors displayed at age 7 years were significant predictors of disordered gambling 30 years later (Shenassa et al. 2012). Comorbidity between disordered gambling and impulse-control disorders is also quite high; a national epidemiological survey conducted in the United States by Kessler et al. (2008) found that 42.7% of American adults who met criteria for pathological gambling as outlined in DSM-IV-TR (American Psychiatric Association 2000) also met criteria for at least one impulse-control disorder. Thus, high trait impulsivity appears to be one personality risk factor for the development of gambling problems. Similarly, conscientiousness, a five-factor model trait that taps into several "non-impulsive" personality characteristics reflecting self-discipline and a tendency to think carefully before acting, has been shown to be inversely related to disordered gambling status, such that low conscientiousness is related to higher problem gambling scores and vice versa (e.g., Brunborg et al. 2016; MacLaren et al. 2011).

Another trait related to impulsivity that has been extensively studied in populations of gamblers is sensation seeking. Sensation seeking is a personality trait characterized by a drive to engage in novel and exciting experiences regardless of risk involved (Zuckerman and Neeb 1979). Although many researchers have hypothesized a relationship between high sensation seeking and disordered gambling, actual results are mixed, with most studies finding no relationship between sensation seeking and gambling severity (see Hammelstein 2004 for a review). In their study investigating the relationship between impulsivity and disordered gambling, Hodgins and Holub (2015) found that whereas impulsivity correlated with disordered gambling scores, sensation seeking was instead correlated with measures of gambling involvement (frequency of casino game play, number of gambling games played). Thus, it may be that high sensation seeking increases an individual's interest in gambling without conferring additional risk of developing gambling-related problems.

Neuroticism has also been linked to the development of gambling problems. Neuroticism is one of the "Big Five" personality dimensions of the five-factor model and broadly refers to a general tendency toward experiencing negative affect (Costa and McCrae 1992). As discussed earlier in the chapter, one of the ways in which gambling behavior can be reinforced is by providing a distraction or temporary relief from negative emotions. Notably, there exists a strong association between the endorsement of gambling as a means of coping with negative affect and problem gambling scores, suggesting that negative reinforcement processes may be particularly pathogenic with respect to disordered gambling (Grubbs and Rosansky 2020; MacLaren et al. 2015; Schellenberg et al. 2016; Stewart and Zack 2008). Thus, it is perhaps unsurprising that neuroticism has been consistently linked to disordered gambling (Bagby et al. 2007; Brunborg et al. 2016; MacLaren et al. 2011).

Personality Disorders and Gambling

In addition to the normative personality traits described above that vary considerably within healthy populations, several personality disorders are highly comorbid with disordered gambling. An epidemiological study conducted by Petry et al. (2005) found that 60.3% of respondents meeting criteria for disordered gambling also met criteria for at least one personality disorder, compared with approximately 15% in the general U.S. adult population (Grant et al. 2004). These high rates of comorbid personality pathology in individuals with disordered gambling have been shown consistently across several studies (e.g., Bagby et al. 2008; Dowling et al. 2015). Cluster B personality disorders (histrionic, borderline, antisocial, and narcissistic personality disorder) have been shown to uniquely predict disordered gambling severity (Brown et al. 2016); notably, two of the four cluster B disorders (borderline and antisocial personality disorder) include impulsive features as diagnostic criteria (American Psychiatric Association 2013), further highlighting the relationship between impulsivity and gambling pathology. This symptom overlap could artificially inflate comorbidity between gambling disorder and these Cluster B disorders; therefore, future research should determine if this high comorbidity persists when the redundant symptoms are removed.

Gambling Motives

Just as personality characteristics of a gambler can influence gambling behaviors, so too can their motivation for gambling. In a study of disordered gambling, Stewart et al. (2008) performed a cluster analysis on participants' reported primary reasons for gambling. This cluster analysis revealed three primary subtypes within the sample: enhancement gamblers (motivated by a desire for fun and/or excitement), coping gamblers (motivated by a desire for escape/relief from negative affect), and low emotion regulation gamblers (not strongly motivated by either enhancement or coping). Gamblers in the coping cluster endorsed the greatest number of disordered gambling symptoms and gambled most frequently, followed by those in the enhancement cluster, with low emotion regulation gamblers scoring the lowest on these variables. Building on these findings, Stewart and Zack (2008) developed the Gambling Motives Questionnaire (GMQ) to measure gamblers' specific motivations for gambling. This measure included subscales for coping and enhancement motives while also introducing a social motives subscale. Replicating their previous findings, the researchers found coping motives to uniquely predict disordered gambling when controlling for gambling behaviors (lifetime variety of games played, lifetime frequency of gambling, maximum spending on gambling in a single day), and enhancement motives predicted gambling behaviors. Additionally, interactions between motives and gender on disordered gambling were observed, such that whereas enhancement motives were more strongly related to disordered gambling in men, coping motives were more strongly related to disordered gambling in women (Stewart and Zack 2008). Many other studies have implicated coping motives as unique predictors of disordered gambling symptoms (see, e.g., MacLaren et al. 2015; Schellenberg et al. 2016). Schellenberg et al. (2016) also introduced a fourth subscale to the GMQ to account for individuals who are motivated to gamble by the prospect of financial gain. Given that a large proportion of self-generated motives for gambling are financial in nature (see, e.g., McGrath et al. 2010), the addition of financial motives to the GMQ is important in ensuring that this measure accounts for the broad range of factors that motivate gambling behavior.

The Pathways Model

Until this point in the chapter, cognitive, behavioral, and personality research has been discussed to provide an overview of the current understanding of the etiology of disordered gambling. One theoretical framework that attempts to link these various threads into a unified model of disordered gambling is known as the pathways model. Formulated by Blaszczynski and Nower (2002), the pathways model posits that there exist three pathways toward disordered gambling, each emphasizing different vulnerabilities shared by subgroups of individuals with disordered gambling.

The first subgroup outlined in the model consists of the behaviorally conditioned gamblers. According to Blaszczynski and Nower (2002), behaviorally conditioned gamblers are otherwise healthy individuals who develop gambling problems after initial gambling exposure through a combination of positive reinforcement and the presence of cognitive biases such as the IOC that distorts their beliefs about winning. After a habitual pattern of gambling is established through these means, behaviorally conditioned gamblers begin to consistently lose money and chase their losses, starting the transition to disordered gambling. Gamblers in the second pathway are drawn to gambling as a means of coping with an underlying and preexisting emotional vulnerability (e.g., mood disorder diagnosis, high trait neuroticism, poor coping skills). This accelerates their behavioral conditioning toward disordered gambling via negative reinforcement. Gamblers in the third group have additional risk factors of high trait impulsivity and impulsive personality pathology (e.g., antisocial or borderline personality disorder) and poor executive functioning. These characteristics are said to further hinder their adaptive coping skills, thereby encouraging excessive gambling and other problem behaviors such as substance abuse in this group.

Several studies have validated the general disordered gambling subtypes proposed by the pathways model (e.g., Moon et al. 2017; Nower et al. 2013). Overall, the pathways model appears to be a valid and useful theoretical framework through which to understand how various cognitive, behavioral, dispositional, and motivational factors interact and contribute to the etiology of disordered gambling.

Conclusion and Future Directions

In this chapter, we have provided an overview of key cognitive, behavioral, dispositional, and motivational research on the etiology of gambling behavior and gambling disorder. If there is any broad conclusion that can be made, it is that no single factor can be pointed to as the direct and unique cause of disordered gambling; rather, a myriad of forces, ranging from operant conditioning and structural features of gambling games to cognitive distortions and underlying personality traits, all contribute in some way toward explaining why some individuals become addicted to gambling. The pathways model provides a useful framework that attempts to account for these heterogeneous causes of disordered gambling by identifying subtypes of gamblers for which different contributing factors may be most etiologically relevant. Still, there is much that we do not know about why some gamble regularly and experience minimal harms but others develop problems. One area in need of future research is longitudinal studies, given the relative paucity of this research compared with correlational studies. Tracking how gamblers' behaviors and cognitions change over time could be invaluable in identifying factors that immediately precede transitions from safe to disordered gambling. Additionally, longitudinal research could be of use in clearing up the impact of certain risk factors with mixed evidence in the extant literature, such as early big wins. Given that the pathways model represents perhaps the most comprehensive and valid existing framework for understanding individuals with disordered gambling, we also recommend that future research aim to expand on our understanding of subtypes of individuals with disordered gambling by testing new hypotheses based on these gambler subtypes. For example, it is theoretically consistent that emotionally vulnerable–subtype gamblers may also be more sensitive to punishment, experience more relief expectancies about gambling, and be more susceptible to the phenomenon of dark flow; similarly, antisocial or impulsive–subtype gamblers may be chronically underaroused and thus more strongly motivated by enhancement. Exploring these types of questions using the pathways model would yield a more complete understanding of the symptomatology of different subtypes of gamblers. Such additional work would be very helpful in informing targets for more tailored prevention programs and treatment plans for different subtypes of problem gamblers.

References

Alcaro A, Huber R, Panksepp J: Behavioral functions of the mesolimbic dopaminergic system: an affective neuroethological perspective. Brain Res Rev 56(2):283–321, 2007

American Psychiatric Association: Diagnostic and Statistical Manual of Mental Disorders, 4th Edition, Text Revision. Washington, DC, American Psychiatric Association, 2000

American Psychiatric Association: Diagnostic and Statistical Manual of Mental Disorders, 5th Edition. Arlington, VA, American Psychiatric Association, 2013

Anderson G, Brown RIT: Real and laboratory gambling, sensation-seeking and arousal. Br J Psychol 75(3):401–410, 1984

Ayton P, Fischer I: The hot hand fallacy and the gambler's fallacy: two faces of subjective randomness? Mem Cognit 32(8):1369–1378, 2004

Bagby RM, Vachon DD, Bulmash EL, et al: Pathological gambling and the five-factor model of personality. Pers Indiv Diff 43(4):873–880, 2007

Bagby R, Vachon D, Bulmash E, Quilty L: Personality disorders and pathological gambling: a review and re-examination of prevalence rates. J Pers Disord 22(2):191–207, 2008

Berridge KC: The debate over dopamine's role in reward: the case for incentive salience. Psychopharmacology (Berl) 191(3):391–431, 2007

Binde P: What are the most harmful forms of gambling? Analyzing problem gambling prevalence surveys. CEFOS Working Paper 12, 2011

Blaszczynski A, Nower L: A pathways model of problem and pathological gambling. Addiction 97(5):487–499, 2002

Boffo M, Smits R, Salmon JP, et al: Luck, come here! Automatic approach tendencies toward gambling cues in moderate-to high-risk gamblers. Addiction 113(2):289–298, 2018

Braunstein L, Kuerbis A, Ochsner K, Morgenstern J: Implicit alcohol approach and avoidance tendencies predict future drinking in problem drinkers. Alcohol Clin Exp Res 40(9):1945–1952, 2016

Braverman J, Shaffer HJ: How do gamblers start gambling: identifying behavioural markers for high-risk internet gambling. Eur J Public Health 22(2):273–278, 2012

Brown M, Oldenhof E, Allen JS, Dowling NA: An empirical study of personality disorders among treatment-seeking problem gamblers. J Gambl Stud 32(4):1079–1100, 2016

Brown RIF: Arousal and sensation-seeking components in the general explanation of gambling and gambling addictions. Int J Addictions 21(9–10):1001–1016, 1986

Brunborg G, Johnsen B, Pallesen S, et al: The relationship between aversive conditioning and risk-avoidance in gambling. J Gambl Stud 26(4):545–559, 2010

Brunborg GS, Johnsen BH, Mentzoni RA, et al: Individual differences in evaluative conditioning and reinforcement sensitivity affect bet-sizes during gambling. Pers Indiv Diff 50(5):729–734, 2011

Brunborg GS, Johnsen BH, Mentzoni RA, et al: Diminished aversive classical conditioning in pathological gamblers. Addiction 107(9):1660–1666, 2012

Brunborg GS, Hanss D, Mentzoni RA, et al: Problem gambling and the five-factor model of personality: a large population-based study. Addiction 111(8):1428–1435, 2016

Capaldi EJ: Partial reinforcement: a hypothesis of sequential effects, Psychol Rev 73(5):459–477, 1966

Clark L, Crooks B, Clarke R, et al: Physiological responses to near miss outcomes and personal control during simulated gambling. J Gambl Stud 28:123–137, 2011

Clark L, Liu R, McKavanagh R, et al: Learning and affect following near-miss outcomes in simulated gambling. J Behav Decis Mak 26(5):442–450, 2013

Costa PT, McCrae RR: Normal personality assessment in clinical practice: the NEO Personality Inventory. Psychol Assess 4(1):5–13, 1992

Cote D, Caron A, Aubert J, et al: Near wins prolong gambling on a video lottery terminal. J Gambl Stud 19(4):433–438, 2003

Cowley E, Briley DA, Farrell C: How do gamblers maintain an illusion of control? Journal of Business Research 68(10):2181–2188, 2015

Crewe-Brown C, Blaszczynski A, Russell A: Prize level and debt size: impact on gambling behaviour. J Gambl Stud 30(3):639–651, 2014

Csikszentmihalyi M: Flow: The Psychology of Happiness. London, Rider, 1992

Custer RL: Profile of the pathological gambler. J Clin Psychiatry 45(12 Pt 2):35–38, 1984

Daruna JH, Barnes PA: A neurodevelopmental view of impulsivity, in The Impulsive Client: Theory, Research, and Treatment. Edited by McCown WG, Johnson JL, Shure MB. Washington, DC, American Psychological Association, 1993, pp 23–37

Daugherty D, MacLin OH: Perceptions of luck: near win and near loss experiences. Anal Gambl Behav 1(2):123–132, 2007

Delfabbro PH, Winefield AH: Poker-machine gambling: an analysis of within session characteristics. Br J Psychol 90:425–439, 1999

Diskin KM, Hodgins DC: Narrowing of attention and dissociation in pathological video lottery gamblers. J Gambl Stud 15(1):17–28, 1999

Diskin KM, Hodgins DC: Narrowed focus and dissociative experiences in a community sample of experienced video lottery gamblers. Can J Behav Sci 33(1):58–64, 2001

Dixon MJ, Harrigan KA, Sandhu R, et al: Losses disguised as wins in modern multi-line video slot machines. Addiction 105:1819–1824, 2010

Dixon MJ, MacLaren V, Jarick M, et al: The frustrating effects of just missing the jackpot: slot machine near-misses trigger large skin conductance responses, but no post-reinforcement pauses. J Gambl Stud 29(4):661–674, 2013

Dixon M, Harrigan K, Santesso D, et al: The impact of sound in modern multiline video slot machine play. J Gambl Stud 30(4):913–929, 2014

Dixon MJ, Collins K, Harrigan KA, et al: Using sound to unmask losses disguised as wins in multiline slot machines. J Gambl Stud 31(1):183–196, 2015

Dixon M, Stange J, Larche M, et al: Dark flow, depression and multiline slot machine play. J Gambl Stud 34(1):73–84, 2018

Dixon MJ, Gutierrez J, Larche CJ, et al: Reward reactivity and dark flow in slot-machine gambling: "light" and "dark" routes to enjoyment. J Behav Addict 8(3):489–498, 2019

Dowling NA, Cowlishaw S, Jackson AC, et al: The prevalence of comorbid personality disorders in treatment-seeking problem gamblers: a systematic review and meta-analysis. J Pers Disord 29(6):735–754, 2015

Ferster CB, Skinner BF: Schedules of Reinforcement. Cambridge, MA, BF Skinner Foundation, 1957

Finlay K, Marmurek HH, Kanetkar V, Londerville J: Casino décor effects on gambling emotions and intentions. Environ Behav 42(4):524–545, 2010

Gillespie MA, Derevensky J, Gupta R: The utility of outcome expectancies in the prediction of adolescent gambling behaviour. Journal of Gambling Issues 19:69–85, 2007

Goddard N: Psychology, in Core Psychiatry. Edited by Wright P, Stern J, Phelan M. London, Elsevier, 2012, pp 63–82

Goodie A, Fortune E: Measuring cognitive distortions in pathological gambling: review and meta-analyses. Psychol Addict Behav 27(3):730–743, 2013

Grant BF, Hasin DS, Stinson FS, et al: Prevalence, correlates, and disability of personality disorders in the United States: results from the National Epidemiologic Survey on Alcohol and Related Conditions. J Clin Psychiatry 65(7):948–958, 2004

Gray JA, McNaughton N (eds): The Neuropsychology of Anxiety: An Enquiry Into the Functions of the Septo-hippocampal System, 2nd Edition. Oxford Psychology Series No 35. Oxford, UK, Oxford University Press, 2000

Graydon C, Stange M, Dixon M: Losses disguised as wins affect game selection on multiline slots. J Gambl Stud 34(4):1377–1390, 2018

Griffiths MD, Parke J: The psychology of music in gambling environments: an observational research note. Journal of Gambling Issues 13:1–12, 2005

Grubbs J, Rosansky J: Problem gambling, coping motivations, and positive expectancies: a longitudinal survey study. Psychol Addict Behav 34(2):414–419, 2020

Habib R, Dixon M: Neurobehavioral evidence for the "near miss" effect in pathological gamblers. J Exp Anal Behav 93(3):313–328, 2010

Hammelstein P: Faites vos jeux! Another look at sensation seeking and pathological gambling. Pers Individ Dif 37(5):917–931, 2004

Hannum R: Casino mathematics. Las Vegas, NV, UNLV Center for Gaming Research, 2012. Available at: https://gaming.unlv.edu/casinomath.html. Accessed July 21, 2020.

Harris A, Griffiths M: The impact of speed of play in gambling on psychological and behavioural factors: a critical review. J Gambl Stud 34(2):393–412, 2018

Hodgins DC, Holub A: Components of impulsivity in gambling disorder. Int J Mental Health Addict 13(6):699–711, 2015

Jacobs DF: A general theory of addictions: a new theoretical model. J Gambl Behav 2:15–31, 1986

Jensen C, Dixon MJ, Harrigan KA, et al: Misinterpreting "winning" in multiline slot machine games. Int Gambl Stud 13(1):112–126, 2012

Jiménez-Murcia S, Fernández-Aranda F, Mestre-Bach G, et al: Exploring the relationship between reward and punishment sensitivity and gambling disorder in a clinical sample: a path modeling analysis. J Gambl Stud 33(2):579–597, 2017

Kahneman D, Tversky A: Subjective probability: a judgment of representativeness. Cogn Psychol 3(3):430–454, 1972

Kassinove J, Schare M: Effects of the "near miss" and the "big win" on persistence at slot machine gambling. Psychol Addict Behav 15(2):155–158, 2001

Kessler RC, Hwang I, LaBrie R, et al: DSM-IV pathological gambling in the national comorbidity survey replication. Psychol Med 38(9):1351–1360, 2008

Koob GF, Le Moal M: Addiction and the brain antireward system. Annu Rev Psychol 59:29–53, 2008

Kyonka EG, Schutte NS: Probability discounting and gambling: a meta-analysis. Addiction 113(12):2173–2181, 2018

Ladouceur R, Walker M: A cognitive perspective on gambling, in Trends in Cognitive and Behavioural Therapies. Edited by Salkovskis PM. Hoboken, NJ, Wiley, 1996, pp 89–120

Ladouceur R, Sévigny S, Blaszczynski A, et al: Video lottery: winning expectancies and arousal. Addiction 98(6):733–738, 2003

Lagorio CH, Winger G: Random-ratio schedules produce greater demand for iv drug administration than fixed-ratio schedules in rhesus monkeys. Psychopharmacology (Berl) 231(15):2981–2988, 2014

Langer EJ: The illusion of control. J Pers Soc Psychol 32(2):311–328, 1975

Laskowski C, Dorchak S, Ward D, et al: Can slot-machine reward schedules induce gambling addiction in rats? J Gambl Stud 35(3):887–914, 2019

Ledgerwood DM, Alessi SM, Phoenix N, Petry NM: Behavioral assessment of impulsivity in pathological gamblers with and without substance use disorder histories versus healthy controls. Drug Alcohol Dependence 105(1–2):89–96, 2009

Ligneul R, Sescousse G, Barbalat G, et al: Shifted risk preferences in pathological gambling. Psychol Med 43(5):1059–1068, 2013

Loba P, Stewart SH, Klein RM, Blackburn JR: Manipulations of the features of standard video lottery terminal (VLT) games: effects in pathological and non-pathological gamblers. J Gambl Stud 17(4):297–320, 2001

Lobbestael J, Arntz A, Wiers RW: How to push someone's buttons: a comparison of four anger-induction methods. Cogn Emot 22:353–373, 2008

Lole L, Gonsalvez CJ: Does size matter? An examination of problem gamblers' skin conductance responses to large and small magnitude rewards. Psychophysiology 54(10):1541–1548, 2017

Lole L, Gonsalvez CJ, Blaszczynski A, Clarke AR: Electrodermal activity reliably captures physiological differences between wins and losses during gambling on electronic machines. Psychophysiology 49(2):154–163, 2012

Lole L, Gonsalvez CJ, Barry RJ, Blaszczynski A: Problem gamblers are hyposensitive to wins: an analysis of skin conductance responses during actual gambling on electronic gaming machines. Psychophysiology 51(6):556–564, 2014

MacKillop J, Anderson EJ, Castelda BA, et al: Divergent validity of measures of cognitive distortions, impulsivity, and time perspective in pathological gambling. J Gambl Stud 22(3):339–354, 2006

MacLaren V: Video lottery is the most harmful form of gambling in Canada. J Gambl Stud 32(2):459–485, 2016

MacLaren VV, Best LA, Dixon MJ, Harrigan KA: Problem gambling and the five-factor model in university students. Pers Individ Dif 50(3):335–338, 2011

MacLaren V, Fugelsang J, Harrigan K, Dixon M: Effects of impulsivity, reinforcement sensitivity, and cognitive style on Pathological Gambling symptoms among frequent slot machine players. Pers Individ Dif 52(3):390–394, 2012

MacLaren V, Ellery M, Knoll T: Personality, gambling motives and cognitive distortions in electronic gambling machine players. Pers Individ Dif 73:24–28, 2015

Madden GJ, Dake JM, Mauel EC, Rowe RR: Labor supply and consumption of food in a closed economy under a range of fixed- and random-ratio schedules: tests of unit price. J Exp Anal Behav 83(2):99–118, 2005

Madden GJ, Ewan E, Lagorio C: Toward an animal model of gambling: delay discounting and the allure of unpredictable outcomes. J Gambl Stud 23(1):63–83, 2007

McGrath DS, Stewart SH, Klein RM, et al: Self-generated motives for gambling in two population-based samples of gamblers. Int Gambl Stud 10(2):117–138, 2010

Mentzoni R, Laberg J, Brunborg G, et al: Effects of sequential win occurrence on subsequent gambling behaviour and urges. Gambl Res 24(1):31–38, 2012

Moon M, Lister J, Milosevic J, Ledgerwood A: Subtyping non-treatment-seeking problem gamblers using the pathways model. J Gambl Stud 33(3):841–853, 2017

Murch W, Clark L: Effects of bet size and multi-line play on immersion and respiratory sinus arrhythmia during electronic gaming machine use. Addict Behav 88:67–72, 2019

Murch W, Chu S, Clark L: Measuring the slot machine zone with attentional dual tasks and respiratory sinus arrhythmia. Psychol Addict Behav 31(3):375–384, 2017

Myrseth H, Pallesen S, Molde H, et al: Personality factors as predictors of pathological gambling. Pers Individ Dif 47(8):933–937, 2009

Nower L, Martins SS, Lin KH, Blanco C: Subtypes of disordered gamblers: results from the National Epidemiologic Survey on Alcohol and Related Conditions. Addiction 108(4):789–798, 2013

Osumi T, Ohira H: Cardiac responses predict decisions: An investigation of the relation between orienting response and decisions in the ultimatum game. Int J Psychophysiol 74:74–79, 2009

Otis E, Yakovenko I, Sherry S, et al: Applicability of the four-factor personality vulnerability model for substance misuse in understanding gambling behaviour and gambling problems. Pers Individ Dif 169:110400, 2021

Parke J, Griffiths M: The psychology of the fruit machine: the role of structural characteristics (revisited). Int J Mental Health Addict 4(2):151–179, 2006

Petry N, Stinson F, Grant B: Comorbidity of DSM-IV pathological gambling and other psychiatric disorders: results from the National Epidemiologic Survey on Alcohol and Related Conditions. J Clin Psychiatry 66(5):564–574, 2005

Ramnerö J, Molander O, Lindner P, Carlbring P: What can be learned about gambling from a learning perspective? A narrative review. Nord Psychol 71(4):303–322, 2019

Rehman I, Mahabadi N, Sanvictores T, Rehman CI: Classical conditioning, in StatPearls. Treasure Island, FL, StatPearls Publishing, August 27, 2020

Reynolds B: A review of delay-discounting research with humans: relations to drug use and gambling. Behav Pharmacol 17(8):651–667, 2006

Rivlin G: The chrome-shiny, lights-flashing, wheel-spinning, touch-screened, Drew-Carey-wisecracking, video-playing, "sound events"-packed, pulse-quickening bandit. New York Times Magazine, May 9, 2004, pp 42–47

Schellenberg BJI, Mcgrath DS, Dechant K: The Gambling Motives Questionnaire financial: factor structure, measurement invariance, and relationships with gambling behaviour. Int Gambl Stud 16(1):1–16, 2016

Schüll ND: Digital gambling: the coincidence of desire and design. Annals of the American Academy of Political and Social Science 597(1):65–81, 2005

Schüll ND: Addiction by Design: Machine Gambling in Las Vegas. Princeton, NJ, Princeton University Press, 2012

Sharpe L, Walker M, Coughlan M, et al: Structural changes to electronic gaming machines as effective harm minimization strategies for non-problem and problem gamblers. J Gambl Stud 21(4):503–520, 2005

Shenassa ED, Paradis AD, Dolan SL, et al: Childhood impulsive behavior and problem gambling by adulthood: A 30-year prospective community-based study. Addiction 107(1):160–168, 2012

Snyder W: Decision-making with risk and uncertainty: the case of horse racing. Am J Psychol 91(2):201–209, 1978

Spenwyn J, Barrett DJ, Griffiths MD: The role of light and music in gambling behaviour: an empirical pilot study. Int J Mental Health Addict 8(1):107–118, 2010

Stacy AW, Wiers RW: Implicit cognition and addiction: a tool for explaining paradoxical behavior. Ann Rev Clin Psychol 6:551–575, 2010

Stewart MJ, Stewart SH, Yi S, Ellery M: Predicting gambling behaviour and problems from implicit and explicit positive gambling outcome expectancies in regular gamblers. Int Gambl Stud 15(1):124–140, 2015

Stewart SH, Zack M: Development and psychometric evaluation of a three-dimensional Gambling Motives Questionnaire. Addiction 103(7):1110–1117, 2008

Stewart SH, Zack M, Collins P, et al: Subtyping pathological gamblers on the basis of affective motivations for gambling: relations to gambling problems, drinking problems, and affective motivations for drinking. Psychol Addict Behav 22(2):257–286, 2008

Stiles M, Hudson A, Ramasubbu C, et al: The role of memory associations in excessive and problem gambling. Journal of Gambling Issues 34:120–139, 2017

St-Pierre RA, Temcheff CE, Gupta R, et al: Predicting gambling problems from gambling outcome expectancies in college student-athletes. J Gambl Stud 30(1):47–60, 2014

Studer B, Limbrick-Oldfield EH, Clark L: "Put your money where your mouth is!" Effects of streaks on confidence and betting in a binary choice task. J Behav Decis Mak 28(3):239–249, 2015

Toce-Gerstein M, Gerstein DR, Volberg RA: A hierarchy of gambling disorders in the community. Addiction 98(12):1661–1672, 2003

Turner NE: Winning. Conference presentation at Alberta Gambling Research Institute 2012: The Causes of Problem Gambling, Banff, AB, Canada, April 13–14, 2012

Walker MB: Irrational thinking among slot machine players. J Gambl Stud 8(3):245–261, 1992

Weatherly JN, Sauter JM, King BM: The "big win" and resistance to extinction when gambling. J Psychol 138(6):495–504, 2004

Wulfert E, Roland B, Hartley J, et al: Heart rate arousal and excitement in gambling: winners versus losers. Psychol Addict Behav 19(3):311–316, 2005

Yakovenko I, Hodgins DC, el-Guebaly N, et al: Cognitive distortions predict future gambling involvement. Int Gambl Stud 16(2):175–192, 2016

Yi R, Mitchell SH, Bickel WK: Delay discounting and substance abuse-dependence, in Impulsivity: The Behavioral and Neurological Science of Discounting. Edited by Madden GJ, Bickel WK. Washington, DC, American Psychological Association, 2010, pp 191–211

Yi S, Stewart M, Collins P, Stewart SH: The activation of reward versus relief gambling outcome expectancies in regular gamblers: relations to gambling motives. J Gambl Stud 31(4):1515–1530, 2015

Zhou Y, Li X, Zhang M, et al: Behavioural approach tendencies to heroin-related stimuli in abstinent heroin abusers. Psychopharmacology (Berl) 221(1):171–176, 2012

Zuckerman M, Neeb M: Sensation seeking and psychopathology. Psychiatry Res 1(3):255–264, 1979

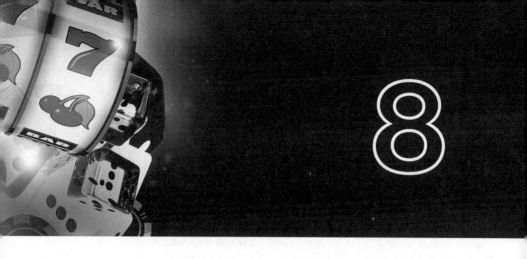

Neurobiology

Luis C. Farhat, M.D.
Marc N. Potenza, M.D., Ph.D.

Gambling disorder is a psychiatric condition characterized by a persistent and recurrent pattern of gambling that is associated with significant distress and impairment (American Psychiatric Association 2013). Originally termed "pathological gambling" in previous editions of the *Diagnostic and Statistical Manual of Mental Disorders* (DSM), gambling disorder had been classified as an impulse-control disorder until the latest edition of DSM in 2013, when it was reclassified within the category of "Substance-Related and Addictive Disorders" (American Psychiatric Association 2013). This change in the classification of gambling disorder in the perspective of the American Psychiatric Association (APA) was strongly related to, among other factors, findings from neurobiological research that indicate there exist important similarities in brain function between gambling disorder and substance use disorders (SUDs). This nosological change in how gambling disorder is conceptualized by the APA underscores the importance of becoming familiar with the neurobiological underpinnings of gambling disorder.

Mental health practitioners and researchers have recognized the limitations of how psychopathology has been characterized over the past 40 years since the seminal work that led to the development of DSM-III (Robins and Guze 1970). Diagnostic categories as determined by DSM are essentially clinically informed theoretical constructs established in accordance with an a priori assumption that a set of symptoms co-occur among individuals due to a latent variable—the psychiatric disorder (Kendler 2009). Yet individuals with the same diagnosis may present with completely nonoverlapping symptoms and respond differently to the same treatments, and this suggests that current diagnostic categories are considerably heterogeneous (Insel et al. 2010). Mental health researchers, including addiction experts, have been investigating neurobiological factors in an attempt to identify characteristics that may aid in developing novel circuit-based treatments, predicting response and determining long-term prognosis, and addressing other matters of clinical relevance (Yücel et al. 2019). However, the impact of neurobiological research in providing valuable contributions to clinical practice in psychiatry remains to be fully achieved (Ross et al. 2015), and additional research is therefore required, particularly for gambling disorder (Potenza et al. 2019).

Given the importance of neurobiology in psychiatry, this chapter considers the neurobiology of gambling disorder. Here, we initially review some of the evidence from both twin and molecular studies to provide an overview of the genetics of gambling disorder. We also review findings from studies using neurocognitive tasks to highlight the roles of impulsivity and compulsivity in gambling disorder, two broad neurocognitive constructs associated with specific neural correlates that could be potential endophenotypes for future research in gambling disorder. We proceed to review findings from neurochemistry studies to highlight possible neurotransmitter systems implicated in the pathophysiology of gambling disorder. Last, we review neuroimaging studies to provide evidence of specific brain functions and structures that have been reported to be altered in gambling disorder compared with healthy control participants and individuals with SUDs, with a special emphasis on alterations in reward processing.

Genetics

Gambling is defined as an activity that involves placing something of value at risk in the hopes of gaining something of greater value in return (Potenza et al. 2001, 2019). Gambling is prevalent, and there exist multiple popular forms of gambling (e.g., casino gambling, internet gambling, lotteries). Nevertheless, relatively few individuals who gamble develop gambling disorder (Hodgins et al. 2011), and this suggests that some individuals may have increased susceptibility to developing gambling disorder. From this perspective, gambling disorder susceptibility, gambling, and gambling-related problems are distributed along a continuum (Toce-Gerstein et al. 2003), with gambling disorder at one extreme end of this spectrum. Although the diagnostic definition of gambling disorder is helpful because clinical decisions are often categorical in nature, understanding individuals along a gambling–problem gambling spectrum is often informative, and it is most helpful for mental health practitioners to understand gambling disorder and problem gambling. With this in mind, data from twin and birth-cohort studies may provide significant insight into genetic factors associated with gambling disorder and gambling disorder vulnerability.

Twin studies are particularly useful because they permit estimation of genetic and environmental contributions to a specific phenotype such as gambling disorder. Given changes over time in the gambling environment (e.g., recent availability of internet gambling [Potenza et al. 2011]), understanding the relative contributions of genetic and environmental factors to gambling disorder may be informative. Available evidence from the Vietnam Twin Era Registry (Eisen et al. 1989), one of the largest twin studies in the United States, suggests that heritable factors (i.e., heritability) explain about 35%–54% of the likelihood of developing gambling disorder (Eisen et al. 1998), which underscores the importance of identifying both genetic and environmental factors that may underlie risk for developing gambling disorder across the lifespan. Evidence from twin studies also indicates that there exists a significant genetic correlation between gambling disorder and SUDs involving tobacco, cannabis, stimulants (Xian et al. 2014), and alcohol (Slutske et al. 2000), suggesting the presence of common underlying etiologic pathways across substance and behavioral addictions. Although this sample was composed of men, similar findings for men and women have been reported, for example, between gambling and alcohol use disorders with respect to genetic and environmental contributions (Slutske et al. 2010). Consistent with gambling disorder's co-occurrence with multiple forms of psychiatric disorders, genetic contributions are also shared between gambling disorder and other non-SUD psychiatric disorders (e.g., depression [Potenza et al. 2005] and anxiety disorders [Giddens et al. 2011]), as well as between gambling disorder and obsessive-compulsive features (Scherrer et al. 2015).

Molecular genetic approaches have also been used to study gambling disorder. Genome-wide association studies (GWASs) may identify genetic variants (e.g., single nucleotide polymorphisms) that are significantly associated with specific phenotypes (Visscher et al. 2012). Other methods used to identify genes associated with phenotypes (e.g., linkage and candidate gene studies) have limitations, including biases and insufficient statistical power. GWASs often need large sample sizes (e.g., tens of thousands of individuals) to identify regions reaching genome-wide significance (e.g., $P < 5 \times 10^{-8}$). Large GWASs evaluating associations between common variants and the gambling disorder phenotype are lacking. To date, there are two GWASs of gambling disorder (Lang et al. 2016; Lind et al. 2013); neither study identified genomic regions reaching genome-wide significance, suggesting collaborative efforts across gambling disorder research centers may be required to characterize the genetic architecture of gambling disorder. After such variants are reliably identified, additional research can then be conducted to clarify the function of each identified variant in the hopes of understanding further the pathophysiology of gambling disorder (Edwards et al. 2013). Additionally, when adequately powered GWASs are available, their summary statistics may be used to calculate polygenic risk scores, which may have clinical value as a tool for risk prediction (Martin et al. 2019). Of note, a polygenic risk score for alcohol use disorder has been linked to gambling disorder (Lang et al. 2016), consistent with findings from twin studies indicating genetic links between these disorders.

Neurocognitive Functioning

Gambling disorder entails the proposed core characteristics of addictions, which it shares with SUDs (Potenza 2006): 1) appetitive urges or craving states immediately prior to engagement in gambling; 2) impaired control, including placement of larger bets, gambling longer than originally intended, and experiencing difficulties quitting gambling; 3) continued engagement despite gambling-related problems; and 4) compulsive engagement as evidenced by habitual gambling. These phenotypic characteristics may relate to neurocognitive functioning associated with impulsivity and compulsivity.

Impulsivity has been defined as a predisposition to rapid reactions to stimuli, either internal or external, often with limited previous forethought or regard for the impact of the negative consequences associated with such reactions on the individual or on others (Moeller et al. 2001). Recent models of impulsivity emphasize the need to account for the multifaceted components of the construct (Fineberg et al. 2014). Indeed, impulsivity may be understood as consisting of several different domains, such as impulsive responses (i.e., failure to suppress prepotent responses) and impulsive choices (i.e., difficulties delaying gratification for larger rewards). Impulsive actions may also involve decision-making in conditions of uncertainty (i.e., risky choices made during unclear scenarios) and diminished reflection (i.e., premature choices when insufficient information has been accumulated), among other factors.

Specific neurocognitive tasks may be used to evaluate different domains of impulsivity and related constructs. For instance, impulsive responses are often assessed through go–no-go or stop-signal tasks. In both cases, individuals are instructed to suppress a predisposed response after they receive the "no-go" or "stop" signal, although the former involves stopping a prepotent response and the latter requires the cessation of an initiated action. Individuals with gambling disorder tend to commit more errors on go–no-go tasks and to show longer stop-signal reaction times on the stop-signal task compared with healthy control subjects, indicating the existence of a deficit in response inhibition in gambling disorder (Ioannidis et al. 2019). Impulsive choices may be evaluated through monetary tasks in which an individual is offered the option to choose a hypothetical smaller dollar amount delivered immediately or a larger amount after a specified delay; the rapid temporal discounting of rewards has been termed *delay discounting*. Individuals with gambling disorder tend to show more rapid temporal discounting than healthy control participants, suggesting difficulties postponing immediate gratification for larger rewards (Ioannidis et al. 2019). Risk-reward decision-making is often evaluated through the Iowa Gambling Task (IGT). During the IGT, individuals are instructed to choose from four deck of cards to maximize their points, with information provided that some decks are better than others. Two of the decks ultimately lead to more points lost than won and are considered disadvantageous; in these decks, wins tend to be bigger than those from advantageous decks, but the losses are even larger. For best performance, participants need to learn not to select from decks with more short-term rewards and larger intermittent losses and to instead choose from advantageous decks that, in the long-run, provide more points being accrued over time. Neurocognitive studies have shown that individuals with gambling disorder are more likely to continue choosing from disadvantageous decks, thus obtaining lower final scores compared with healthy control subjects (Ioannidis et al. 2019).

Compulsivity has been defined as a tendency to perform repetitive overt or covert behaviors in a habitual manner that lead to functional impairment despite being done to prevent perceived negative consequences (Fineberg et al. 2010, 2014). Compulsivity has been understudied compared with impulsivity, and some have argued that although it might be a useful concept for clinicians, it may be "too ambiguous and confusing for research studies" (Yücel and Fontenelle 2012). Yet researchers (Fineberg et al. 2014) have proposed theoretical frameworks that may be used to subdivide compulsivity into four different cognitive domains: contingency-related cognitive flexibility (i.e., learning and unlearning behavior based on contingencies), set shifting (i.e., reorienting attention to different characteristics to achieve goals), attentional bias (i.e., attending to or avoiding relevant stimuli), and habit learning (i.e., repeating complex, familiar learned behaviors with limited forethought).

Different cognitive tasks may be used to evaluate specific domains of compulsivity. Card-playing tasks (CPTs) and probabilistic reversal learning tasks (PRLTs) have been used to evaluate contingency-related cognitive flexibility. In CPTs, individuals learn that progressive decreases in win-to-loss ratios during the game should lead to quitting the card game; continuing to play when win-to-loss ratios are not favorable indicates impairment of contingency-related cognitive flexibility. In PRLTs, individuals adapt to new rules that reverse good and bad options in a game that requires them to choose the better of two stimuli; the number of bad choices after the rule change indicates impairment of contingency-related cognitive flexibility. Individuals with gambling disorder have demonstrated poorer performance relative to healthy control subjects on CPTs but not PRLTs, although heterogeneity across studies using PRLTs is considerably high (van Timmeren et al. 2018). Among individuals with gambling disorder, measures of cognitive flexibility have been associated with problem gambling severity (Leppink et al. 2016) and treatment outcomes (Grant et al. 2010). The Wisconsin Card Sorting Test (WCST) has traditionally been used to measure set shifting, another form of cognitive flexibility, because individuals are required to continuously sort cards according to classification rules that change. Numbers of preservation errors are frequently employed as an index of set shifting performance. Individuals with gambling disorder perform worse than healthy control subjects on the WCST (van Timmeren et al. 2018). Variants of the Stroop task have been used to evaluate attentional biases. In the traditional Stroop task, individuals are presented with names of ink colors printed in the same or a different color from the word spelled; individuals are instructed to read the names of ink colors, and the length of the reaction time when a mismatch is presented is used as an index measure of attentional bias. Individuals with gambling disorder demonstrate longer reaction times than healthy control subjects on the Stroop task (van Timmeren et al. 2018).

A conceptual difference between impulsivity and compulsivity may involve reward-seeking versus punishment-avoidance motivations; thus, some have hypothesized that impulsivity and compulsivity are diametrically opposed constructs (Stein and Hollander 1995). However, both impulsive and compulsive behaviors may relate to deficits in self-regulation and inhibitory control (Fineberg et al. 2010). Consistently, both impulsivity and compulsivity have been found to be elevated in individuals with gambling disorder (el-Guebaly et al. 2012) and other addictions (Leeman and Potenza 2012). Translational research has associated both impulsive and compulsive acts with segregated, but intercommunicating, cortico-striatal-thalamic circuits (CSTCs). Compulsive behaviors may be driven by the caudate nucleus and inhibited by the orbitofrontal cortex, whereas impulsive behaviors may be driven by the ventral striatum or nucleus accumbens and inhibited by the ventromedial prefrontal cortex (Fineberg et al. 2010). These CSTCs have been implicated in neuroimaging studies of individuals with gambling disorder.

Neurochemistry

Four main neurotransmitter systems have been hypothesized to contribute to the pathophysiology of gambling disorder: serotonin with respect to impulse control, dopamine with respect to reward-related behaviors, norepinephrine with respect to arousal and excitement, and opioids with respect to motivations and urges (Bullock and Potenza 2012; Potenza 2013b).

Serotonin, or 5-hydroxytryptamine (5-HT), is a neurotransmitter derived from the amino acid tryptophan. Serotonergic neurons are located in the raphe nucleus of the brain stem and send ascending projections that terminate in cortical, limbic, and midbrain regions. Serotonin has been implicated in multiple processes relating to mood, perception, reward, anger, aggression, appetite, memory, sexuality, and attention, among others (Berger et al. 2009). Several lines of evidence suggest serotonergic processes contributing to gambling disorder. Low levels of metabolites of 5-HT and of platelet monoamine oxidase activity (a peripheral marker of 5-HT) have been found in cerebrospinal fluid (CSF) and serum samples of individuals with gambling disorder (Nordin and Eklundh 1999). Altered 5-HT receptor sensitivity has been documented in individuals with gambling disorder because administration of meta-chlorophenylpiperazine (m-CPP), a partial agonist at 5-HT$_1$/5-HT$_2$ receptors, produces different behavioral and biochemical responses among individuals with gambling disorder compared with individuals without gambling disorder (Pallanti et al. 2006). Specifically, whereas individuals with gambling disorder reported feeling euphoric, individuals without gambling disorder frequently reported experiencing unpleasant sensations; individuals with gambling disorder also showed increased prolactin responses after administration of m-CPP. However, randomized, placebo-controlled trials (RCTs) have provided mixed results as to whether selective serotonin reuptake inhibitors may be effective in the treatment of gambling disorder (Bartley and Bloch 2013; Kraus et al. 2020). Additional research is required to further clarify the role of serotonin in gambling disorder.

Dopamine is a catecholamine neurotransmitter derived from the amino acid tyrosine. Dopaminergic brain pathways, such as the mesolimbic pathway, have been traditionally implicated in rewarding and reinforcing behaviors (Everitt and Robbins 2005). Elevated levels of dopamine have been found in the CSF of individuals with gambling disorder (Bergh et al. 1997), although this finding was no longer significant when CSF flow rate was controlled for (Nordin and Eklundh 1999). In a small sample, D_3 receptor levels correlated with impulsivity and problem gambling severity in gambling disorder (Boileau et al. 2013). However, availability of $D_{2/3}$ receptors did not differ between individuals with gambling disorder and healthy control subjects (Boileau et al. 2013). Additionally, antipsychotic medications such as olanzapine or haloperidol with D_2-like dopamine receptor antagonism properties have not demonstrated efficacy over placebo in gambling disorder treatment (Fong et al. 2008; McElroy et al. 2008) or have increased gambling-related motivations and behaviors in individuals with gambling disorder (Zack and Poulos 2007). Thus, a role for dopamine in gambling disorder has been questioned (Potenza 2013a, 2018).

Norepinephrine is a catecholamine derived from dopamine and associated with stress-induced responses ("fight-or-flight" reactions) (Moore and Bloom 1979). Norepinephrine has been implicated in arousal and excitement-seeking behavior. Elevated concentrations of norepinephrine or its metabolites have been found in both the urine and CSF of individuals with gambling disorder (Roy et al. 1988). Increased adrenergic function observed among individuals with gambling disorder may contribute to the "high" associated with gambling; consistently, individuals with gambling disorder show an increased activation of the sympathetic nervous system during casino gambling, as measured by increased heart rates and serum norepinephrine levels (Meyer et al. 2004).

Opioid systems have been implicated in individuals with gambling disorder. Both opioidergic peptides and receptors contribute to opioid systems. Challenge studies with oral amphetamine showed a blunted opioid response in those with gambling disorder (Mick et al. 2016), a transdiagnostic finding that is also observed among individuals with SUDs (Gorelick et al. 2005). Clinical trials implicate opioids in gambling disorder pathophysiology because RCTs show opioid antagonists such as naltrexone and naloxone may be more efficacious than placebo (Potenza et al. 2019). However, much of this evidence comes from older studies with potential biases (Bartley and Bloch 2013). Specific subgroups (e.g., individuals with gambling disorder and a family history of addictions or strong gambling urges) may be particularly inclined to respond favorably to opioid receptor antagonists (Grant et al. 2008). Additional research is warranted to clarify the roles of opioid systems in gambling disorder.

Neuroimaging

Multiple neuroimaging studies of individuals with gambling disorder have been published over the past two decades, with results that are consistent with understandings of psychiatric conditions as brain disorders arising from alterations in brain circuitries (Insel et al. 2010). Conceptualizations of gambling disorder as an addiction without a drug provide a framework for investigating mechanisms underlying addictions without confounding effects of substance-related brain changes (Balodis and Potenza 2020). In this section, we review evidence from neuroimaging studies of gambling disorder, with an emphasis on magnetic resonance imaging (MRI) studies.

Dual-process models posit important roles for reward and control systems in gambling disorder (Antons et al. 2020). Reward systems of the brain are associated with reinforcement of reward-related behaviors and learning with the goal of stimulating adaptive behaviors. Reward processing involves interconnected networks of cortical and subcortical structures, such as the prefrontal cortex, striatum (including the nucleus accumbens), amygdala, and ventral tegmental area. Natural reinforcers such as food, sexual activity, and maternal behavior often activate these regions, which ultimately helps to promote survival of the species by stimulating engagement in and reinforcement of these behaviors (Fauth-Bühler et al. 2017). Neuroscientific models of reinforcement learning implicate frontostriatal neurocircuitry of the reward system. Discrepancies between expected and actual rewards (prediction errors) serve to update expected values of rewards, which involves additional brain regions such as the insula (Schultz et al. 1997). These reward-related systems have been implicated in gambling disorder by MRI studies.

Reward sensitivity dysfunction may be central to the pathophysiology of gambling disorder. Many functional MRI (fMRI) studies in gambling disorder to date have focused on evaluating reward processing with monetary cues and rewards (reviewed by Balodis and Potenza 2020). These studies indicate a blunted activation of frontostriatal circuits involving the striatum and ventromedial prefrontal cortex during the reward anticipation and outcome phases (Luijten et al. 2017). Blunted frontostriatal activity has also been reported among individuals with SUDs (Allain et al. 2015), especially during reward anticipation (Luijten et al. 2017), suggesting a transdiagnostic construct relevant to addictions. Diminished frontostriatal activity may reflect a deficit of reward sensitivity in gambling disorder and other addictive states. For example, individuals with gambling disorder may gamble to compensate for a general insensitivity to natural rewards such as food and sexual activity, which is consistent with some theoretical models of addiction such as the reward deficiency syndrome theory (Blum et al. 2000). Given that monetary cues are relevant to gambling, additional studies using non–gambling-related stimuli are required to indicate whether this hypo-sensitivity to reward is a global function associated with stimuli related to other reinforcement-based behaviors (e.g., food, sexual activity). Relatively few stud-ies have examined frontostriatal activity in the context of nonmonetary cues. One such study used erotic cues instead of monetary ones, and individuals with gambling disorder showed decreased frontostriatal activity compared with healthy control subjects; furthermore, differences in activity in frontostriatal circuitry in individuals with gambling disorder correlated with problem gam-bling severity (Sescousse et al. 2013). Additional research should seek to repli-cate and extend these findings.

Reward-learning dysfunctions may also contribute to gambling disorder. Monetary task–based fMRI studies have suggested increased activation of areas within a salience network, including the dorsal anterior cingulate cortex (ACC) and the anterior insula, in gambling disorder during gambling urges (see Balodis and Potenza 2020 for a review). The salience network, which comprises differ-ent brain areas, such as the bilateral insula, dorsal ACC, and subcortical areas, has been implicated in the allocation of attention to salient events (Seeley et al. 2007). Increased activation of the salience network could reflect recruitment of attentional resources in response to gambling-related cues in gambling disor-der, which could be associated with urges to gamble and maintenance of gam-bling behavior. Among individuals with SUDs, the insula has been implicated in tobacco cravings because individuals who smoked tobacco and sustained damage to the insula were 100 times more likely than individuals who smoked tobacco and sustained damage to other brain regions to stop smoking without experienc-ing urges to smoke (Naqvi et al. 2007). Further evidence of a reward-learning dysfunction in people with gambling disorder comes from studies that used ex-perimental gambling tasks to evaluate correlates of loss-chasing behavior; in one such study, individuals with gambling disorder showed diminished activation of the amygdala relative to control subjects prior to ceasing loss-chasing behavior (Worhunsky et al. 2017). Given the amygdala has been implicated in cost-benefit analyses with a goal of avoiding losses (Shohamy et al. 2009), reduced activation of the amygdala may reflect impaired probabilistic learning (i.e., acquiring in-formation that is based on the likelihood of prior events that have been paired with specific outcomes). However, alternative possibilities (e.g., involving poorer signaling of negative emotional states) also warrant consideration.

Additional circuitry involved primarily in other psychological processes may also influence reward and loss processing. For instance, investigations have focused on "near-miss effects" involving losses perceived as "close wins" (re-viewed by Balodis and Potenza 2020). These studies suggest neural mechanisms for how slot machines may facilitate gambling and promote cognitive distor-tions. Additional research is warranted to investigate other domains of psycho-logical phenomena in gambling disorder.

Data suggest functional brain differences and similarities between individ-uals with gambling disorder and healthy control subjects and individuals with SUDs, with data on volumetric differences arguably more mixed (reviewed by

Balodis and Potenza 2020). Although smaller studies have reported increased ventral striatum volumes among individuals with gambling disorder (Koehler et al. 2015), large voxel-based morphometry studies have failed to identify significant volumetric differences between individuals with gambling disorder and healthy control subjects, although they have found significant differences among individuals with SUDs related to cocaine versus those with gambling disorder and healthy control subjects (Yip et al. 2018). These findings suggest that volumetric brain alterations in SUDs may be associated with neurotoxic effects of substance use, and this speculation warrants further direct study. Given the relative scarcity of available data, additional research remains necessary, especially considering that few neuroimaging studies in gambling disorder have controlled for the co-occurrence of substance use.

Conclusion

The neurobiological underpinnings of gambling disorder are complex. Findings from twin studies indicate that gambling disorder is a heritable condition. Impulsivity and compulsivity, "neurocognitive endophenotypes" that are associated with changes in discrete neural systems, have been found to be elevated in individuals with gambling disorder. Four main neurotransmitter systems—namely, serotonin, dopamine, norepinephrine, and endogenous opioids—and functional alterations in reward-related brain systems have been implicated in gambling disorder. Nonetheless, there is still much to learn. The extent to which the underlying heritability of gambling disorder is solely attributed to underlying genetic factors or to epigenetic interactions of shared environmental exposures remains unknown; to date, GWAS studies have failed to identify common variants associated with the gambling disorder phenotype, but larger sample sizes are required to achieve adequate statistical power. Also, it remains unclear whether the proposed neurocognitive endophenotypes or functional brain alterations will play any role in improving public health and clinical outcomes. As the understanding grows, it is hoped that there will be more tangible gains with respect to developing improved policy, prevention, and treatment efforts.

References

Allain F, Minogianis EA, Roberts DC, Samaha AN: How fast and how often: the pharmacokinetics of drug use are decisive in addiction. Neurosci Biobehav Rev 56:166–179, 2015

American Psychiatric Association: Diagnostic and Statistical Manual of Mental Disorders, 5th Edition. Arlington, VA, American Psychiatric Association, 2013

Antons S, Brand M, Potenza MN: Neurobiology of cue-reactivity, craving, and inhibitory control in non-substance addictive behaviors. J Neurol Sci 415:116952, 2020

Balodis IM, Potenza MN: Common neurobiological underpinnings of gambling and substance use disorders. Progress Neuropsychopharm Biol Psychiatry 99:109847, 2020

Bartley CA, Bloch MH: Meta-analysis: pharmacological treatment of pathological gambling. Expert Rev Neurother 13(8):887–894, 2013

Berger M, Gray JA, Roth BL: The expanded biology of serotonin. Annu Rev Med 60:355–366, 2009

Bergh C, Eklund T, Sodersten P, Nordin C: Altered dopamine function in pathological gambling. Psychol Med 27(2):473–475, 1997

Blum K, Braverman ER, Holder JM, et al: Reward deficiency syndrome: a biogenetic model for the diagnosis and treatment of impulsive, addictive, and compulsive behaviors. J Psychoactive Drugs 32 (suppl 1):1–112, 2000

Boileau I, Payer D, Chugani B, et al: The D2/3 dopamine receptor in pathological gambling: a positron emission tomography study with [11C]-(+)-propyl-hexahydro-naphtho-oxazin and [11C]raclopride. Addiction 108(5):953–963, 2013

Bullock SA, Potenza MN: Pathological gambling: neuropsychopharmacology and treatment. Curr Psychopharmacology 1(1):24349964, 2012

Edwards SL, Beesley J, French JD, Dunning AM: Beyond GWASs: illuminating the dark road from association to function. Am J Hum Genet 93(5):779–797, 2013

Eisen S, Neuman R, Goldberg J, et al: Determining zygosity in the Vietnam Era Twin Registry: an approach using questionnaires. Clin Genet 35(6):423–432, 1989

Eisen SA, Lin N, Lyons MJ, et al: Familial influences on gambling behavior: an analysis of 3359 twin pairs. Addiction 93(9):1375–1384, 1998

el-Guebaly N, Mudry T, Zohar J, et al: Compulsive features in behavioral addictions: the case of pathological gambling. Addiction 107:1726–1734, 2012

Everitt BJ, Robbins TW: Neural systems of reinforcement for drug addiction: from actions to habits to compulsion. Nat Neurosci 8(11):1481–1489, 2005

Fauth-Bühler M, Mann K, Potenza MN: Pathological gambling: a review of the neurobiological evidence relevant for its classification as an addictive disorder. Addict Biol 22(4):885–897, 2017

Fineberg NA, Potenza MN, Chamberlain SR, et al: Probing compulsive and impulsive behaviors, from animal: models to endophenotypes: a narrative review. Neuropsychopharmacology 35(3):591–604, 2010

Fineberg NA, Chamberlain SR, Goudriaan AE, et al: New developments in human neurocognition: clinical, genetic, and brain imaging correlates of impulsivity and compulsivity. CNS Spectr 19(1):69–89, 2014

Fong T, Kalechstein A, Bernhard B, et al: A double-blind, placebo-controlled trial of olanzapine for the treatment of video poker pathological gamblers. Pharmacol Biochem Behav 89(3):298–303, 2008

Giddens JL, Xian H, Scherrer JF, et al: Shared genetic contributions to anxiety disorders and pathological gambling in a male population. J Affective Dis 132:406–412, 2011

Gorelick DA, Kim YK, Bencherif B, et al: Imaging brain mu-opioid receptors in abstinent cocaine users: time course and relation to cocaine craving. Biol Psychiatry 57(12):1573–1582, 2005

Grant JE, Kim SW, Hollander E, Potenza MN: Predicting response to opiate antagonists and placebo in the treatment of pathological gambling. Psychopharmacology (Berl) 200:521–527, 2008

Grant JE, Odlaug BL, Chamberlain SR, et al: Open-label memantine treatment of pathological gambling reduces gambling severity and cognitive inflexibility. Psychopharmacology (Berl) 212:603–612, 2010

Hodgins DC, Stea JN, Grant JE: Gambling disorders. Lancet 378(9806):1874–1884, 2011

Insel T, Cuthbert B, Garvey M, et al: Research domain criteria (RDoC): toward a new classification framework for research on mental disorders. Am J Psychiatry 167(7):748–751, 2010

Ioannidis K, Hook R, Wickham K, et al: Impulsivity in gambling disorder and problem gambling: a meta-analysis. Neuropsychopharmacology 44(8):1354–1361, 2019

Kendler KS: An historical framework for psychiatric nosology. Psychol Med 39(2):1935–1941, 2009

Koehler S, Hasselmann E, Wustenberg T, et al: Higher volume of ventral striatum and right prefrontal cortex in pathological gambling. Brain Struct Funct 220(1):469–477, 2015

Kraus SW, Etuk R, Potenza MN: Advances in pharmacotherapy for gambling disorder: a systematic review. Expert Opin Pharmacotherapy 21(3):287–296, 2020

Lang M, Leménager T, Streit F, et al: Genome-wide association study of pathological gambling. Eur Psychiatry 36:38–46, 2016

Leeman RF, Potenza MN: Similarities and differences between pathological gambling and substance use disorders: a focus on impulsivity and compulsivity. Psychopharmacology (Berl) 219:469–490, 2012

Leppink EW, Redden SA, Chamberlain SR, Grant JE: Cognitive flexibility correlates with gambling severity in young adults. J Psychiatr Res 81:9–15, 2016

Lind PA, Zhu G, Montgomery GW, et al: Genome-wide association study of a quantitative disordered gambling trait. Addict Biol 18(3):511–522, 2013

Luijten M, Schellekens AF, Kühn S, et al: Disruption of reward processing in addiction: an image-based meta-analysis of functional magnetic resonance imaging studies. JAMA Psychiatry 74(4):387–398, 2017

Martin AR, Daly MJ, Robinson EB, et al: Predicting polygenic risk of psychiatric disorders. Biol Psychiatry 86(2):97–109, 2019

McElroy S, Nelson EB, Welge JA, et al: Olanzapine in the treatment of pathological gambling: a negative randomized placebo-controlled trial. J Clin Psychiatry 69(3):443–440, 2008

Meyer G, Schwertfeger J, Exton MS, et al: Neuroendocrine response to casino gambling in problem gamblers. Psychoneuroendocrinology 29(10):1272–1280, 2004

Mick I, Myers J, Ramos AC, et al: Blunted endogenous opioid release following an oral amphetamine challenge in pathological gamblers. Neuropsychopharmacology 41(7):1742–17450, 2016

Moeller FG, Barrat ES, Dougherty DM, et al: Psychiatric aspects of impulsivity. Am J Psychiatry 158(11):1783–1793, 2001

Moore RY, Bloom FE: Central catecholamine neuron systems: anatomy and physiology of the norepinephrine and epinephrine systems. Annu Rev Neurosci 2:113–168, 1979

Naqvi NH, Rudrauf D, Damasio H, Bechara A: Damage to the insula disrupts addiction to cigarette smoking. Science 315(5811):531–534, 2007

Nordin C, Eklundh T: Altered CSF 5-HIAA disposition in pathologic male gamblers. CNS Spectr 4(12):25–33, 1999

Pallanti S, Bernardi S, Quercioli L, et al: Serotonin dysfunction in pathological gamblers: increased prolactin response to oral m-CPP versus placebo. CNS Spectr 11(12):956–964, 2006

Potenza MN: Should addictive disorders include non-substance-related conditions? Addiction 1:142–151, 2006

Potenza MN: How central is dopamine to pathological gambling or gambling disorder. Front Behav Neurosci 7:206, 2013a

Potenza MN: Neurobiology of gambling behaviors. Curr Opin Neurobiol 23(4):660–667, 2013b

Potenza MN: Searching for replicable dopamine-related findings in gambling disorder. Biol Psychiatry 83:984–986, 2018

Potenza MN, Kosten TR, Rounsaville BJ: Pathological gambling. JAMA 286(2):141–144, 2001

Potenza MN, Xian H, Shah KR, et al: Shared genetic contributions to pathological gambling and major depression in men. Arch Gen Psychiatry 62:1015–1021, 2005

Potenza MN, Wareham JD, Steinberg MA, et al: Correlates of at-risk/problem internet gambling in adolescents. J Am Acad Child Adolesc Psychiatry 50(2):150–159, 2011

Potenza MN, Balodis IM, Derevensky J, et al: Gambling disorder. Nat Rev Dis Primers 5(1):51, 2019

Robins E, Guze SB: Establishment of diagnostic validity in psychiatric illness: its application to schizophrenia. Am J Psychiatry 126(7):983–987, 1970

Ross DA, Travis MJ, Arbuckle MR: The future of psychiatry as clinical neuroscience: why not now? JAMA Psychiatry 72(5):413–414, 2015

Roy A, Pickar D, De Jong J, et al: Norepinephrine and its metabolites in cerebrospinal fluid, plasma, and urine: relationship to hypothalamic-pituitary-adrenal axis function in depression. Arch Gen Psychiatry 45(9):849–857, 1988

Scherrer JF, Xian H, Slutske WS, et al: Associations between obsessive-compulsive classes and pathological gambling in a national cohort of male twins. JAMA Psychiatry 72(4):342–349, 2015

Schultz W, Dayan P, Montague PR: A neural substrate of prediction and reward. Science 275(5306):1593–1599, 1997

Seeley WW, Menon V, Schatzberg AF, et al: Dissociable intrinsic connectivity networks for salience processing and executive control. J Neurosci 27(9):2349–2356, 2007

Sescousse G, Barbalat G, Domenech P, Dreher JC: Imbalance in the sensitivity to different types of rewards in pathological gambling. Brain 136 (Pt 8):2527–2538, 2013

Shohamy D, Myers CE, Hopkins RO, et al: Distinct hippocampal and basal ganglia contributions to probabilistic learning and reversal. J Cogn Neurosci 21(9):1821–1833, 2009

Slutske WS, Eisen S, True WR, et al: Common genetic vulnerability to pathological gambling and alcohol dependence in men. Arch Gen Psychiatry 57(7):666–673, 2000

Slutske WS, Zhu G, Meier MH, Martin NG: Genetic and environmental influences on disordered gambling in men and women. Arch Gen Psychiatry 67(6):624–630, 2010

Stein DJ, Hollander E: Obsessive-compulsive spectrum disorders. J Clin Psychiatr 56(6):265–266, 1995

Toce-Gerstein M, Gerstein DR, Volberg RA: A hierarchy of gambling disorders in the community. Addiction 98(12):1661–1672, 2003

van Timmeren T, Daams JG, van Holst RJ, Goudriaan AE: Compulsivity-related neurocognitive performance deficits in gambling disorder: a systematic review and meta-analysis. Neurosci Biobehav Rev 84:204–217, 2018

Visscher PM, Brown MA, McCarthy MI, Yang J: Five years of GWAS discovery. Am J Hum Genet 90(1):7–24, 2012

Worhunsky PD, Potenza MN, Rogers RD: Alterations in functional brain networks associated with loss-chasing in gambling disorder and cocaine-use disorder. Drug Alcohol Depend 178:363–371, 2017

Xian H, Giddens JL, Scherrer JF, et al: Environmental factors selectively impact co-occurrence of problem/pathological gambling with specific drug-use disorders in male twins. Addiction 109(4):635–644, 2014

Yip, SW, Worhunsky PD, Xu J, et al: Gray-matter relationships to diagnostic and trans-diagnostic features of drug and behavioral addictions. Addict Biol 23(1):394–402, 2018

Yücel M, Fontenelle LF: Compulsivity as an endophenotype: the search for a hazy moving target. Addiction 107(10):1735–1736, 2012

Yücel M, Oldenhof E, Ahmed SH, et al: A transdiagnostic dimensional approach towards a neuropsychological assessment of addiction: an international Delphi consensus study. Addiction 114(6):1095–1109, 2019

Zack M, Poulos CX: A D2 antagonist enhances the rewarding and priming effects of a gambling episode in pathological gamblers. Neuropsychopharmacol 32:1678–1686, 2007

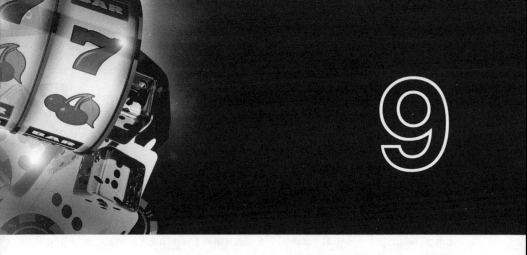

Screening and Assessment Instruments

Randy Stinchfield, Ph.D.

This chapter describes instruments currently available for the assessment of problem gambling and gambling disorder and provides information on the development, content, intended purpose, psychometric properties (reliability, validity, and classification accuracy), norms, administration methods, scoring, and interpretation of each instrument. See the appendix at the end of this chapter for a quick reference for instrument psychometric information.

Screening and Diagnostic Instruments

The South Oaks Gambling Screen (SOGS; Lesieur and Blume 1987) is a 20-item self-report screening instrument for pathological gambling (see Appendix D in this volume). DSM-III (American Psychiatric Association 1980) and DSM-III-R (American Psychiatric Association 1987) diagnostic criteria were used in the development and validation of the SOGS (Culleton 1989; Lesieur and Blume 1987). The SOGS is scored by summing selected items, with a score of 5 or more indicating probable pathological gambling. The SOGS has demonstrated excellent internal consistency (Cronbach α=0.97) and 1-month test-retest reliability (r=0.71). Validity was examined by correlating the SOGS with counselors' independent assessments (r=0.86), family member assessments (r=0.60), and DSM-III-R pathological gambling diagnosis (r=0.94). The SOGS was compared with the DSM-III-R diagnosis of pathological gambling and demonstrated satisfactory overall diagnostic accuracy among members of Gamblers Anonymous (GA) (98.1%), university students (95.3%), and hospital employees (99.3%). The original SOGS is based on lifetime gambling activity and does not differentiate pathological gamblers in remission from those actively gambling problematically.

Little systematic research has been conducted on the psychometric properties of the SOGS under varying conditions of use, such as estimating the prevalence of pathological gambling in the general population. Also, psychometric data obtained in the development of the SOGS arc now over 30 years old, and diagnostic criteria for pathological gambling have undergone revision, raising questions regarding the psychometric properties of the SOGS within a current context.

The SOGS demonstrated satisfactory reliability and validity for a 1-year time frame (Stinchfield 2002). Satisfactory reliability was demonstrated in general (Cronbach α=0.69) and treatment samples (Cronbach α=0.86). Satisfactory validity was observed between the SOGS and DSM-IV criteria (American Psychiatric Association 1994) (r=0.77 in the general sample and r=0.83 in the treatment sample). Correlations with other gambling problem severity measures in the gambling treatment sample were moderate to high (ranging from r=0.33 to r=0.65). The SOGS demonstrated high overall diagnostic accuracy (0.96), high sensitivity (0.99), modest specificity (0.75), high positive predictive power (0.96), high negative predictive power (0.90), low false-positive rate (0.04), and low false-negative rate (0.10). The SOGS showed poorer classification accuracy in the general population, with a modest sensitivity rate of 0.67 and a high false-positive rate of 0.50 (Stinchfield 2002), further raising questions regarding its widespread use in prevalence estimate studies. The SOGS overestimated the number of pathological gamblers in the general population compared with DSM-IV criteria.

Ladouceur and colleagues (2000) examined the accuracy of the SOGS in terms of how well children, adolescents, and adults understand the items and the effect that misunderstanding item content has on scores. Most participants misunderstood some SOGS items, leading to higher scores. Clarification of misunderstood items resulted in lower SOGS scores and in fewer respondents being classified as probable pathological gamblers.

Gamblers Anonymous 20 Questions

GA disseminates 20 questions (GA-20) for the purpose of identifying problem gamblers (view questions: www.gamblersanonymous.org/20questions.html). A score of 7 or more affirmative answers indicates that the respondent is a problem gambler. Although the GA-20 correlates with gambling frequency (Kuley and Jacobs 1988), only two studies have reported psychometric information. In one, the GA-20 demonstrated high internal consistency (Cronbach $\alpha=0.94$) and correlation with the SOGS ($r=0.94$) (Ursua and Uribelarrea 1998). The GA-20 differentiated between problem gamblers and social gamblers with a sensitivity of 0.98, specificity of 0.99, and overall diagnostic accuracy of 0.99. These findings are based on a sample with a base rate of approximately 50, inflating classification accuracy indices.

Massachusetts Gambling Screen

The Massachusetts Gambling Screen (MAGS) was designed to screen for gambling problems and assess problem gambling among adolescents and adults (Shaffer et al. 1994). The MAGS measures past-year behavior and includes 14 items adapted from the Short Michigan Alcoholism Screening Test (Selzer et al. 1975). The MAGS classifies respondents as nonproblem, in-transition, or pathological gamblers using a weighted scoring derived from a discriminant function analysis. In terms of validity, the MAGS total discriminant score correlated ($r=0.83$) with the total DSM-IV score.

DSM-IV Multiple Response

Fisher (2000b) developed a 10-item questionnaire, the DSM-IV Multiple Response (DSM-IV-MR), to measure DSM-IV diagnostic criteria for pathological gambling in adults. There is one item for each criterion, and items are paraphrased from DSM-IV criteria. Most items have four response options: 1) never, 2) once or twice, 3) sometimes, and 4) often. Each item is allocated 1 point, and scores range from 0 to 10. A person with a score of 3 or 4, including at least 1 point from criterion 8, 9, or 10, is classified as a problem gambler, and a person with a score of 5 or more is classified as a severe problem gambler. The DSM-IV-MR has satisfactory internal consistency reliability (Cronbach $\alpha=0.79$). In terms of validity, significantly different mean scores were found between regular and nonregular gamblers and between self-identified problem gamblers and social gamblers.

Diagnostic Interview for Gambling Schedule

The Diagnostic Interview for Gambling Schedule (DIGS) is a structured clinical interview (Winters et al. 2002). In addition to 20 diagnostic symptom items (lifetime and past year), the DIGS evaluates gambling treatment history, onset of gambling, and family and social functioning. The DSM-IV diagnostic criteria items demonstrated good internal consistency (Cronbach $\alpha = 0.92$). The total diagnostic score (range, 0–10) exhibited moderate correlations with the following measures of gambling severity: gambling frequency ($r = 0.39$), highest amount gambled in 1 day ($r = 0.42$), current gambling debt ($r = 0.47$), number of financial problems ($r = 0.40$), number of borrowing sources ($r = 0.31$), and legal problems ($r = 0.50$).

National Opinion Research Center DSM-IV Screen for Gambling Problems

A U.S. national gambling survey was conducted in 1998 by the National Opinion Research Center (1999) using the National Opinion Research Center DSM-IV Screen for Gambling Problems (NODS). The NODS includes 17 questions reflecting DSM-IV diagnostic criteria. Interpretation of NODS scores for respondents who have gambled and lost more than $100 is as follows: a score of 0 designates a low-risk gambler, a score of 1 or 2 indicates an at-risk gambler, a score of 3 or 4 designates a problem gambler, and a score of 5 or greater indicates a pathological gambler. In a clinical sample of 40 individuals in outpatient problem gambling treatment, the NODS demonstrated high test-retest coefficients for lifetime ($r = 0.99$) and past-year gambling ($r = 0.98$).

Gambling Assessment Module

The Gambling Assessment Module (GAM-IV) is in the early stages of testing, and little psychometric information is available (Cunningham-Williams et al. 2003). Multiple versions of the GAM-IV exist for different administration methodologies, including interview with paper and pencil, interview with computer, and self-administration. The GAM-IV generates DSM-IV diagnoses for seven different types of gambling. Good agreement exists between the GAM-IV and clinician ratings for five diagnostic criteria ($\kappa = 0.5–0.7$), but the remaining five criteria had poor agreement ($\kappa = 0.0–0.3$) (Cunningham-Williams et al. 2003).

Gambling Behavior Interview

The Gambling Behavior Interview (GBI) is a 76-item instrument assessing past-year pathological gambling (Stinchfield 2002, 2003; Stinchfield et al. 2005, 2016). The GBI consists of eight content domains: 1) gambling attitudes (4 items), 2) frequency of different types of gambling (15 items), 3) time and money spent gambling (4 items), 4) gambling frequency at different venues (7 items), 5) the SOGS (25 items), 6) DSM-IV diagnostic criteria (10 items), 7) research diagnostic items (32 items), and 8) demographics (9 items).

The GBI has excellent internal consistency (Cronbach $\alpha=0.92$), and all 10 diagnostic criteria have high corrected item–total correlations (ranging from $r=0.52$ to $r=0.82$). DSM-IV criteria also exhibited construct validity, with good discrimination between the general population and gambling treatment samples. Convergent validity of DSM-IV criteria was exhibited by generally high correlations with concurrent problem gambling severity measures (ranging from $r=0.27$ to $r=0.90$). Discriminant validity was exhibited by low correlations with variables unrelated to problem gambling (ranging from $r=-0.02$ to $r=-0.16$).

Although the standard DSM-IV cutoff score of 5 yielded respectable overall diagnostic accuracy (0.91), sensitivity was low (0.83), and the false-negative rate was high (0.13). A cutoff score of 4 yielded better classification accuracy, including higher overall diagnostic accuracy (0.95), sensitivity (0.93), and specificity (0.96) and a lower false-negative rate (0.06). The discriminant function analysis yielded better classification accuracy than either cutoff score, with an overall diagnostic accuracy of 0.97, sensitivity of 0.94, and specificity of 0.99.

Early Intervention Gambling Health Test

The Early Intervention Gambling Health Test (EIGHT) is an eight-item screening instrument (see Appendix B) designed for use by general practitioners (Sullivan 1999; Sullivan et al., in press). If four or more questions are answered affirmatively, the person may meet criteria for pathological gambling. EIGHT scores correlated with SOGS scores ($r=0.75$) and were in good to excellent agreement with counselor-based ratings and diagnoses of pathological gambling (S. Sullivan, personal communication, May 6, 2003). When administered to 100 prison inmates, the EIGHT correlated with the SOGS ($r=0.83$), had high sensitivity (0.91) with DSM-IV diagnostic criteria, and had low specificity (0.50) and low positive predictive value (PPV) (0.59) (Sullivan et al., in press).

Timeline Follow-Back

The Timeline Follow-Back (TLFB; Sobell et al. 1985) has been adapted for assessing gambling (Hodgins and Makarchuk 2003; Stinchfield et al. 2007; Weinstock et al. 2004). The TLFB assesses the number of days and the amount of money spent gambling over a 6-month period. The TLFB has adequate 3-week test-retest reliability, with intraclass correlations (ICCs) of 0.61 to 0.98. Agreement with collaterals was fair to good, with ICCs of 0.46 to 0.65.

Stinchfield et al. (2007) adapted the TLFB to assess gambling over a 4-week period. The TLFB correlated with other measures of gambling frequency ($r=0.24$ to $r=0.53$). Weinstock and colleagues (2004) similarly generated a TLFB (G-TLFB) to evaluate young adult frequent gamblers. The G-TLFB demonstrated adequate to excellent 2-week test-retest reliability ($r=0.73$ to $r=0.93$), and scores correlated with daily self-monitoring reports ($r=0.59$ to $r=0.87$). Dimensions of frequency and duration demonstrated concurrent validity with other gambling assessments, and the G-TLFB demonstrated discriminant validity with demographic variables and a measure of positive impression management.

Addiction Severity Index for Pathological Gamblers and the Gambling Severity Index

The Addiction Severity Index (ASI) was modified for pathological gambling (ASI-PG) by Lesieur and Blume (1992) to include six gambling items that are scored to create a composite score, the Gambling Severity Index (GSI). The GSI exhibited satisfactory reliability (Cronbach $\alpha=0.73$) and validity ($r=0.57$ with the SOGS). The GSI seems to be particularly well suited for problem gamblers with substance use problems.

Structured Clinical Interview for Pathological Gambling

The Structured Clinical Interview for Pathological Gambling (SCI-PG) is a clinician-administered, DSM-IV-based diagnostic interview that is compatible with the Structured Clinical Interview for DSM-IV (Grant et al. 2004). The SCI-PG assesses both the 10 inclusion criteria and the exclusionary criterion ("not better accounted for by a manic episode") of pathological gambling. The SCI-PG demonstrated excellent reliability, validity, and classification accuracy in preliminary testing of individuals with gambling problems. Further testing is needed to examine its suitability for other populations.

Canadian Problem Gambling Index and Problem Gambling Severity Index

The Canadian Problem Gambling Index (CPGI; Ferris and Wynne 2001) is a problem gambling assessment tool developed in Canada for the purpose of conducting population-based surveys. It arose out of dissatisfaction with using existing clinical screens for epidemiological purposes. The goal in developing the CPGI was to provide a more meaningful measure of problem gambling with more indicators of the social and environmental context of gambling and problem gambling. Although the CPGI includes 31 items, 9 of them make up a measure of problem gambling that is the Problem Gambling Severity Index (PGSI).

The nine-item PGSI is commonly administered as a stand-alone scale that uses four response options: 0, never; 1, sometimes; 2, most of the time; and 3, almost always. The nine items are summed, with a score range from 0 to 27. PGSI scores are interpreted as follows: 1) score of 0 and no reported gambling indicates nongambling, 2) score of 0 and reported gambling indicates nonproblem gambling, 3) score of 1–2 indicates low-risk gambling, 4) score of 3–7 indicates moderate-risk gambling, and 5) score of 8 or more indicates problem gambling.

The PGSI psychometric properties were computed from a general population of 3,120 Canadian adults, and this included a temporal stability subsample of 417 respondents from the general population. Evidence of validity and classification accuracy was derived from clinical interviews with a subsample of 143 respondents from the general population survey. PGSI internal consistency was 0.84 (Cronbach α), and the 4-week test-retest correlation was 0.78. An estimate of PGSI validity was computed from correlations with measures of problem gambling, including the SOGS ($r=0.83$), DSM-IV ($r=0.83$), and clinical interviews ($r=0.48$). These correlations with the SOGS and DSM-IV diagnostic criteria should be interpreted with caution, given the similarity in items between the PGSI and the DSM-IV and SOGS, as noted by Svetieva and Walker (2008). Specifically, eight of the nine PGSI items share content with the SOGS and DSM-IV. Classification accuracy was computed using DSM-IV as the reference standard: sensitivity was 0.83, and specificity was 1.00. These classification accuracy coefficients need to be interpreted cautiously because of the similarity of content between the PGSI and DSM-IV diagnostic criteria. The PGSI prevalence rate for problem gambling among the sample drawn from the Canadian general population was 0.9%, the SOGS problem and pathological gambling rate was 1.3%, and the DSM-IV pathological gambling rate was 0.7% for the same sample. The two interpretation categories of low-risk gambling and moderate-risk gambling should be considered preliminary given that little empirical evidence has been provided to justify their use. (See Svetieva and Walker 2008 for a comprehensive critical review of the CPGI and PGSI.)

Sydney Laval Universities Gambling Screen

The Sydney Laval Universities Gambling Screen (SLUGS) is a seven-item screen developed to measure prevalence rates and estimate the need for treatment services in population-based surveys. The SLUGS is a result of collaboration between Australian and Canadian researchers (Blaszczynski et al. 2008). The developers define pathological gambling with three key features: 1) impaired control, 2) severity of harm, and 3) self-identified need for treatment. These three key features served as the conceptual framework for developing a new screen. Nevertheless, some of the seven items are similar to existing items found in other measures of problem gambling. Three items measure the first key feature of impaired control: 1) "unable to resist urge to gamble," 2) "gamble more money than intended," and 3) "spend more time gambling than intended." Three items measure the second key feature of severity of harm: 4) "spent more disposable income than intended," 5) "spent more leisure time than intended," and 6) "degree of problems caused by gambling." One item measures the third key feature of self-identified need for treatment: 7) "degree to which help was required for gambling." In terms of psychometric properties, the SLUGS had a Cronbach α of 0.85, indicating good internal consistency, and the SLUGS was correlated with the SOGS; however, given the similarity of item content, these correlations are not surprising. Other limitations include a lack of evidence of temporal stability; a lack of evidence of classification accuracy; and a lack of scoring instructions, cut scores, and interpretation of scores.

Victorian Gambling Screen

The Victorian Gambling Screen (VGS) is 21-item screen measuring three factors: 1) harm to self (HS) (15 items), 2) harm to partner (3 items), and 3) enjoyment of gambling (3 items) (Ben-Tovim et al. 2001). The authors concluded that only the 15-item HS scale is useful for measuring problem gambling. The HS scale items have 0- to 4-point response options: 0, never; 1, rarely; 2, sometimes; 3, often; and 4, always. The HS scale's 15 items are summed, for a score range of 0 to 60. The HS scale shows excellent internal consistency (Cronbach $\alpha=0.96$) (Ben-Tovim et al. 2001). The HS scale showed evidence of convergent validity, with a high correlation with the SOGS ($r=0.87$). The HS scale is interpreted with the following cut scores and categories: 1) 21+ for "problem gambler," 2) 9+ for "borderline or problem gambler," and 3) 14+ for "pathological gambler." These cut scores were determined using ROC (receiver operator characteristics) analysis to optimize the balance between sensitivity and specificity. A cross-validation study by other researchers has shown satisfactory internal consistency (Cronbach $\alpha=0.89$) and evidence for convergent validity, including correlation with the SOGS ($r=0.41$) (Tolchard and Battersby 2010). The HS scale is not so much a new scale as it is a new combination of existing items.

Brief Screens

There are some settings in which only a brief screen, such as five items or fewer, can be administered. There have been limited empirical investigations of the classification accuracy of brief screens and few investigations beyond those related to their development. Therefore, there are few empirical data on which to base a decision about what brief pathological gambling screen to use for a given sample and setting.

Lie/Bet Questionnaire

The Lie/Bet Questionnaire is a two-item screen for pathological gambling (Johnson et al. 1997): 1) "Have you ever had to lie to people important to you about how much you gambled?" and 2) "Have you ever felt the need to bet more and more money?" This two-item screen has demonstrated a sensitivity of 0.99, specificity of 0.91, positive predictive power of 0.92, and negative predictive power of 0.99 in comparing GA members and control subjects who were not problem gamblers. In a second study, the questionnaire demonstrated a sensitivity of 1.00, specificity of 0.85, positive predictive power of 0.78, and negative predictive power of 1.00 (Johnson et al. 1998).

National Opinion Research Center Diagnostic Screen for Gambling Disorders, Loss of Control, Lying, and Preoccupation

The National Opinion Research Center Diagnostic Screen for Gambling Disorders, Loss of Control, Lying, and Preoccupation (NODS-CLiP) is a three-item screen derived from the NODS (Toce-Gerstein et al. 2009). The 17-item NODS was administered to a sample of 8,867 participants in eight separate surveys. The full NODS was used as the "gold standard" to determine group membership as either pathological gambling or nonpathological gambling. The following three NODS items were the best set for identifying pathological gamblers: 1) Have you ever tried to stop, cut down, or control your gambling? 2) Have you ever lied to family members, friends, or others about how much you gamble or how much money you lost on gambling? and 3) Have there ever been periods lasting 2 weeks or longer when you spent a lot of time thinking about your gambling experiences or planning out future gambling ventures or bets? The NODS-CLiP uses a lifetime time frame and can be administered in 1 minute. The investigators found that this three-item screen had a sensitivity of 0.99, specificity of 0.88, false-positive rate of 0.01, and false-negative rate of 0.12 when the full NODS was used as the gold standard. Answering yes to one or more items is indicative of pathological gambling.

The NODS-CLiP was tested in a clinical sample and was found to have a sensitivity of 0.98, specificity of 0.30, PPV of 0.87, negative predictive value (NPV) of 0.80, and diagnostic efficiency of 0.86 (Volberg et al. 2011). The NODS-CLiP was developed from general population samples, but it did not perform as well in a clinical sample. A strength of the NODS-CLiP is that it is derived from a measure of the standardized DSM-IV, which has shown evidence of classification accuracy. Limitations of the NODS-CLiP include 1) a lifetime time frame rather than a "current" time frame, thus increasing the false-positive rate for current pathological gambling, and 2) a lack of independence between the NODS-CLiP and the full NODS "gold standard" or criterion from which the items were selected. Further research is needed to cross-validate these classification accuracy estimates.

National Opinion Research Center Diagnostic Screen for Gambling Disorders, Preoccupation, Escape, Risked Relationships, and Chasing

Given that the NODS CLiP did not perform well in a clinical sample, another brief screen was developed from the NODS for clinical settings. The National Opinion Research Center Diagnostic Screen for Gambling Disorders, Preoccupation, Escape, Risked Relationships, and Chasing (NODS-PERC) is a four-item screen derived from the full NODS, a longer 17-item measure of the 10 DSM-IV diagnostic criteria (Volberg et al. 2011). The NODS-PERC was developed by administering the lifetime and past-12-month time-frame NODS to 375 participants in a study of brief interventions for problem and pathological gambling at the University of Connecticut Health Center. The full NODS was used as the "gold standard" to determine group membership as either pathological gambling or nonpathological gambling. The authors found that the following four NODS items were the best set to identify pathological gamblers: 1) Have there ever been periods lasting 2 weeks or longer when you spent a lot of time thinking about your gambling experiences, or planning out future gambling ventures or bets? 2) Have you ever gambled as a way to escape from personal problems? 3) Has there ever been a period when, if you lost money gambling one day, you would return another day to get even? and 4) Has your gambling ever caused serious or repeated problems in your relationships with any of your family members or friends? The NODS-PERC uses a lifetime time frame, can be administered in 1 minute, and uses response options of yes or no. A response of yes to one or more questions indicates the need for further assessment. The NODS-PERC yielded a sensitivity of 0.997, specificity of 0.394, PPV of 0.885, NPV of 0.963, and diagnostic efficiency of 0.891. The NODS-PERC is intended for use in clinical settings. Again, there is a lack of independence between the screen and the criterion in the development of this new screen. That is, the 17-item NODS is used as the criterion in order to select the four NODS items for the screen. Further research is needed to cross-validate these classification accuracy estimates. A strength of the NODS-PERC is that it is based on a measure of the standardized DSM-IV that has shown evidence of classification accuracy. Limitations of the NODS-PERC include 1) a lack of independence between the NODS-PERC and the full NODS "gold standard" or criterion from which the items were selected and 2) use of a lifetime time frame rather than a "current" time frame, thus increasing the false-positive rate for current pathological gambling.

Brief Biosocial Gambling Screen

The Brief Biosocial Gambling Screen (BBGS) is a three-item screen derived from DSM-IV diagnostic criteria for pathological gambling as measured in the National Epidemiologic Survey on Alcohol and Related Conditions (NESARC) that uses the Alcohol Use Disorder and Associated Disabilities Interview Schedule (AUDADIS) to measure DSM-IV diagnostic criteria for pathological gambling (Gebauer et al. 2010). The authors tested two-, three-, and four-item models and found that a three-item screen yielded satisfactory classification accuracy. The three items in the BBGS were 1) During the past 12 months, have you become restless, irritable, or anxious when trying to stop and (or) cut down on gambling? 2) During the past 12 months, have you tried to keep your family or friends from knowing how much you gambled? and 3) During the past 12 months, did you have such financial trouble as a result of gambling that you had to get help with living expenses from family, friends, or welfare?

The BBGS time frame is the past 12 months, and the screen can be administered in 1 minute. Classification accuracy of the BBGS was measured from the original NESARC database, and the authors reported a sensitivity of 0.96 and specificity of 0.99. There is a lack of independence between the screen and the criterion in the development of this new screen. That is, the AUDADIS is used as the criterion from which to select the three BBGS items for the screen. Further research is needed to cross-validate these classification accuracy estimates.

Strengths of the BBGS include use of a current time frame of the past 12 months and the fact that it is based on a measure of the standardized DSM-IV criteria set, which has shown evidence of classification accuracy. A limitation of the BBGS is the lack of independence between the BBGS and the AUDADIS "gold standard" or criterion from which the items were selected and against which the BBGS classification accuracy was tested.

Short SOGS

The Short SOGS is a five-item screen derived from the 20-item SOGS (Room et al. 1999). The five items are as follows: In the past 12 months, 1) Was there ever a time when you gambled more than you intended to? 2) Have people criticized your gambling? 3) Have money arguments centered on your gambling? 4) Have you felt guilty about the way you gamble or what happens when you gamble? and 5) Have you claimed to be winning money gambling when you were not? These five items were selected out of the 20 SOGS items based on an item analysis from a 1995 Ontario province survey. The score from the Short SOGS items was highly correlated with the full 20-item SOGS score ($r=0.87$). All respondents who scored in the probable pathological gambling range on the 20-item SOGS also scored 2 or more on the Short SOGS. The Short SOGS has a time frame of the previous 12 months. A score of 2 or more is indicative of problem or pathological gambling. No further reliability, validity, or classification accuracy information was provided. Strengths of the Short SOGS include use of a current time frame of the past 12 months and the fact that it was derived from the SOGS, a standardized scale with satisfactory psychometric properties, including classification accuracy. A limitation of the Short SOGS is that it was derived from the SOGS, which has the known limitations described earlier.

One-Item Screen for Problem Gambling

The One-Item Screen for Problem Gambling includes the following item: "Have you ever had an issue with your gambling?" (Thomas et al. 2008). This item is nearly identical to the SOGS item "Do you feel you have ever had a problem with gambling?" (Lesieur and Blume 1987). The time frame is the past 12 months, and response options are yes and no. This screen was developed in Australia for medical practice. When compared with the PGSI (Ferris and Wynne 2001), the One-Item Screen was found to yield a false-positive rate of 0.04 and a false-negative rate of 0.21, which is high (Thomas et al. 2008). A cross-validation of the screen was conducted by Rockloff et al. (2011), who reported a sensitivity of 0.21, specificity of 0.98, and false-negative rate of 0.79, which is exceedingly high. A strength of this screen is its brevity of one item; however, this also appears to be the cause of the low sensitivity and false-negative rate.

Instruments for Evaluation of Treatment Efficacy

Gambling Treatment Outcome Monitoring System

The Gambling Treatment Outcome Monitoring System (GAMTOMS) is a multidimensional assessment system that includes the following instruments: 1) Gambling Treatment Admission Questionnaire, 2) Primary Discharge Questionnaire, 3) Client Follow-up Questionnaire, 4) Staff Discharge Form, 5) Significant Other Intake Questionnaire, and 6) Significant Other Follow-up Questionnaire (Stinchfield 1999; Stinchfield and Winters 2001; Stinchfield et al. 2007). Reliability and validity of the GAMTOMS have been evaluated in a treatment sample of more than 1,000 patients from a Minnesota gambling treatment outcome study (Stinchfield 1999; Stinchfield and Winters 2001; Stinchfield et al. 2007). The GAMTOMS has also been evaluated for reliability, validity, classification accuracy, and validity of self-reporting with a sample of 74 gambling treatment patients (Stinchfield et al. 2007). The GAMTOMS gambling frequency section demonstrated modest correlations with the gambling TLFB ($r=0.53$), the SOGS ($r=0.47$), and DSM-IV criteria ($r=0.36$).

Pathological Gambling Modification of the Yale-Brown Obsessive Compulsive Scale

The Yale-Brown Obsessive Compulsive Scale was modified to measure severity of pathological gambling and change in symptoms in response to treatment (PG-YBOCS) (Hollander et al. 1998) (see Appendix E of this volume). Inter-rater agreement on Urge and Behavior scores was high, with ICCs of 0.99 and 0.98, respectively. In terms of validity, the PG-YBOCS correlated with the Clinical Global Impression (CGI) pathological gambling scale ($r=0.89$) and the SOGS ($r=0.86$).

Gambling Symptom Assessment Scale

The Gambling Symptom Assessment Scale (G-SAS) was developed to assess gambling symptoms during treatment (Kim et al. 2001) (see Appendix C of this volume). The G-SAS measures past-week gambling urges and thoughts and includes 12 items with response options ranging from 0 to 4. Responses are summed, and the total score range is 0–48, with a score of 31 or above signifying severe symptoms, scores of 21–30 signifying moderate symptoms, and a score of 20 or less signifying mild symptoms. In 58 patients, the G-SAS demonstrated satisfactory 1-week test-retest reliability ($r=0.70$) and internal consistency (Cronbach $\alpha=0.89$). In terms of validity, G-SAS scores correlated with those of the CGI Improvement ($r=0.78$) and Severity ($r=0.81$) subscales.

Clinical Global Impression Scale—Pathological Gambling

The CGI Scale was developed for treatment studies of schizophrenia (Guy 1976). It contains three items that the clinician rates: severity of illness, global improvement, and treatment efficacy. The CGI Scale has been adapted by gambling researchers (Hollander et al. 1998; Kim et al. 2001) to assess severity of pathological gambling and to measure "global gambling improvement" in psychopharmacological studies. The CGI Severity and Improvement items have 7-point response options. No psychometric information on the adaptation of this scale to pathological gambling is available.

Youth Gambling Assessment Instruments

South Oaks Gambling Screen—Revised for Adolescents

The South Oaks Gambling Screen—Revised for Adolescents (SOGS—RA) is a 12-item screen for youth adapted by Winters and colleagues (1993, 1995) from the adult SOGS by using a past-year time frame, changing the wording of items and response options to better reflect adolescent gambling and reading levels, eliminating two items considered to have poor content validity for adolescents, and giving only 1 point for any source of borrowed money rather than the 9 possible points for separate sources as in the SOGS. A score of 4 or more indicates problem gambling; a score of 2–3, at-risk gambling; and a score of 0–1, nonproblem gambling (Winters et al. 1995). The SOGS-RA has shown evidence of reliability (e.g., Cronbach $\alpha=0.80$). Evidence of validity includes correlations with gambling participation ($r=0.54$) and amount of money gambled in the past year ($r=0.42$). Classification accuracy estimates of 97% true positive, 0.5% false negative, and 2.4% false positive compared with the DSM-IV-J (J for juvenile; see below) as the criterion (Derevensky and Gupta 2000). The SOGS-RA has a number of weaknesses, including that it was adapted from an adult instrument and does not take into account all of the developmental issues unique to youth; and the cut score is set lower than in the adult SOGS, which has the effect of identifying more youth as having problem gambling.

DSM-IV-J and DSM-IV-MR-J

The DSM-IV-J and DSM-IV-MR-J are 12-item questionnaires developed to measure 9 of the 10 DSM-IV diagnostic criteria of pathological gambling in juveniles (Fisher 1992, 2000a). The items are adapted from the DSM-IV criteria to reflect the developmental stage of youth. Fisher simplified the language, omitted details that were less relevant for youth, and excluded criterion 10 ("relies on others to provide money to relieve a desperate financial situation caused by gambling"). Eight of the nine scored items have four response options: 1) never, 2) once or twice, 3) sometimes, and 4) often. Scores range from 0 to 9, and a score of 4 or more identifies problem gambling. Internal consistency was found to be 0.75 (Cronbach α). Validity evidence includes correlations with the SOGS-RA ($r=0.67$) and GA-20 ($r=0.68$) (Derevensky and Gupta 2000). Weaknesses include that it was adapted from adult content and therefore does not take into account youth developmental issues related to gambling, there is a lack of evidence of classification accuracy, and it has not been updated for DSM-5 (American Psychiatric Association 2013).

Canadian Adolescent Gambling Inventory

The Canadian Adolescent Gambling Inventory (CAGI; Tremblay et al. 2010) is a 44-item assessment instrument designed specifically for adolescents that represents multiple domains of problem gambling and measures a continuum of gambling problem severity from low to high problem severity. The CAGI has 19 items that measure gambling frequency (using 6-point response options) and time spent gambling in a typical week on 19 forms of gambling, and 2 items to measure money and items of value lost gambling. The second half of the CAGI measures five problem gambling–related domains: 1) severity, as measured by the Gambling Problem Severity Scale (GPSS; 9 items); 2) psychological consequences (6 items); 3) social consequences (5 items); 4) financial consequences (6 items); and 5) loss of control (4 items). Each of these items has a 4-point response option, assigned a score of 0 to 3, and the scores are then summed for each scale. The 9-item GPSS score range is from 0 to 27, and scores of 0–1 are "no problem," 2–5 are "low to moderate severity," and 6 or more indicates "high severity." Estimates of reliability, validity, and classification accuracy are satisfactory, including reliability coefficient α values ranging from 0.83 to 0.90, temporal stability coefficient values ranging from 0.77 to 0.90, and convergent validity coefficient values ranging from 0.14 to 0.67; for the GPSS, sensitivity is 0.93 and specificity is 0.93 (Tremblay et al. 2010). Weaknesses of the CAGI include that it is long (44 items); however, the 9-item GPSS scale can be administered as a stand-alone screen.

Brief Adolescent Gambling Screen

The Brief Adolescent Gambling Screen (BAGS; Stinchfield et al. 2017) is a three-item screen derived from the nine-item GPSS of the CAGI. The BAGS has three items with 4-point response options that are coded as 0–3, for a total score range of 0–9. A cut score of 4 or more indicates a positive screen for problem gambling. The BAGS demonstrates satisfactory estimates of reliability, validity, and classification accuracy. Estimates of classification accuracy using DSM-5 gambling disorder as the reference standard include a hit rate of 0.95, sensitivity of 0.88, specificity of 0.98, false-positive rate of 0.02, and false-negative rate of 0.12. Because these classification estimates are preliminary, derived from a relatively small sample size, and based on the same sample from which the items were selected, it will be important to cross-validate the BAGS with larger and more diverse samples. Weaknesses include the fact that the BAGS is only three items, and like most brief screens, it may be too short and may miss cases because of its brevity.

Conclusion

Multiple instruments have been developed in response to the need to detect and measure problem gambling. Existing instruments require additional psychometric evaluation, particularly with regard to specific population groups (e.g., seniors), for which new or modified instruments might be optimal. Information generated from these studies will enable clinicians and researchers to make more informed decisions as to how, within specific settings and for specific purposes, to best identify, assess, and monitor individuals with gambling problems.

References

American Psychiatric Association: Diagnostic and Statistical Manual of Mental Disorders, 3rd Edition. Washington, DC, American Psychiatric Association, 1980

American Psychiatric Association: Diagnostic and Statistical Manual of Mental Disorders, 3rd Edition, Revised. Washington, DC, American Psychiatric Association, 1987

American Psychiatric Association: Diagnostic and Statistical Manual of Mental Disorders, 4th Edition. Washington, DC, American Psychiatric Association, 1994

American Psychiatric Association: Diagnostic and Statistical Manual of Mental Disorders, 5th Edition. Washington, DC, American Psychiatric Association, 2013

Ben-Tovim D, Esterman A, Tolchard B, Battersby MW: The Victorian Gambling Screen: Project Report. Melbourne, Victorian Research Panel, 2001

Blaszczynski A, Ladouceur R, Moodie C: The Sydney Laval Universities Gambling Screen: preliminary data. Addict Res Theor 16(4):401–411, 2008

Boudreau B, Poulin C: The South Oaks Gambling Screen—Revised Adolescent (SOGS-RA) revisited: a cut-point analysis. J Gambl Stud 23:299–308, 2007

Culleton RP: The prevalence rates of pathological gambling: a look at methods. J Gambl Behav 5:22-41, 1989

Cunningham-Williams R, Books SJ, Cottler LB: Diagnostic concordance between the GAM-IV-12 and clinician ratings among pathological gamblers in St. Louis. Paper presented at the 3rd annual conference of the National Center for Responsible Gaming, Las Vegas, NV, December 2–5, 2003

Derevensky JL, Gupta R: Prevalence estimates of adolescent gambling: a comparison of the SOGS-RA, DSM-IV-J, and the GA 20 questions. J Gambl Stud 16:227–251, 2000

Ferris J, Wynne H: The Canadian Problem Gambling Index: Final Report. Ottawa, ON, Canadian Centre on Substance Abuse, 2001

Fisher SE: Measuring pathological gambling in children: the case of fruit machines in the UK. J Gambl Stud 8:263–285, 1992

Fisher S: Developing the DSM-IV-DSM-IV criteria to identify adolescent problem gambling in non-clinical populations. J Gambl Stud 16:253–273, 2000a

Fisher S: Measuring the prevalence of sector-specific problem gambling: a study of casino patrons. J Gambl Stud 16:25–51, 2000b

Gebauer L, LaBrie R, Shaffer HJ: Optimizing DSM-IV-TR classification accuracy: a brief biosocial screen for detecting current gambling disorders among gamblers in the general household population. Can J Psychiatry 55(2):82–90, 2010

Grant JE, Steinberg M, Kim SW, et al: Preliminary validity and reliability testing of a Structured Clinical Interview for Pathological Gambling (SCI-PG). Psychiatr Res 28:79–88, 2004

Guy W: Clinical Global Impressions, in ECDEU Assessment Manual for Psychopharmacology—Revised. DHEW Publ No ADM 76–338. Edited by Guy W. Rockville, MD, National Institute of Mental Health, Psychopharmacology Research Branch, 1976, pp 218–222

Hodgins DC, Makarchuk K: Trusting problem gamblers: reliability and validity of self-reported gambling behavior. Psychol Addict Behav 17:244–248, 2003

Hollander E, DeCaria CM, Mari E, et al: Short-term single-blind fluvoxamine treatment of pathological gambling. Am J Psychiatry 155:1781–1783, 1998

Johnson EE, Hamer R, Nora RM, et al: The Lie/Bet Questionnaire for screening pathological gamblers. Psychol Rep 80:83–88, 1997

Johnson EE, Hamer RM, Nora RM: The Lie/Bet Questionnaire for screening pathological gamblers: a follow-up study. Psychol Rep 83:1219–1224, 1998

Kim SW, Grant JE, Adson DE, Shin YC: Double-blind naltrexone and placebo comparison study in the treatment of pathological gambling. Biol Psychiatry 49:914–921, 2001

Kuley NB, Jacobs DF: The relationship between dissociative-like experiences and sensation seeking among social and problem gamblers. J Gambl Behav 4:197–207, 1988

Ladouceur R, Bouchard C, Rheaume N, et al: Is the SOGS an accurate measure of pathological gambling among children, adolescents and adults? J Gambl Stud 16:1–24, 2000

Lesieur HR, Blume SB: The South Oaks Gambling Screen (SOGS): a new instrument for the identification of pathological gamblers. Am J Psychiatry 144:1184–1188, 1987

Lesieur HR, Blume SB: Modifying the Addiction Severity Index for use with pathological gamblers. Am J Addict 1:240–247, 1992

National Opinion Research Center: Gambling Impact and Behavior Study: Report to the National Gambling Impact Study Commission. Chicago, IL, National Opinion Research Center at the University of Chicago, 1999. Available at: www.norc.org/PDFs/Publications/GIBSFinalReportApril1999.pdf. Accessed February 20, 2021.

Pallanti S, DeCaria CM, Grant JE, et al: Reliability and validity of the pathological gambling adaptation of the Yale-Brown Obsessive-Compulsive Scale (PG-YBOCS). J Gambl Stud 21:431–443, 2005

Poulin C: Problem gambling among adolescent students in the Atlantic provinces of Canada. J Gambl Stud 16:53–78, 2000

Rockloff M, Ehrich J, Themessl-Huber M, Evans LG: Validation of a one item screen for problem gambling. J Gambl Stud 27:701–707, 2011

Room R, Turner NE, Ialomiteanu A: Community effects of the opening of the Niagara casino. Addiction 94(10):1449–1466, 1999

Selzer ML, Vinokur A, van Rooijen L: A self-administered Short Michigan Alcoholism Screening Test (SMAST). J Stud Alcohol 36:117–126, 1975

Shaffer HJ, LaBrie R, Scanlan KM, Cummings TN: Pathological gambling among adolescents: Massachusetts Gambling Screen (MAGS). J Gambl Stud 10:339–362, 1994

Sobell LC, Sobell MB, Maisto SA: Time-Line Follow-Back assessment method, in Alcoholism Treatment Assessment Research Instruments. NIAAA Treatment Handbook Series, Vol 2; DHHS Publ No 85–1380. Edited by Lettieri DJ, Nelson JE, Sayers MA. Rockville, MD, National Institute on Alcoholism and Alcohol Abuse, 1985, pp 530–534

Stinchfield R: Gambling treatment outcome monitoring system, in Behavioral Outcomes and Guidelines Sourcebook. Edited by Coughlin KM. New York, Faulkner and Gray, 1999, pp 173–174, 464–466

Stinchfield R: Reliability, validity, and classification accuracy of the South Oaks Gambling Screen (SOGS). Addict Behav 27:1–19, 2002

Stinchfield R: Reliability, validity, and classification accuracy of a measure of DSM-IV diagnostic criteria for pathological gambling. Am J Psychiatry 160:180–182, 2003

Stinchfield R, Winters KC: Outcome of Minnesota's gambling treatment programs. J Gambl Stud 17:217–245, 2001

Stinchfield R, Govoni R, Frisch GR: DSM-IV diagnostic criteria for pathological gambling: reliability, validity, and classification accuracy. Am J Addict 14:73–82, 2005

Stinchfield R, Winters KC, Botzet A, et al: Development and psychometric evaluation of the Gambling Treatment Outcome Monitoring System (GAMTOMS). Psychol Addict Behav 21:174–184, 2007

Stinchfield R, McCready J, Turner N, et al: Reliability, validity, and classification accuracy of the DSM-5 diagnostic criteria for gambling disorder and comparison to DSM-IV. J Gambl Stud 32(3):905–922, 2016

Stinchfield R, Wynne H, Wiebe J, Tremblay J: Development and psychometric evaluation of the Brief Adolescent Gambling Screen (BAGS). Front Psychol 8:2204, 2017

Sullivan S: Development of the "EIGHT" Problem Gambling Screen. Unpublished doctoral thesis, Auckland Medical School, Auckland, New Zealand, 1999

Sullivan S, Brown R, Skinner B: Development of a problem gambling screen for use in a prison inmate population. eGambling: The Electronic Journal of Gambling Issues (in press)

Svetieva E, Walker M: Inconsistency between concept and measurement: the Canadian Problem Gambling Index (CPGI). Journal of Gambling Issues 22:157–173, 2008

Thomas SA, Piterman L, Jackson AC: Problem gambling: what do general practitioners need to know and do about it? Med J Aust 189(3):135–136, 2008

Toce-Gerstein M, Gerstein DR, Volberg RA: The NODS-CLiP: a rapid screen for adult pathological and problem gambling. J Gambl Stud 25:541–555, 2009

Tolchard B, Battersby MW: The Victorian Gambling Screen: reliability and validation in a clinical population. J Gambl Stud 26(4):623–638, 2010

Tremblay J, Stinchfield R, Wiebe J, Wynne H: Canadian Adolescent Gambling Inventory (CAGI): Phase III Final Report. Canadian Consortium on Gambling Research (CCGR), 2010. Available at: https://prism.ucalgary.ca/handle/1880/48158. Accessed February 20, 2021.

Ursua MP, Uribelarrea LL: 20 questions of Gamblers Anonymous: a psychometric study with population of Spain. J Gambl Stud 14:3–15,1998

Volberg RA, Munck IM, Petry NM: A quick and simple screening method for pathological and problem gamblers in addiction programs and practices. Am J Addict 20:220–227, 2011

Weinstock J, Whelan JP, Meyers AW: Behavioral assessment of gambling: an application of the timeline followback method. Psychol Assess 16:72–80, 2004

Welte JW, Barnes GM, Tidwell MO, Hoffman JH: The prevalence of problem gambling among U.S. adolescents and young adults: Results from a national survey. J Gambl Stud 24:119–133, 2008

Winters KC, Stinchfield R, Fulkerson J: Toward the development of an adolescent gambling problem severity scale. J Gambl Stud 9:63–84, 1993

Winters KC, Stinchfield R, Kim L: Monitoring adolescent gambling in Minnesota. J Gambl Stud 11:165–183, 1995

Winters KC, Specker S, Stinchfield R: Measuring pathological gambling with the Diagnostic Interview for Gambling Severity (DIGS), in The Downside: Problem and Pathological Gambling. Edited by Marotta D, Cornelius JA, Eadington WR. Reno, NV, University of Nevada, 2002, pp 143–148

Appendix

Instruments for the Assessment of Gambling Disorder

Instrument	Content areas	Number and type of items	Administration time and method	Scoring instructions, score range, cut scores, and interpretation of scores
South Oaks Gambling Screen (SOGS) (Lesieur and Blume 1987)	Games played; signs and symptoms of problem gambling; negative consequences; sources of money to gamble	20 scored items; true/false	10- to 20-minute paper-and-pencil questionnaire	1 point for each item; score range, 0–20; score of 5 or more indicates probable pathological gambler
Gamblers Anonymous 20 questions (GA-20) (Ursua and Uribelarrea 1998)	Signs and symptoms of compulsive gambling; negative consequences	20 items; true/false	10-minute paper-and-pencil questionnaire or interview	1 point for each item; score of 7 or more indicates compulsive gambler
Massachusetts Gambling Screen (MAGS) (Shaffer et al. 1994)	Signs and symptoms of PG; psychological and social problems associated with gambling; a 12-item measure of DSM-IV diagnostic criteria	14-item MAGS (7 MAGS items are scored); yes or no; past year	5- to 10-minute self-administered paper-and-pencil questionnaire or clinician-administered interview	7 MAGS items are scored by multiplying each item by a discriminant function coefficient; then sum and add a constant; score 0–2, transitional or probable pathological gambler; score >2, pathological gambler

| Instrument (continued) | Psychometrics | | Classification accuracy indices |
	Reliability	Validity	Sample characteristics, criterion, base rate, sensitivity, specificity, and hit rate
South Oaks Gambling Screen (SOGS) (continued)	Cronbach α=0.97; 1-month test-retest reliability r=0.71	Correlated with counselor assessments (r=0.86), family member assessment (r=0.60), and DSM-III-R PG diagnosis (r=0.94)	GA members (n=213), university students (n=384), and hospital employees (n=152); criterion was DSM-III-R diagnosis of PG Hit rates among GA members (0.98), university students (0.95), and hospital employees (0.99)
Gamblers Anonymous 20 Questions (GA-20) (continued)	Cronbach α=0.94	Yielded high correlations with frequency of gambling and with dissociative experiences (Kuley and Jacobs 1988); was highly correlated with the SOGS (r=0.94) (Ursua and Uribelarrea 1998)	Criterion is group membership; 127 problem gamblers; 142 nonproblem social gamblers Base rate=0.47; sensitivity=0.98; specificity=0.99; hit rate=0.99 Note that these classification accuracy indices are based on a sample with a base rate of about 50%, which inflates classification accuracy indices
Massachusetts Gambling Screen (MAGS) (continued)	MAGS 7-item scale Cronbach α=0.84 DSM-IV 12-item scale Cronbach α=0.89	MAGS total discriminant score was correlated with total DSM-IV score (r=0.83)	NA

Instrument	Content areas	Number and type of items	Administration time and method	Scoring instructions, score range, cut scores, and interpretation of scores
DSM-IV Multiple Response (DSM-IV-MR) (Fisher 2000b)	DSM-IV diagnostic criteria	10 items, 1 item for each criterion; 4-point response options for most items	5-minute questionnaire	1 point for each item; score range, 0–10; score of 3–4 (including at least 1 point from criterion 8, 9, or 10) indicates problem gambler; score of 5 or more indicates severe problem gambler
Diagnostic Interview for Gambling Schedule (DIGS) (Winters et al. 2002)	Demographics, gambling involvement, treatment history, onset of gambling, gambling frequency, amounts of money bet and lost, sources of borrowed money, financial problems, legal problems, mental health screen, medical status, family and social functioning, and diagnostic symptoms (lifetime and past year)	20 diagnostic symptom items to measure the 10 DSM-IV diagnostic criteria; 2 items for each criterion	30-minute interview	If respondent endorses either of the 2 items per criterion, the criterion is considered endorsed; 1 point for each of the 10 criteria; score range, 0–10; cut score of 5 or more indicates PG

| Instrument (continued) | Psychometrics | | Classification accuracy indices |
	Reliability	Validity	Sample characteristics, criterion, base rate, sensitivity, specificity, and hit rate
DSM-IV Multiple Response (DSM-IV-MR) (continued)	Cronbach $\alpha = 0.79$	Discriminated between regular and nonregular gamblers and between problem and social gamblers	NA
Diagnostic Interview for Gambling Schedule (DIGS) (continued)	Cronbach $\alpha = 0.92$	Total diagnostic score (0–10) exhibited significant correlations with the following measures of gambling problem severity: gambling frequency ($r = 0.39$); highest amount gambled in one day ($r = 0.42$); current gambling debt ($r = 0.47$); number of financial problems ($r = 0.40$); number of borrowing sources ($r = 0.31$); and legal problems ($r = 0.50$)	NA

Instrument	Content areas	Number and type of items	Administration time and method	Scoring instructions, score range, cut scores, and interpretation of scores
National Opinion Research Center DSM-IV Screen for Gambling Problems (NODS) (National Opinion Research Center 1999)	DSM-IV diagnostic criteria for diagnosing PG including lifetime and past-year time frames; a filtering question of losing $100 or more used prior to administration of NODS	17 items	5- to 10-minute interview for NODS	1 point for each DSM criterion; score range is 0–10; score of 0, low-risk gambler; 1 or 2, at-risk gambler; 3 or 4, problem gambler; and 5 or more, pathological gambler
Gambling Assessment Module (GAM) (Cunningham-Williams et al. 2003)	Structured gambling diagnostic interview of gambling frequency and DSM-IV diagnostic criteria for 11 different gambling activities	Demographics section has 27 items; gambling section has 40 items; interviewer observation section has 7 items	30–60 minutes; interview (paper and pencil, or computerized)	Score of 5 or more DSM-IV diagnostic criteria indicates PG; 11 algorithms provided for the activity-specific diagnoses

| Instrument (continued) | Psychometrics | | Classification accuracy indices |
	Reliability	Validity	Sample characteristics, criterion, base rate, sensitivity, specificity, and hit rate
National Opinion Research Center DSM-IV Screen for Gambling Problems (NODS) (continued)	2- to 4-week test-retest correlation: $r=0.99$ and 0.98 for lifetime and past year, respectively	Administered to 40 individuals in outpatient problem gambling treatment programs; of these 40, 38 scored 5 or more on the lifetime NODS, and 2 obtained scores of 4; for past-year NODS, 30 scored 5 or more, 5 scored 3 or 4, and 5 scored 2 or less	NA
Gambling Assessment Module (GAM-IV) (continued)	DSM-IV diagnosis of PG 1 week test-retest with two interviewers: $\kappa=0.79$; game-specific $\kappa=0.51-0.77$	Concordance with clinician ratings was fair for five diagnostic criteria ($\kappa=0.5-0.7$) and poor for the other five criteria ($\kappa=0.0-0.3$)	NA

Instrument	Content areas	Number and type of items	Administration time and method	Scoring instructions, score range, cut scores, and interpretation of scores
Gambling Behavior Interview (GBI) (Stinchfield et al. 2007)	Clinical interview to measure signs and symptoms of PG, including gambling frequency, amount of time and money spent gambling, the SOGS, DSM-IV diagnostic criteria, and 32 research items with a past-year time frame	76 items, including 20 SOGS, 10 DSM-IV diagnostic criteria, and 32 research items	30- to 60-minute interview	DSM score of 5 or more indicates PG; 20-item research scale uses item weights; 5-item screen score of 2 or more indicates probable PG
Early Intervention Gambling Health Test (EIGHT) (Sullivan 1999)	Problem gambling signs and symptoms	8 items	5 minutes; questionnaire and interview	Each item=1 point; cut score of 4+ indicates that gambling is affecting patient's health

Instrument (continued)	Psychometrics		Classification accuracy indices
	Reliability	Validity	Sample characteristics, criterion, base rate, sensitivity, specificity, and hit rate
Gambling Behavior Interview (GBI) (continued)	DSM-IV: Cronbach α=0.95 20-item research scale: Cronbach α=0.96 5-item screen: Cronbach α=0.95	20-item research scale and 5-item screen were correlated with DSM-IV diagnostic criteria (r=0.90; r=0.92), and with SOGS score (r=0.82; r=0.85)	Group membership was criterion: gambling treatment patients (n=121) and general population who had gambled in the past year (n=138) Classification accuracy was computed for discriminating between the two groups Base rate was 0.47 DSM-IV using standard cut score of 5+: hit rate=0.91; sensitivity=0.83; specificity=0.98; false-positive rate=0.03; and false-negative rate=0.13 20-item research scale, using item weights: hit rate=1.00; sensitivity=1.00; specificity=1.00; false-positive rate=0.00; and false-negative rate=0.00 5-item screen with cut score of 2+: hit rate=0.99; sensitivity=0.99; specificity=0.99; false-positive rate=0.02; and false-negative rate=0.01
Early Intervention Gambling Health Test (EIGHT) (continued)	NA	Correlated with SOGS (r=0.75); good to excellent agreement with counselor ratings and diagnosis	Sample of prison inmates (n=100); compared with DSM-IV diagnosis of PG: sensitivity=0.91; specificity=0.50; PPV=0.59

Instrument	Content areas	Number and type of items	Administration time and method	Scoring instructions, score range, cut scores, and interpretation of scores
Timeline Follow-Back (TLFB) adapted for gambling (G-TLFB) (Hodgins and Makarchuk 2003; Stinchfield et al. 2007)	A calendar or diary to measure gambling days and time and money spent gambling each day	Adapted for different time periods; 1 year, 6 months, or past 4 weeks	Varies by time period assessed; but a few minutes each day	Count days of gambling and days abstinent; sum the amount of time spent gambling; sum the amount of money lost gambling
Addiction Severity Index—Pathological Gambling (ASI-PG) and Gambling Severity Index (GSI) (Lesieur and Blume 1992)	Modification of ASI for PG by adding gambling frequency and problems associated with gambling	6 items in GSI	Additional 10 minutes to administer gambling items	Composite score range, 0–1; no specific interpretations given for scores; however, comparable to ASI indices
Structured Clinical Interview for Pathological Gambling (SCI-PG) (Grant et al. 2004)	DSM-IV diagnostic criteria for PG	11 screening items; 33 PG diagnostic items	10- to 20-minute interview; clinician-administered	Endorsement of 5 or more of the 10 DSM-IV diagnostic criteria and evidence that the gambling is not better accounted for by a manic episode indicate PG

Instrument *(continued)*	Psychometrics			Classification accuracy indices
	Reliability	Validity		Sample characteristics, criterion, base rate, sensitivity, specificity, and hit rate
Time-Line Follow-Back (TLFB) adapted for gambling (G-TLFB) *(continued)*	3-week test-retest (ICC = 0.61–0.98); 2-week test-retest (r = 0.74–0.96)	Agreement with collaterals: ICC = 0.46–0.65; correlation with other measure of gambling frequency (r = 0.53); G-TLFB correlation with SOGS (r = 0.30) and MAGS (r = 0.28)		NA
Addiction Severity Index—Pathological Gambling (ASI-PG) and Gambling Severity Index (GSI) *(continued)*	Cronbach α = 0.73	Correlated with SOGS (r = 0.57)		NA
Structured Clinical Interview for Pathological Gambling (SCI-PG) *(continued)*	Interrater agreement, κ = 1.0; test-retest reliability, r = 0.97	Convergent validity: correlated with SOGS (r = 0.78) and with PG-YBOCS (r = 0.38); discriminant validity: correlated with HAM-A (r = 0.23) and HAM-D (r = 0.19)		Longitudinal course of 20 gambling treatment patients was the criterion: sensitivity = 0.88; specificity = 1.00; PPV = 1.00; and NPV = 0.67

Instrument	Content areas	Number and type of items	Administration time and method	Scoring instructions, score range, cut scores, and interpretation of scores
Canadian Problem Gambling Index (CPGI) and Problem Gambling Severity Index (PGSI) (Ferris and Wynne 2001)	Gambling involvement, problem gambling, adverse consequences, family history of gambling, comorbid disorders, and distorted cognitions	31 total; 9-item PGSI	15-minute interview	Each item is 1 point, and score range is 0–9; score of 0 indicates nonproblem gambling; score of 1–2 indicates low-risk gambling; score of 3–7 indicates moderate-risk gambling; and score of 8 or more indicates problem gambling
Sydney Laval Universities Gambling Screen (SLUGS) (Blaszczynski et al. 2008)	Loss of control, negative consequences, and self-identified need for treatment	7 items; Likert scale from 0 to 100	Self-administered via paper and pencil	NA
Victorian Gambling Screen (VGS) (Ben-Tovim et al. 2001)	Harm to self	15 items; 5-point response options	Self-administered or interview	Scores range from 0 to 60; three cut scores

| Instrument (continued) | Psychometrics | | Classification accuracy indices |
	Reliability	Validity	Sample characteristics, criterion, base rate, sensitivity, specificity, and hit rate
Canadian Problem Gambling Index (CPGI) and Problem Gambling Severity Index (PGSI) (continued)	9-item problem gambling scale Cronbach $\alpha=0.84$; 4-week test-retest correlation of 0.78	Discriminating between different groups; correlated with the SOGS ($r=0.83$), DSM-IV ($r=0.83$), and results of clinical interviews ($r=0.48$)	DSM-IV was the criterion; sensitivity=0.83; specificity=1.00
Sydney Laval Universities Gambling Screen (SLUGS) (continued)	Cronbach $\alpha=0.85$	Each SLUGS item correlated with SOGS score ($r=0.41-0.70$)	SLUGS development sample included 2,069 participants, and the majority were college students; the authors did not provide any information about a cut score or classification accuracy in the development article
Victorian Gambling Screen (VGS) (continued)	Cronbach $\alpha=0.96$ and 0.89	Correlated with SOGS ($r=87$ and 0.41)	Authors did not provide any information about classification accuracy

Instrument	Content areas	Number and type of items	Administration time and method	Scoring instructions, score range, cut scores, and interpretation of scores
Brief Screens				
Lie/Bet (Johnson et al. 1997)	Lie to people about your gambling; bet more and more money	2 items	1-minute interview	Answering "Yes" to one or both items indicates PG
National Opinion Research Center Diagnostic Screen for Gambling Disorders, Loss of Control, Lying, and Preoccupation (NODS CLiP) (Toce-Gerstein et al. 2009)	3 DSM-IV items from NODS: loss of control, lying, and preoccupation	3 items; yes/no; lifetime	1-minute interview	"Yes" response to any one of the three items is considered positive for PG and indicates need for further assessment

| Instrument (continued) | Psychometrics | | Classification accuracy indices |
	Reliability	Validity	Sample characteristics, criterion, base rate, sensitivity, specificity, and hit rate
Brief Screens (continued)			
Lie-Bet (continued)	κ=0.81	NA	Classification accuracy indices were computed on 191 male GA members and 171 male non–problem gambling controls; sensitivity=0.99, specificity=0.91, positive predictive power=0.92, and NPV=0.99; a second study that included women reported sensitivity=1.00, specificity=0.85, PPV=0.78, and NPV=1.00
National Opinion Research Center Diagnostic Screen for Gambling Disorders, Loss of Control, Lying, and Preoccupation (NODS-CLiP) (continued)	NA	NA	Sensitivity=0.99; specificity=0.88; false-positive rate=0.01; false-negative rate=0.12 NODS-CLiP was tested in a clinical sample and was found to have sensitivity=0.98; specificity=0.30; positive predictive power=0.87; NPV=0.80; and diagnostic efficiency=0.86 (Volberg et al. 2011)

Brief Screens (continued)

Instrument	Content areas	Number and type of items	Administration time and method	Scoring instructions, score range, cut scores, and interpretation of scores
National Opinion Research Center Diagnostic Screen for Gambling Disorders, Preoccupation, Escape, Risked Relationships, and Chasing (NODS- PERC) (Volberg et al. 2011)	4 DSM-IV items from NODS: preoccupation, escape, risked relationships, and chasing	4 items; yes/ no; lifetime	1-minute interview	"Yes" response to any one of the 4 items indicates a need for further PG assessment
Brief Biosocial Gambling Screen (BBGS) (Gebauer et al. 2010)	3 DSM-IV items: withdrawal, lying about gambling, financial difficulties caused by gambling	3 items; yes/ no; past year	1-minute interview	"Yes" response to any one of the 3 items is indicative of PG pending further assessment
Short SOGS (Room et al. 1999)	5 SOGS items: gambled more than you intended to, people criticized your gambling, money arguments centered on your gambling, felt guilty, and claimed to be winning money gambling when you were not	5 items; yes/ no; past year	1-minute self-administered	"Yes" response to 2 or more items is interpreted as problem gambling

	Psychometrics		Classification accuracy indices
Instrument *(continued)*	Reliability	Validity	Sample characteristics, criterion, base rate, sensitivity, specificity, and hit rate
Brief Screens *(continued)*			
National Opinion Research Center Diagnostic Screen for Gambling Disorders, Preoccupation, Escape, Risked Relationships, and Chasing (NODS-PERC) *(continued)*	NA	NA	Sensitivity=0.997; specificity=0.39; PPV=0.89; NPV=0.96; and diagnostic efficiency=0.89
Brief Biosocial Gambling Screen (BBGS) *(continued)*	NA	NA	Sensitivity=0.96; specificity=0.99
Short SOGS *(continued)*	NA	Correlated with 20-item SOGS (*r*=0.87)	Research participants who scored 5 or more on the SOGS also scored 2 or more on the Short SOGS

Instrument	Content areas	Number and type of items	Administration time and method	Scoring instructions, score range, cut scores, and interpretation of scores
Brief Screens (continued)				
One-Item Screen for Problem Gambling (Thomas et al. 2008)	1 item: Have you ever had an issue with your gambling?	1 item; yes/no; past year;	1-minute interview intended for screening in a medical practice	"Yes" response is interpreted as problem gambling
Instruments for Evaluation of Treatment Efficacy				
Gambling Treatment Outcome Monitoring System (GAMTOMS) (Stinchfield et al. 2007) (includes Gambling Treatment Admission Questionnaire [GTAQ])	GTAQ includes a 10-item measure of DSM-IV diagnostic criteria for PG, as well as other measures of gambling problem severity, including the SOGS, gambling frequency, gambling-related financial problems, and legal problems	142-item GTAQ has a 10-item measure of DSM-IV diagnostic criteria	30- to 45-minute paper-and-pencil questionnaire	DSM-IV diagnostic criteria items are 1 point each and are summed; score range, 0–10; cut score of 5 or more indicates PG

Instrument *(continued)*	Psychometrics		Classification accuracy indices
	Reliability	Validity	Sample characteristics, criterion, base rate, sensitivity, specificity, and hit rate

Brief Screens *(continued)*

One-Item Screen for Problem Gambling *(continued)*	NA	NA	Compared with the PGSI (Ferris and Wynne 2001), it was found to yield a false-positive rate of 0.04 and a false-negative rate of 0.21 (Thomas et al. 2008); a cross-validation yielded sensitivity=0.21; specificity=0.98; false-negative rate=0.79 (Rockloff et al. 2011)

Instruments for Evaluation of Treatment Efficacy *(continued)*

Gambling Treatment Outcome Monitoring System (GAMTOMS) (includes Gambling Treatment Admission Questionnaire [GTAQ]) *(continued)*	Internal consistency reliability: DSM-IV diagnostic criteria (Cronbach α=0.89), SOGS (Cronbach α=0.85), and financial problems (Cronbach α=0.78); 1-week test-retest yielded correlations of r=0.74 for DSM-IV; r=91 for SOGS	Validity of the DSM-IV diagnostic criteria was measured by correlations with the following measures of gambling problem severity: SOGS (r=0.83); gambling frequency (r=0.43); and number of financial problems (r=0.40)	DSM-IV diagnosis of PG was used to classify clinical vs. nonclinical cases: base rate=0.20; hit rate=0.96; sensitivity=0.96; specificity=0.95; false-positive rate=0.01; and false-negative rate=0.14 DSM-IV diagnosis of PG was used to classify SOGS PPG vs. non-PPG cases: base rate=0.79; hit rate=0.98; sensitivity=0.97; specificity=1.00; false-positive rate=0.00; and false-negative rate=0.10

Instruments for Evaluation of Treatment Efficacy *(continued)*

Instrument	Content areas	Number and type of items	Administration time and method	Scoring instructions, score range, cut scores, and interpretation of scores
Pathological Gambling Modification of the Yale-Brown Obsessive Compulsive Scale (PG-YBOCS) (Hollander et al. 1998)	Severity of PG symptoms over a recent time period (usually within the past 1 or 2 weeks); gambling thoughts or urges and behavior	10 items; rated on a 5-point Likert scale ranging from least severe (0) to most severe (4)	Clinician-administered interview that takes about 10 minutes	Each set of questions is totaled separately; one total score is also obtained; the authors did not provide interpretations of scores because the scale is used as a measure of change
Gambling Symptom Assessment Scale (G-SAS) (Kim et al. 2001)	Gambling urges, thoughts, feelings, and behavior	10 items; 4-point Likert response options	Clinician-administered interview that takes about 10 minutes	Scores range from 0 to 40; authors did not provide interpretation of scores

Instrument (continued)	Psychometrics		Classification accuracy indices
	Reliability	Validity	Sample characteristics, criterion, base rate, sensitivity, specificity, and hit rate
Instruments for Evaluation of Treatment Efficacy (continued)			
Pathological Gambling Modification of the Yale-Brown Obsessive Compulsive Scale (PG-YBOCS) (continued)	Cronbach α=0.97; test-retest correlation: r=0.29–0.56; interrater agreement: ICC=0.97	Exhibited significantly different scores between a PG and a control sample; change score was correlated with SOGS (r=0.90) and uncorrelated with anxiety (r=−0.01) and depression (r=0.08)	Pallanti et al. (2005) recruited 188 pathological gamblers and 149 healthy control subjects; no information was provided about classification accuracy
Gambling Symptom Assessment Scale (G-SAS) (continued)	Cronbach α=0.89; test-retest correlation: r=0.70	Correlated with CGI (r=0.78)	Authors did not provide information about classification accuracy

Instrument	Content areas	Number and type of items	Administration time and method	Scoring instructions, score range, cut scores, and interpretation of scores
Instruments for Evaluation of Treatment Efficacy *(continued)*				
Clinical Global Impressions—Pathological Gambling (CGI-PG) (Guy 1976)	3 items: 1) severity of illness, 2) rating of improvement, and 3) efficacy index; used primarily in psychopharmacological treatment studies	Three items; improvement item is rated on a 7-point Likert scale from very much improved to very much worse	Clinician-administered interview that takes about 5 minutes	NA
Youth Gambling Assessment Instruments				
South Oaks Gambling Screen—Revised for Adolescents (SOGS-RA) (Winters et al. 1993)	Signs and symptoms of adolescent problem gambling, including negative consequences and loss of control	12 items; yes/no; past year	10 minutes; self-administered via paper-and-pencil questionnaire	1 point for each of the 12 items; score range, 0–12; 0, no problem; 2–3, at-risk gambling; 4 or more, problem gambling

	Psychometrics		Classification accuracy indices
Instrument *(continued)*	Reliability	Validity	Sample characteristics, criterion, base rate, sensitivity, specificity, and hit rate
Instruments for Evaluation of Treatment Efficacy *(continued)*			
Clinical Global Impressions— Pathological Gambling (CGI-PG) *(continued)*	NA	CGI correlated with PG-YBOCS ($r=0.89$)	NA
Youth Gambling Assessment Instruments *(continued)*			
South Oaks Gambling Screen—Revised for Adolescents (SOGS-RA) *(continued)*	Cronbach $\alpha=0.80$; 2-week test-retest $\kappa=0.57$ and Cronbach $\alpha=0.81$ and 0.76 for male and female subjects, respectively (Poulin 2000); Cronbach $\alpha=0.74$ (Welte et al. 2008)	Gambling activity, $r=0.39$; gambling frequency, $r=0.54$; and amount of money gambled in past year, $r=0.42$	Using the criterion of DSM-IV-J: 97% true positive; 0.5% false negative; and 2.4% false positive (Derevensky and Gupta 2000); using two criteria of self-identified need for help and receipt of help, 96% were correctly classified; however, sensitivity was about 60%, and specificity was 96% for both proxies (Boudreau and Poulin 2007); hit rate=0.59; sensitivity=0.87; specificity=0.31 (Stinchfield et al. 2017)

Youth Gambling Assessment Instruments (*continued*)

Instrument	Content areas	Number and type of items	Administration time and method	Scoring instructions, score range, cut scores, and interpretation of scores
DSM-IV-J and DSM-IV-MR-J (Fisher 1992, 2000a)	Nine DSM-IV diagnostic criteria	Nine criteria measured with 12 items; yes/no (DSM-IV-J); multiple-response options (DSM-IV-MR-J); past year	5- to 10-minute self-administered paper-and-pencil questionnaire	1 point for each of the nine criteria; score range, 0–9; score of 4 or more indicates problem gambling
Canadian Adolescent Gambling Inventory (CAGI) and Gambling Problem Severity Scale (GPSS) (Tremblay et al. 2010)	Gambling frequency, time and money spent gambling, gambling problem severity of behavior and negative consequences	44 items; multiple-response options; past 3 months	10–20 minutes; self-administered paper-and-pencil questionnaire	9-item gambling problem severity scale; score range, 0–27; scores of 0–1, "no problem"; 2–5, "low to moderate severity"; and 6 or more, "high severity"

Youth Gambling Assessment Instruments (continued)

| Instrument (continued) | Psychometrics | | Classification accuracy indices |
	Reliability	Validity	Sample characteristics, criterion, base rate, sensitivity, specificity, and hit rate
DSM-IV-J and DSM-IV-MR-J (continued)	Cronbach α=0.75	DSM-IV-J correlated with the SOGS-RA (r=0.67) and GA-20 (r=0.68) (Derevensky and Gupta 2000)	NA
Canadian Adolescent Gambling Inventory (CAGI) and Gambling Problem Severity Scale (GPSS) (continued)	Cronbach α: 0.83–0.90; temporal stability coefficients: 0.77–0.90	Correlated with gambling frequency (r=0.32–0.55) and money spent gambling (r=0.12–0.50); convergent validity coefficients: 0.14–0.67	GPSS sensitivity=0.93 and specificity=0.93 (Tremblay et al. 2010); GPSS hit rate=0.89; sensitivity=1.00; specificity=0.85 (Tremblay et al. 2010)

Instrument	Content areas	Number and type of items	Administration time and method	Scoring instructions, score range, cut scores, and interpretation of scores
Youth Gambling Assessment Instruments (continued)				
Brief Adolescent Gambling Screen (BAGS) (Stinchfield et al. 2017)	Three items drawn from the CAGI GPSS on gambling problem severity	Three items; 4-point multiple-response options (0–3); past 3 months	1-minute; self-administered or clinician administered	3 items with a score range of 0 to 9; score of 4 or more indicates problem gambling

| Instrument *(continued)* | Psychometrics | | Classification accuracy indices |
	Reliability	**Validity**	**Sample characteristics, criterion, base rate, sensitivity, specificity, and hit rate**
Youth Gambling Assessment Instruments *(continued)*			
Brief Adolescent Gambling Screen (BAGS) *(continued)*	Coefficient α: 0.72; McDonald's coefficient omega: 0.79	Convergent validity coefficient for BAGS and SOGS-RA: 0.67	Hit rate = 0.95; sensitivity = 0.88; specificity = 0.98

Note. HAM-A = Hamilton Rating Scale for Anxiety; HAM-D = Hamilton Rating Scale for Depression; ICC = intraclass correlation; NA = not available, not provided, or unknown; NPV = negative predictive value; PG = pathological gambling; PPG = problem and pathological gambling; PPV = positive predictive value.

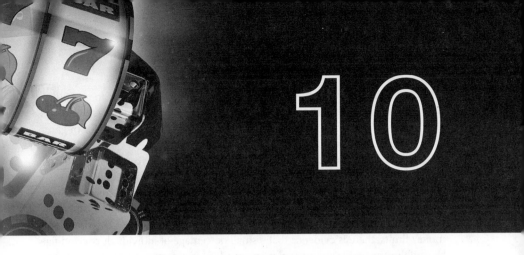

Understanding Youth Gambling Problems

Prevention and Treatment Strategies

Jeffrey L. Derevensky, Ph.D.
Lynette Gilbeau, B.Ed.

There is little doubt that the landscape of gambling on an international level has dramatically changed over the past several decades. With the exception of the temporary closing of land-based gambling venues because of coronavirus disease 2019 (COVID-19), the availability and accessibility of diverse gambling opportunities during the past decade have dramatically increased, with gambling being recognized as a socially acceptable recreational activity (Grande-Gosende et al. 2019; Nowak and Aloe 2018). Today's gambling opportunities include traditional forms of gambling—casinos, lotteries, horse and dog tracks, poker, and sports wagering—with newer activities being devoted to online gambling (traditional forms of gambling but done remotely, skill-based slots, and esports wagering). As gambling venues continue to reopen after the COVID-19 shutdown, there has been a renewed interest in gambling, with some casinos reporting increased year-over-year revenues despite travel restrictions, social distancing measures, and reductions in the number of gamblers permitted in casinos.

Gambling has traditionally been viewed as an adult activity, yet there is ample evidence that it is also a popular, socially acceptable activity among adolescents (Calado and Griffiths 2016; Derevensky 2012; Productivity Commission 2010; U.K. Gambling Commission 2019; Volberg et al. 2010). Although most people generally gamble in a responsible manner, setting and maintaining both time and money limits, there is evidence that a small percentage of individuals overindulge by gambling excessive amounts of money and get into serious gambling-related financial, mental health, and interpersonal difficulties (Black and Shaw 2019). Adolescents are no exception. A number of factors are associated with prevalence rates of problem gambling (including accessibility, availability, age, gender, cultural factors, and advertising). Notwithstanding measurement issues and controversies, studies of adolescents and young adults have typically reported that youth have among the highest prevalence rates of problem or disordered gambling (Derevensky 2012; Shaffer and Hall 2001; Volberg et al. 2010; Welte et al. 2008).

There has been overwhelming support by the general public for most forms of gambling. The glitz and glamour associated with casino gambling as well as televised world championship poker events and entertaining movies with gambling themes have heightened the excitement for young people. Research studies throughout North and South America, Europe, Asia, and Australasia all suggest gambling's popularity among adolescents. Survey and prevalence findings examining youth gambling behavior have consistently revealed that adolescents have managed to participate, to some degree, in practically all forms of social, government-regulated, and nonregulated forms of gambling despite age prohibitions (Derevensky 2012; Molinaro et al. 2014; Volberg et al. 2010). Although the prevalence rates of gambling disorder vary from jurisdiction to jurisdiction and there is variability in factors such as the minimum age at which individuals can gamble and the types of available gambling activities and their accessibility, past-year prevalence rates of problem and disordered gambling among adolescents and young adults have been reported to range between 0.2% and 12.3%, notwithstanding differences among assessment instruments, cutoff scores, and time frames (Calado and Griffiths 2016). Interestingly, these rates are two to six times the prevalence rates reported for adults, with young adults (ages 18–25 years) experiencing the highest prevalence rates among adults (National Research Council 1999; Productivity Commission 2010; Volberg et al. 2010). Equally important to note is that despite the increased diversity of gambling activities, increased legalization, and increased availability of gambling opportunities, the prevalence rates of gambling and problem gambling among adolescents have generally not increased. There is also evidence to suggest that problem gambling may be temporal and that individuals fluctuate between "safe gambling" and "problem gambling" over their lifetimes (Williams et al. 2015). This should not be misinterpreted to suggest that problems may only be short-lived, without significant long-term negative consequences. There is strong evidence to suggest that youth experiencing gambling disorder experience multiple long-lasting negative mental health, academic, social, financial, familial, employment, and legal consequences (Blinn-Pike et al. 2010; Derevensky 2012; Derevensky and Gupta 2011; Derevensky et al. 2011; Hansen and Rossow 2008; St-Pierre et al. 2017; Volberg et al. 2010).

Understanding Adolescent Gambling

As previously noted, although gambling is most often considered an adult activity, numerous research studies reveal gambling's popularity among adolescents (Calado and Griffiths 2016; Delfabbro et al. 2016; Derevensky 2012; Volberg et al. 2010). Irrespective of the fact that most jurisdictions have statutes restricting underage access to regulated forms of gambling (casino, lottery play, and so on), prevalence studies consistently reveal that youth ages 12–17 years participate to some degree in most forms of gambling (Derevensky and Gilbeau 2019).

Ample research suggests that a large majority of teens have gambled for money well before the age of 18 years, yet most do so only occasionally with few gambling or gambling-related problems. Similar to adults, gambling behaviors among adolescents exist on a continuum from nongambling to social, occasional, or recreational gambling to at-risk gambling (gambling excessively and experiencing some gambling-related problems without reaching the clinical criteria for disordered gambling) to problem, compulsive, or disordered gambling (Derevensky 2012). As one moves along the continuum, the number and severity of gambling-related problems (psychosocial, behavioral, financial, interpersonal, academic, mental health, and legal difficulties) increase.

Understanding the gambling behaviors of adolescents helps lay the foundation for effective prevention and treatment programs. Typical gambling behaviors include purchasing lottery tickets (primarily scratch tickets as opposed to large lottery draws), betting on games of skill (videogames, sports), sports wagering (pro, college, or amateur events), fantasy sports and sports pools, social casino gambling, and poker and other card games, with a new interest in gambling on esports. As children get older, they gain greater access to gambling venues and are more prone to gamble on a diverse number of different restricted activities. As gaming and gambling are starting to merge, a growing number of youth gamble (e.g., the use of loot boxes) while simultaneously gaming. Zendle (2019) has argued that there are clear parallels in both psychological and legal terms between real-money video gaming and gambling. Other concerns about the interplay between excessive video gaming and gambling have been raised by Derevensky et al. (2013), Hollingshead et al. (2016), Kim et al. (2015), Marchica et al. (2019), and Parke et al. (2012). The primary motivations stated by youth include gambling for enjoyment, to make money, excitement, social involvement, relaxation, to escape daily problems, to minimize depression, and to help deal with loneliness (Derevensky 2012).

Adolescent Problem or Disordered Gambling

As previously described, most adolescents can best be described as occasional, recreational, or social gamblers, engaging in this behavior relatively infrequently. They are, in general, capable of setting and to a large extent maintaining both financial and time limits. Yet for some individuals, their gambling escalates and progresses to a point at which gambling-related problems begin. These problems include a preoccupation with gambling; a need to gamble with increasing amounts of money to maintain the desired level of excitement and enjoyment; becoming restless or irritable when attempting to reduce or stop gambling; making repeated unsuccessful attempts at reducing or stopping gambling; repeatedly trying to win back money lost; using gambling as a way of escaping daily problems or reducing dysphoric moods; increasing lying to family members, peers, and friends as a way of hiding gambling losses; losing or jeopardizing significant relationships; sacrificing employment or educational opportunities; committing illegal acts to finance gambling; and relying on others for financial assistance (Fisher 2000). Yet it is important to note that adolescents with severe gambling disorder are not a homogeneous group. For example, not all individuals endorse all the characteristics previously mentioned. As well, differences in motivations for gamblers and the types of gambling activities preferred are apparent. For example, sports gamblers are typically different from card and machine gamblers. As such, when clinicians are attempting to provide intervention strategies, it is often important to consider the severity of the gambling disorder, the underlying motivations for gambling, the types of games played, differences in gambling triggers, and other psychosocial and mental health disorders concomitant with the gambling disorder. Although the motivations for gambling differ, there is often an underlying reason prompting individuals' continued gambling despite repeated losses. For some adolescents, self-esteem is enhanced during their winning phase; for others, depressive symptoms disappear while gambling; and for others, a new peer group of fellow gamblers develops. Yet there is ample evidence that for a vast majority of adolescent problem gamblers, gambling provides a psychological form of escape (e.g., from peers, parents, academic tasks, daily problems). While gambling, these youth go into a dissociative state in which they lose track of time and repress feelings of helplessness and loneliness (see Derevensky 2012 for a comprehensive list of risk and protective factors). There is also neurobiological evidence suggesting adolescents have a bias toward immediate gains rather than long-term ones (Galvan et al. 2006). Compared with the adult amygdala, the adolescent amygdala is activated more easily by reward cues and is less sensitive to potential harm (Ernst et al. 2005).

Preventing Youth Problem Gambling

Given both short- and long-term negative harms associated with problem gambling, multiple prevention initiatives aimed at harm minimization or harm reduction have been developed. The application of these strategies for gambling often emanates from prevention initiatives initially developed in the field of substance abuse. Besides governmental age restrictions and prohibitions for regulated forms of gambling, such prevention efforts have traditionally focused on issues of personal responsibility, controlled use, and healthy choices (Petry et al. 2009). Data from jurisdictions in which strict efforts to prevent problem gambling have been instituted has been associated with comparatively low (and seemingly decreasing) prevalence estimates of disordered gambling (Bullock and Potenza 2012; Potenza et al. 2019). Nevertheless, the majority of prevention programs, either in land-based or online gambling operations, have typically targeted adults because of youth age prohibitions.

Given the age restrictions impacting adolescent gambling, we will not focus on prevention initiatives established for adults such as self-exclusion or third-party exclusions, behavioral tracking, personalized normative feedback or personal messaging, precommitment or limit setting, regulations concerning game speed, removal of bill acceptors, reducing denomination of bills accepted in electronic gambling machines, changes in game speed, establishment of breaks in play, and pop-up messaging restrictions of certain forms of gambling, among others. (For a more comprehensive approach for adult prevention programs, see Derevensky 2020; Potenza et al. 2019.) However, it is important to note that in research from Finland, raising the age for legalized gambling from 15 to 18 years was reportedly associated with fewer gambling problems among adolescents and young adults (Hodgins et al. 2001). Assuming a harm minimization strategy, the ultimate goal of gambling-related prevention programs is to reduce, minimize, or eliminate the potential harmful consequences concomitant with gambling in general and problem or disordered gambling in particular.

Prevention Paradigms: Harm Minimization vs. Abstinence

Prevention intervention programs typically fall into two general categories: harm minimization or abstinence (Derevensky 2012, 2020; Derevensky and Gilbeau 2019). Abstinence-based programs emphasize that because underage youth are legally prohibited from accessing gambling establishments, purchasing lottery products, or gambling in general, they therefore should not gamble until they are of legal age (Derevensky 2012; Floros 2018). In contrast, harm reduction or harm minimization initiatives incorporate policies, programs, or strategies that aim to reduce the negative harmful consequences of engaging in risky behaviors without necessitating abstinence (Ariyabuddhiphongs 2013; Derevensky 2020; Dickson et al. 2004).

Concerns have been raised that the abstinence model may not be effective for youth because the majority of adolescents report having gambled in the past year and report gambling on unregulated (non-government-controlled gambling) activities with friends and family members at an early age (Derevensky 2012, 2020). Blaszczynski (2001) makes the point that negative harmful consequences of gambling are not necessarily limited to pathological or problem gamblers, but they may also impact recreational, occasional, or social gamblers, thereby suggesting that prevention programs should not only target youth experiencing gambling problems but recreational, occasional, or social gamblers as well.

Derevensky and Gupta (2011) have long argued that a harm minimization approach makes sense given that gambling is pervasive, historically part of our culture (Schwartz 2006), socially acceptable, and government sanctioned (in some cases, government owned and operated). There is research showing that children as young as age 9 or 10 years have gambled for money (Derevensky 2012; Productivity Commission 2010). Still further, adopting a harm minimization approach is also consistent with a public health framework (Messerlian et al. 2004).

Types of Prevention Programs

Although there is a growing emphasis on the development of gambling prevention programs for young adults (ages 18–25 years), a number of existing prevention programs have been educational initiatives targeting school-age children (typically those at the primary or secondary school level). These existing educational programs typically provide a universal prevention strategy and are conceptualized as being a protective factor. They are designed to increase the individual's knowledge about the risks associated with excessive gambling, address erroneous cognitive beliefs, and sometimes emphasize mathematical concepts such as probability, with some programs addressing issues related to motivations for gambling (Grande-Gosende et al. 2019).

Primary Prevention (Universal Prevention)

Primary prevention programs target the general public or whole population groups, such as children and adolescents, regardless of identified risk or need (Dickson-Gillespie et al. 2008). These prevention programs do not specifically target children or youth deemed to be at risk for a gambling problem and can be community-based programs or school-based prevention programs (Kourgiantakis et al. 2016). Most of the primary prevention programs, which are relatively low-cost, attempt to prevent the onset of gambling behavior or curtail individuals' gambling (Williams et al. 2012). The goal is to increase awareness of the risks and consequences associated with excessive problem gambling (Messerlian and Derevensky 2005; Messerlian et al. 2004). Although primary prevention programs for youth are often available for substance use or abuse, drinking and driving, sex education, bullying, smoking, eating disorders, and other mental health issues, there are a limited number of programs for gambling prevention. Even in jurisdictions where programs exist, schools are often reluctant to devote time to these programs because they perceive there are more pressing mental health and education issues (Derevensky 2012). Most existing gambling prevention programs fall under the rubric of universal prevention targeting all individuals rather than just those considered at high risk for developing a gambling problem (Derevensky 2012). Jurisdictions such as Florida, Massachusetts, and Oregon have developed such statewide programs and made them available to school districts.

Secondary Prevention (Selective Prevention)

Secondary prevention programs target youth at high risk of developing problem gambling behaviors (e.g., children of parents with problem gambling, those with substance abuse issues) (Dowling and Brown 2010) and are developed to identify, assess, and provide appropriate rapid interventions for children in order to prevent more severe problem gambling from developing (Calado et al. 2020; Dowling and Brown 2010; Kourgiantakis et al. 2016; Messerlian et al. 2004). Other goals of secondary prevention strategies include equipping individuals with more effective coping skills, enhancing problem solving abilities, and fostering engagement in healthier activities while reducing substance use (Messerlian and Derevensky 2005). Secondary prevention programs also reduce the social normalization of gambling or positive gambling expectancies and can address other co-occurring disorders (Dowling and Brown 2010). Secondary prevention programs can be offered in specialized schools (e.g., children with conduct and behavioral disorders) or through community or social service settings (Dowling and Brown 2010; Kourgiantakis et al. 2016).

Tertiary Prevention (Indicated Prevention)

Tertiary prevention programs, also referred to as treatment or intervention programs, target youth presenting signs and symptoms of problem gambling behavior (Derevensky 2012; Messerlian et al. 2004). Effective treatment strategies for both adolescents and adults are designed to not only address gambling-related issues but also help individuals experiencing a wide variety of mental health disorders (Derevensky 2012; Dowling and Brown 2010).

Youth Gambling Prevention Initiative: From Research to Prevention

In the past two decades, a number of educational initiatives have been developed to promote responsible gambling decision-making or prevent the onset of gambling activities (Williams et al. 2012). Because the age at onset of gambling represents a significant risk factor for later gambling involvement, delaying the onset of gambling experiences is considered important (Derevensky and Gilbeau 2019; Derevensky and Gupta 2011).

Risk and Protective Factors

A number of intervention programs have been developed by applying a risk or protective factor model to identify both the risk and protective factors associated with adolescent gambling to minimize risk factors and maximize protective factors (Calado et al. 2020; Dickson et al. 2002; Shek and Sun 2011). St-Pierre and Derevensky (2016) classified gambling prevention programs as either psychoeducational programs or comprehensive psychoeducational and skills training prevention programs. Most school-based youth gambling prevention programs have incorporated multiple objectives, including 1) highlighting the difference between games of skill and games of chance; 2) educating youth about erroneous cognitions, statistical probability, and the independence of events; 3) dispelling myths surrounding the "illusion of control" and the randomness of events; 4) articulating the warning signs of problem gambling; and 5) providing resources for youth at risk of a gambling problem (Derevensky 2012; Derevensky and Gilbeau 2019; Ladouceur et al. 2013; Turner et al. 2008).

Using a systematic review procedure, called PRISMA (Preferred Reporting Items for Systematic Reviews and Meta-Analyses), Grande-Gosende and colleagues (2019) examined nine studies targeting prevention programs for young adults, with all studies being done in North America. They concluded that the majority of the studies were built as secondary prevention programs for college students who displayed signs of being at-risk (exhibiting signs of problem gambling but not reaching the clinical criteria for disordered gambling) or problem gamblers. As such, these programs were designed to help young adults reduce their gambling to a "safe" level or at the very least to ensure their gambling did not increase. Several of these programs have been initiated to encourage the development of interpersonal skills, foster coping strategies, provide examples of positive decision-making, educate youth about the short- and long-term risks associated with problem gambling, provide strategies to reduce the influence of peer pressure, and increase resilience (Derevensky 2012, 2020; Derevensky and

Gilbeau 2017). Research has shown that youth respond best to prevention programs that are interactive in nature (Oh et al. 2017). Additionally, prevention programs delivered by trained staff rather than untrained teachers may be more effective (Donati et al. 2014; Todirita and Lupu 2013). Given the technology-based nature of gambling (online casino and sports gambling), more recently, a number of online prevention programs have begun to be developed.

The lack of awareness of youth problem gambling issues among parents (Campbell et al. 2011), educators (Castren et al. 2017), and mental health professionals (Sansanwal et al. 2016; Temcheff et al. 2014) has curtailed the development and implementation of adolescent gambling prevention programs. (It should be noted that many programs have been developed in the absence of a clear theoretical framework describing the expected causal mechanism by which the programs exert their effects [St-Pierre and Derevensky 2016].) Parental involvement in both supervision and education about gambling and gambling-related harm is also important. Studies conducted by Derevensky and colleagues have shown that parents, educators, and even mental health professionals view gambling as the least concerning activity compared with other adolescent risky behaviors (i.e., smoking, substance use, alcohol use, drinking and driving) (Campbell et al. 2011; Derevensky and Gilbeau 2019; Derevensky and Gupta 2011). Another complementary approach is using positive youth development strategies that focus on adolescents' strengths, talents, and future potential with goals including the promotion of competencies such as self-confidence, resilience, and self-determination (Shek and Sun 2011).

Longitudinal Challenges

Although some initiatives have been evaluated by examining short-term changes in behaviors, few have incorporated a longitudinal design. In a recent meta-analysis of 20 research articles concerning school-based gambling education programs, Keen and colleagues (2017) reported that only 9 of the studies attempted to measure intervention effects on behavioral outcomes, with 5 reporting significant changes in gambling behavior. Although some evaluations of these prevention programs have shown these programs to be effective in the short term for increasing knowledge and modifying or reducing erroneous beliefs about gambling (Grande-Gosende et al. 2019; Ladouceur et al. 2013; Todirita and Lupu 2013), the long-term effects have not been assessed (yet the theory that as accessibility and availability increase, so does problem gambling has not been realized among youth). School-based prevention initiatives based on unique determinants of behavior have shown positive results in increasing gambling knowledge and reducing gambling misperceptions (Calado et al. 2020; Ladouceur et al. 2013), both of which are thought to ultimately impact gambling behavior. Complicating the long-term assessment of these programs has been a general lack of follow-up because of restricted funding (Derevensky 2012; Derevensky and Gupta 2011).

Emerging Adults as a High-Risk Group

Nowak and Aloe (2018) suggested probable pathological gambling among college students ranges from 3% to 32%, with an average estimated rate of 10% for serious gambling problems (Grande-Gosende et al. 2019). This population group is more likely to engage in multiple risky behaviors, including excessive alcohol use, and to exhibit more gambling-related harms (Engwall et al. 2004; Karlsson and Håkansson 2018). As a group, college students typically are experiencing a newfound independence from their families, often attending college away from home, and reaching the legal age for gambling and drinking (Grande-Gosende et al. 2019). There is also evidence suggesting that among adults, the 18- to 25-year-old age group has the highest prevalence rates of gambling-related problems (Derevensky 2012; Volberg et al. 2010). These factors underline the importance of prevention initiatives for this cohort.

In a report by the Task Force on College Gambling Policies (Emerson et al. 2009), the authors made numerous recommendations regarding college gambling and alcohol abuse prevention as guidelines for college administrators, including:

- Establishing a committee to develop and monitor gambling policy
- Ensuring that college policies are in compliance with local, state, and federal laws regarding gambling, including promoting awareness of the laws and encouraging enforcement of existing statutes
- Striving to ensure the application of gambling or alcohol use prohibitions at special events
- Developing relationships with local gambling operators to encourage restrictions on advertising and ensure that the gambling laws are enforced
- Promoting awareness about problem gambling signs and symptoms
- Promoting responsible gambling principles (i.e., setting and maintaining time and money limits)
- Making accommodations for students recovering from problem gambling
- Surveying students, such as by incorporating measures into existing campus health surveys, to determine their attitudes, involvement, and problems with gambling
- Strengthening the capacity of counseling services

Public Health or Regulatory Policies and the Impact of Advertising

Gambling-related advertising has been shown to have an impact on adolescent gambling activity (Derevensky 2012). As such, public policy regarding targeted gambling advertisement content may be important. (Strict rules concerning the promotion of gambling have been established in Italy and Australia.) While online, youth report being bombarded with gambling-related pop-up messages typically depicting happy individuals who are "living the dream" (Derevensky and Gilbeau 2019). These ads do not depict the downside, risks, or potential difficulties associated with gambling (Derevensky and Gilbeau 2019). Furthermore, many of these pop-up messages are intended to entice viewers to gamble online or sign up for bonuses. A growing number of online gaming operators have used social media to advertise and invite individuals to gamble money or play for free on their sites (Gainsbury et al. 2015).

Treating Adolescent Problem Gamblers

What happens when adolescents or young adults gamble excessively? Management of individuals with gambling problems requires consideration of multiple factors, including the presence or absence of comorbid psychiatric and mental health disorders as well as the level of individuals' motivation to change their behavior. Although few treatment facilities provide specialized treatment for adolescent gambling disorder, it is important to note that youth with gambling disorder experience a number of other concomitant mental health disorders. Thus, one must ask if the gambling disorder is in fact the primary or a secondary disorder. (See Figure 10-1, in which any of the outer circles could be inserted in the middle.)

If one assumes a biopsychosocial approach, then treatment must take into consideration a large number of factors, including biological, psychological, and social factors. It should also be noted that environmental factors must also be addressed (e.g., gambling accessibility, availability, advertising).

Treatment-Seeking Individuals

It is difficult to treat individuals with gambling disorder if they fail to seek help. Hodgins et al. (2011), acknowledging study limitations, have concluded that only 10% of adult problem gamblers seek any form of treatment. Based on stud-

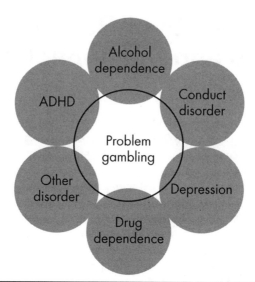

FIGURE 10–1.   Is youth problem gambling a primary disorder?

ies in the United States (Kessler et al. 2008; Slutske 2006; Volberg et al. 2006), Canada (Suurvali et al. 2008), and Australia (Slutske et al. 2009), Hodgins often refers to non-treatment-seeking individuals as the "lost 90%." He has suggested that the most frequent motivators for seeking treatment among adults are financial difficulties, relationship impacts, and negative emotions (stress, anxiety, depression). Other related research suggests that treatment seeking increases as problem severity increases (Slutske 2006).

Adolescents with gambling problems typically do not present themselves for treatment of their own accord. There are likely many reasons that they fail to seek treatment, including 1) fear of being identified, 2) the belief that they can control their behavior, 3) the need to maintain self-perceptions of invincibility and invulnerability, 4) the general negative perceptions associated with therapy, 5) guilt associated with their gambling problems, 6) a lack of recognition and acceptance that they have a gambling problem despite scoring high on gambling severity screens, and 7) their belief in natural recovery and self-control (Hardoon et al. 2003).

Referrals from parents, friends, teachers, the court system, and local helplines become the primary sources through which a treatment population is often acquired. As part of an effective outreach program, posters and brochures are distributed to schools, and workshops are provided for school psychologists, guidance counselors, teachers, and directly to children and adolescents. As a result of these types of outreach programs, adolescents sometimes directly request treatment. Our clinical experience has been that adolescent problem gamblers develop a social network consisting of other problem gamblers. This results in clients recommending their friends for treatment. After adolescents realize and accept that they have a serious gambling problem, they become astutely aware of gambling problems among their friends. Eventually, some successfully convince their peers to seek help as well.

Because adolescents with gambling problems have little access to "extra discretionary money" and many initially seek treatment without their parents' knowledge, it is important to provide treatment at no cost. Although this is not practical for treatment providers in independent practice, state or provincial funding (or support by insurance providers when available) is fundamental when treating adolescents with serious gambling problems.

There are currently no data on the prevalence of adolescents seeking treatment for gambling disorder. What we know is the percentage of youth seeking treatment is considerably lower than the 10% of adults seeking help. Many gambling helplines report very few adolescents calling for help, but some call because they may have a parent or relative with gambling disorder (Derevensky 2019). Adolescents in general think they do not need "professional" help and typically do not perceive themselves as having a problem. As an illustration, we provide the following example. Outside our offices, we have a poster with the title "This may be the most important quiz you take." Listed below the title are the characteristics of an adolescent with problem gambling exemplified by the DSM-IV-MR-J (Fisher 2000). At the bottom of the poster, it suggests that if the individual endorses five or more of nine gambling-related items, she or he may have a gambling problem. One young man, age 18 years, read the poster and reported he endorsed all the items but did not think he had a gambling problem, even though his parents, grandparents, girlfriend, and peers thought he had a problem.

Stages of Change

The first step in any therapeutic treatment approach is getting the individual to acknowledge a problem exists. To this end, DiClemente et al. (2000) suggested a transtheoretical model of intentional behavior change for adolescent problem gambling. The three dimensions of the transtheoretical model represent distinct aspects of the process of change. Based on earlier work by DiClemente and Prochaska (1982), the stages of change model represents the motivational, temporal, and developmental nature of the process of change. DiClemente and colleagues suggest that individuals move from precontemplation (not considering initiating change) to contemplation (seriously considering changing one's behavior) to preparation (a commitment and plan to change the behavior) to action (performing the actual behavior change) to maintenance (sustaining the behavior change over time) to termination (the point at which there is no longer a temptation to gamble). Adolescents often vary widely on this continuum when seeking treatment.

Psychosocial Interventions

A number of psychosocial interventions have been proposed for working with both adults and youth experiencing gambling problems or gambling disorder. The following represents several approaches for helping individuals experiencing gambling-related problems.

Self-Help Groups

Gamblers Anonymous (GA), with chapters established internationally, is the most common self-help group for individuals with gambling disorder, although more recently, multiple internet-based groups have emerged. Modeled on the work of Alcoholics Anonymous (AA) and primarily designed for adults, these self-help groups often welcome adolescents with gambling disorder. Despite widespread availability, GA may not resonate equally with all cultural groups (Potenza et al. 2019). GA is a 12-step fellowship program involving regular attendance at group meetings, with individuals having gambling disorder obtaining a "sponsor" with whom they maintain regular contact. Some chapters provide peer assistance with managing financial problems related to gambling. The basic premise is that gambling disorder are similar to other forms of addictive disorders, requiring considerable social support, and abstinence is the desired goal. Unfortunately, little research has been done examining GA's overall long-term efficacy, with even less research related to adolescents. Our clinical experience has shown that adolescents with gambling disorder have generally not fared well within GA self-help groups. This may be primarily because there are very few adolescent meetings and youth attending adult meetings typically do not perceive themselves as having the same severity (consequences) of their gambling behaviors as is found among long-term adult gamblers (e.g., they have not lost their home, job, or spouse; their financial indebtedness is generally lower).

Cognitive Therapies

Cognitive therapies primarily address gambling-related cognitive distortions, erroneous beliefs (e.g., one can control or predict outcomes of chance events), and the "gambler's fallacy" (winning is around the corner). Several studies (Abler et al. 2009; Grant et al. 2007; Nordin et al. 2007) incorporated randomized trials with individuals either receiving cognitive therapy focusing on correcting irrational thoughts or being assigned to a wait-list control group. The results suggest that although some benefits occurred in terms of reducing gambling-related urges and problems, there is no evidence that cognitive therapy yields long-term benefits or that cognitive-behavioral therapy (CBT) outcomes are better than those with other forms of treatment. A more recent systematic review of psychosocial treatments of gambling problems that used PRISMA to identify 21 randomized controlled trials (11 with multi-session, in-person therapies) reported that most therapies had short-term immediate benefits, yet few demonstrated long-term, sustained benefits (Sander and Peters 2009).

Cognitive-Behavioral Therapy

CBT has been reported to be the most common treatment approach for helping individuals with gambling problems (Potenza et al. 2019). CBT addresses the cognitive components associated with gambling (e.g., cognitive distortions, illusions of control, independence of events), along with addressing gambling-related emotions and cravings or urges, identifying external triggers for gambling, practicing alternative responses to triggers, and promoting alternatives to gambling [Grant and Kim 2001]). CBT approaches, although typically done in a traditional individual face-to-face context with a therapist, can also be done via online programs, telehealth, workbooks, or a combination of these (Carlbring and Smit 2008). Ledgerwood and Petry (2004), working with adults with gambling problems, provided an 8-week CBT approach delivered over the internet along with phone calls and email contacts. CBT, compared with a wait-list control group, was found to significantly reduce gambling-related problems during the sessions.

In yet another study, Petry et al. (2006) found that adults who participated in a CBT group (with or without support from GA) had significantly greater reductions in number of days gambling and fewer gambling-related problems than those assigned to only attend GA meetings. Petry et al. (2006) also noted that CBT gains were maintained throughout a 12-month follow-up. They also reported that professionally delivered CBT was superior to a CBT-based workbook group in terms of reducing the amount of money gambled. Patients who completed CBT, independent of the presentation format, reported better outcomes than the GA-meeting-only group, with face-to-face interactions being superior. Larimer et al (2012), using CBT, demonstrated reductions in illusions of control and gambling consequences.

In one of the few empirically based treatment studies with adolescents, Ladouceur et al. (1994), working with four adolescent male pathological gamblers, implemented a CBT program. Within their program, five components were included: information about gambling, cognitive interventions, problem-solving training, relapse prevention, and social skill training. Cognitive therapy was provided individually for approximately 3 months (mean, 17 sessions). Ladouceur et al. (1994) reported clinically significant improvements with respect to the individuals' beliefs about the perception of control when gambling and a significant reduction in the severity of gambling problems. One month after termination of treatment, one adolescent was reported to have relapsed. At 3 and 6 months after treatment, the remaining three adolescents had sustained therapeutic treatment gains and were abstinent, with none of the adolescents having symptoms that met the DSM criteria for pathological gambling at the last follow-up assessment. Ladouceur et al. (1994) concluded that the treatment duration necessary for adolescents was relatively short compared with that required for adults and that the positive gains resulting from CBT represent "promising new avenues for treatment." Ladouceur and his colleagues' therapeutic approach was predicated on the belief 1) that adolescents persist in their gambling behavior despite repeated losses as a result of their erroneous beliefs and perceptions and 2) that winning money is central to their continued efforts. Others have suggested that winning money may not be the central reason why adolescents get overly involved in gambling, but rather they do so for the excitement and physiological arousal derived from their gambling or they use gambling as a maladaptive way to cope with a host of mental health issues (Gupta and Derevensky 1998). It is important to note that in the Ladouceur et al. treatment study, the adolescents were reported to have no other mental health issues, a rare phenomenon among treatment samples.

Motivational Interviewing

Motivational interviewing (MI) is predicated on understanding and resolving ambivalence toward changing one's gambling behaviors. It is primarily guided by five principles: 1) expression of empathy (acceptance of the individual and recognition that one's ambivalence to changing one's behavior is normal); 2) the development and articulation of discrepancies among one's current behavior, goals, and self-image; 3) avoidance of confrontational situations; 4) understanding resistance (identifying opportunities to reinforce accurate perceptions rather than merely correcting inaccurate perceptions); and 5) support of the individual's ability to change (Miller and Rollnick 2002). Similar in some respects to the work of DiClemente et al. (2000), there is an understanding that many individuals fail to seek therapeutic interventions of their own accord, with a large number of individuals who do begin a program failing to complete treatment (Scherrer et al. 2005). A number of systematic reviews and meta-analyses have suggested that MI has been associated with a significant overall reduction in gambling (Yakovenko et al. 2015). Among college students, Larimer and colleagues (2012) reported that a single MI session was equally as effective as 4–6 weeks of CBT and suggested that patient populations with high rates of problem gambling would likely benefit from brief MI. Derevensky (2020) concluded that MI is relatively brief, easy to administer, and cost-effective and seemingly reduces the treatment dropout rate. Therefore, he suggested that this might be a useful approach with adolescents.

Pharmacological Treatment

Over the past 20 years, pharmacological approaches have been tested for the treatment of adults with problem gambling. One review and meta-analysis reported that across three types of medications (antidepressants, opiate antagonists, and mood stabilizers), individuals appeared to improve with medications relative to placebo or no-treatment groups (Potenza et al. 2019). Based on the available neurochemical, neurocognitive, and neuroimaging evidence for the pathophysiology of gambling disorder, several medications have been investigated: serotonergic antidepressants, lithium, glutamatergic agents, catechol-O-methyltransferase (COMT) inhibitors, neuroleptics, dopamine D_1 and D_2 receptor antagonists, and opioid receptor antagonists (Grant et al. 2012; Potenza et al. 2019). Although multiple studies have shown promising results for adults, other studies have shown no significant changes in behavior. Currently, no pharmacological agents have been approved in any country by a regulatory board for the express treatment of gambling disorder (Potenza et al. 2019), and very few trials are assessed for adolescents.

Online Forms of Treatment

Given that the vast majority of adolescents and young adults have access to a smartphone (95% of teens have access to a smartphone, and 45% report being online "almost constantly") (Pew Research Center 2018), there is an increased likelihood that youth can gamble online but also that they may use online chats or programs to help with gambling-related problems. The internet has rapidly become a major source of health information for adolescents and young adults (Gainsbury 2012). The high rates of internet use among adolescents and young adults have prompted trials of online interventions for a wide range of substance use and abuse problems. Gainsbury and Blaszczynski (2012) have argued that there are several reasons that online interventions may be potentially advantageous for reducing high-risk behaviors among youth. The benefits of computerized programs include increased self-disclosure due to confidentiality or anonymity reducing fears about being personally identifiable, a nonjudgmental approach, and the ability to access a large and vulnerable population in a cost-effective and confidential manner without issues related to travel and the potential discomfort of walking into a clinic or therapist's office. This type of intervention may encourage youth to seek treatment and divulge personally relevant information. Still further, online treatment allows individuals to access online screening instruments in private at their own convenience and receive automatic and personalized feedback.

A growing body of evidence suggests that brief online feedback that compares an individual's gambling behavior against normative behaviors results in significant behavioral changes. This approach attempts to modify a person's gambling behavior by facilitating a behavioral change through addressing misperceptions of typical gambling behaviors, as well as providing the individual with a look at their gambling behavior compared with actual norms (Celio and Lisman 2014; Lewis and Neighbors 2006). In fact, Grande-Gosende et al. (2019) found that the majority of prevention studies among college students incorporated a personalized normative feedback (PNF) approach. Many of these studies only used a single session to elicit a behavior change (Hopper 2008; Larimer et al. 2012; Neighbors et al. 2015). The principles of PNF have also been applied as a harm minimization strategy for adults participating in online casino gambling (Auer and Griffiths 2015, 2016). Derevensky and his colleagues at McGill University recently developed an application for smartphone use to help young adults track and modify their gambling behavior. Such approaches may also minimize treatment dropout rates among problem gamblers (Melville et al. 2007) while increasing the number of individuals seeking help.

McGill University's Treatment Approach

Our clinical experience suggests that for an adolescent with a gambling problem, a good day is when the money lasts all day while gambling. A bad day is when the same amount of money is lost quickly after only a short time. After all money is lost, their preexisting problems (e.g., parental, familial, academic, legal, vocational, mental health, peer, personal) reappear, with additional gambling-related financial problems only compounding existing problems. The initial claim by adolescents with gambling problems is that they gamble primarily for the excitement and enjoyment, with the goal of winning money also being a highly endorsed response. Yet in discussions with young problem gamblers, they quickly realize money won is used merely as a means to continue gambling. Even after a "big" win and recouping of losses, few adolescents with gambling problems can resist the urge to stop gambling. As one adolescent said, "There is nothing in the world that is as exciting as gambling to me, not drugs, not alcohol, or even sex."

The clinical treatment approach itself needs to be predicated on empirical research and clinical data. Ample research suggests that gambling problems frequently develop as a result of the need to escape other underlying problems (e.g., attentional problems, conduct disorder, oppositional defiant disorder, learning problems, anxiety disorders, poor problem solving and coping skills, relational and familial problems, low self-esteem, and legal difficulties) (Derevensky 2012). Therefore, it is important to address the mental health issues of youth. It is also important to note that some youths enter treatment immediately after stopping their gambling, requesting assistance in maintaining abstinence and dealing with the concomitant gambling-related problems.

The clinical information provided next, based on the empirical research, is designed to help practitioners and clinicians working with adolescents with serious gambling problems. A more thorough description can be found in a book chapter by Derevensky et al. (2011).

Intake assessment includes a semistructured interview covering the DSM-5 criteria for gambling disorder as well as other pertinent gambling behaviors (e.g., preferred activities, frequency, wagering patterns, accumulated losses). Questionnaires, screening instruments, and surveys provide information on the adolescent's current familial situation, academic or work status, social functioning, alcohol or drug use, risk-taking behaviors, self-esteem, coping skills, personality traits, levels of depression and anxiety, suicide ideation or attempts, and readiness for change.

The therapeutic process and fostering motivation for change include establishment of mutual trust, the client's acceptance of the problem, identification of underlying problems, psychotherapy addressing personal issues, understanding of the client's motivation for changing behavior, development of effective coping skills, restructuring of free time (sports and leisure activities), and development of a healthy lifestyle. Ensuring involvement of family members, using cognitive restructuring, dispelling illusions of control, acknowledging gambling "triggers," providing warning signs of gambling problems, and establishing a debt repayment plan (when necessary) are essential. Overarching goals for therapy are set at the beginning of treatment and are revised several times during the therapeutic process. Smaller weekly goals that are objective and measurable are also a crucial part of creating a space where clients can feel supported and motivated and can track progress through their healing process. It is important that goals be tailored to the client's priorities, gambling severity, and comorbid disorders. For example, a client with a comorbid personality or anxiety disorder is not approached in the same way as a client with gambling addiction without depressive symptomatology. In most cases, multiple therapeutic goals are addressed simultaneously over many sessions while tailoring the time allocated to each goal to the needs of the client.

After a youth has been identified as being a liar or thief among family members or friends, it becomes difficult for them to regain the trust of others and to resume healthy relationships. This becomes one of the more difficult challenges faced by problem gamblers. They have typically lied numerous times about having quit gambling; however, when they actually stop their gambling, they want to be trusted almost immediately. Although on a cognitive level, they understand the lack of trust by significant others, they have great difficulty with being repeatedly questioned as to their daily activities. We often remind youths that it took quite some time to destroy the trust and will likely take even longer to rebuild it. One parent asked his son to bring receipts for all expenses to help account for his money. This proved both embarrassing and difficult, such as when asking friends for a receipt when they purchased a coffee for him. This type of situation requires some intervention on behalf of the therapist. One needs to explain to family members and friends that these deceptive actions are part of the constellation of problematic behaviors exhibited by individuals who cannot control their gambling. Consequently, when the gambling is under control, family members and friends can anticipate being treated with honesty and respect. Family members, peers, and significant others become important support personnel to help ensure abstinence and can take an active role in relapse prevention. Youth with gambling problems are likely to be happier and more apt to abstain from gambling if they feel they belong to a peer group and are supported by family members and friends. As a result, the periodic inclusion of family members and friends in therapy sessions has proven to be beneficial. Nevertheless, the process of rebuilding relationships can be long and arduous and is often met with only partial success. Although this is highly dependent on circumstances, some friends or family members may not be willing to forgive the problem gambler or reestablish contact.

Adolescents struggling to overcome a gambling problem experience more positive outcomes when not faced with large amounts of unstructured time. Some adolescents in treatment are still in school or have a job, and thus their free time consists mainly of evenings and weekends. Others have dropped out of school and may have a part-time job, but others are not working. For these youth, structuring their time becomes paramount because they initially find it exceedingly difficult to resist urges to gamble when they are bored. We frequently ask adolescents to carry a notepad or use their smartphones to keep track of daily schedules. Spending time with friends or family and doing school- or work-related activities are beneficial. Other suggested activities include participating in organized sports activities, engaging in a hobby, watching movies, and performing volunteer work. Adolescents' weekly success is evaluated on how well they achieve weekly agreed-on goals, with their gambling-related behaviors (reduction or abstinence) being one part of the program. Thus, if an individual fails to meet his or her goals surrounding gambling behavior, he or she still may achieve success in other areas. This approach tends to help keep the clients from being discouraged and motivates them to attain a balanced lifestyle and to continue treatment.

Effective money management skills are typically lacking in adolescents who have a gambling problem. As such, therapeutic goals involve educating them as to the value of money (because they tend to lose perspective after gambling large sums), building money management skills, and helping them develop and maintain a reasonable debt repayment plan. Interestingly, problem gamblers often view purchases in terms of gambling expenses. When one teenager was asked the cost of traveling to the casino, he replied, "Half a hand." He went on further to explain that he typically waged $25 per hand on blackjack, and taxi fare to the casino was only $13. Having youths carry less money, in small denominations (carrying large bills enhances their stature and self-image as the "big shot"), is also important.

As previously noted, our clinical work suggests that abstinence from gambling is the optimal goal. Abstinence among our clinical sample reduces the likelihood of relapse of gambling problems. It should be noted that small, occasional relapses (we tend to refer to them as "slips") throughout the treatment process are to be expected. However, when gambling has ceased for an extended period of time (i.e., 6 months), an effective relapse prevention program should help individuals remain free of gambling.

Given that gambling treatment usually continues over an extended period of time, it is important to gradually end therapy. This allows adolescents to have increasingly longer stretches without therapeutic support during which they must autonomously take control of maintenance of therapeutic gains. Difficulties encountered during this phasing-out process provide useful information and can be dealt with while the adolescent is still actively engaged in therapy. Relapse prevention after termination may include continued access to their primary therapist for "booster" sessions, the existence of a good social support network, engagement in either school or work, the practice of a healthy lifestyle, and avoidance of powerful triggers. Youths are contacted periodically via telephone, text messages, or email for 1 year after treatment to ensure they are maintaining their abstinence and doing well in general. Where necessary, additional support is provided.

Conclusion

Treatment studies in general and adolescent treatment studies in particular have typically consisted of case studies and small sample sizes and have been criticized for not being subjected to rigorous scientific standards (Blaszczynski and Silove 1995; National Gambling Impact Study Commission 1999). With the exception of some online interventions, there are likely several reasons why more stringent criteria, scientifically validated methodological procedures, and experimental analyses concerning the efficacy of treatment programs for youth have not been implemented. Several plausible reasons include the following: 1) there are difficulties in attracting both adolescents in treatment and control groups; 2) adolescent gamblers are not a homogeneous group; 3) treatment program providers differ widely in terms of theoretical orientation and level of expertise; 4) high dropout rates are common; 5) age, gender, and severity of gambling and concomitant mental health disorders are important factors in the frequency, duration, and types of treatments provided; and 6) treatment programs for adolescents with multiple addictions require broader and likely different outcome measures.

The resulting treatment paradigms have in general incorporated a rather restrictive and narrow focus depending on one's theoretical treatment orientation (see Blaszczynski and Silove 1995 for their analyses of the limitations of each approach). Blaszczynski and Silove (1995) further suggest that there is ample empirical support for the supposition that gambling involves a complex and dynamic interaction among ecological, psychophysiological, developmental, cognitive, and behavioral components. Given this complexity, a plan to address each of these components should be adequately incorporated into a successful treatment paradigm. Although Blaszczynski and Silove addressed their concerns with respect to programs for adults with problem gambling, a similar multidimensional approach may be necessary to address the multitude of problems facing adolescent problem gamblers (Derevensky 2012).

Understanding that adolescents with gambling problems are not a homogeneous group suggests the importance of treatment flexibility. Although there are no empirically derived data showing effectiveness, clinical work suggests that at the very least short-term gains are possible. Problem gambling in adolescents varies in frequency, type of activity, and gambling severity. Those with severe gambling problems exhibit a number of dissociative behaviors that allow them to escape into another world, often with altered egos, and to repress unpleasant daily events. When gambling, adolescents report that all their problems disappear, albeit temporarily. They report that betting on the outcome of a sports event or watching the reels of an electronic gambling machine spin makes their adrenaline flow, their heart rate increase, and their excitement intensify. Interestingly, these same physiological responses are reported whether they win or lose (the near-miss phenomenon).

The McGill treatment program's outcome has not been formally empirically validated using the standards necessary for a rigorous, scientifically controlled study. As such, more clinical research is necessary before definitive conclusions can be drawn. Nevertheless, based on clinical criteria established for success (i.e., abstinence for 6 months after treatment; return to school or work; no longer meeting the DSM criteria for gambling disorder; improved peer and family relationships; improved coping skills; and no marked signs of depressive symptomatology, delinquent behavior, or excessive use of alcohol or drugs), the treatment program appears to have reached its goals and objectives in successfully working with youth with serious gambling problems.

Gambling problems among youth continue to raise important public health and social policy issues. With new technological forms of gambling (including social casino games and loot boxes) being developed, and gambling's increased availability, status as a recognized and socially acceptable form of entertainment, and ease of access, adolescents will continue to gamble, with an identifiable number getting into more severe gambling and gambling-related problems. Greater emphasis on outreach, awareness, and prevention programs remains essential. The lack of awareness concerning youth gambling problems among parents, educators, and mental health professionals is a concern. We have long argued that the search for best practices in the prevention and treatment of adolescent gambling problems is only beginning in earnest. Empirically validated prevention and treatment programs still require refinement and evaluation. Our governments have been the recipients of huge gambling-related revenues. There remains a need for funding for the prevention and treatment of gambling disorder. The prevention and treatment of problem gambling in young people is a complex, multidimensional process. As we have previously noted, the long-term benefits to the individual and society outweigh the immediate costs of funding such programs.

Youth gambling and problem gambling will not disappear on their own. Although there are many competing demands and concerns, the issues surrounding youth gambling should not be dismissed. Legislators, parents, and treatment providers have important roles in helping minimize problems.

References

Abler B, Hahlbrock R, Unrath A, et al: At-risk for pathological gambling: imaging neural reward processing under chronic dopamine agonists. Brain 132(9):2396–2402, 2009

Ariyabuddhiphongs V: Problem gambling prevention: before, during, and after measures. Int J Ment Health Addict 11(5):568–582, 2013

Auer M, Griffiths M: The use of personalized behavioral feedback for online gamblers: an empirical study. Front Psychol 6:1406, 2015

Auer M, Griffiths M: Personalized behavioral feedback for online gamblers: a real world empirical study. Front Psychol 7:1875, 2016

Black D, Shaw M: The epidemiology of gambling disorder, in Gambling Disorder. Edited by Heinz A, Romanczuk-Seiferth N, Potenza M. Berlin, Springer, 2019, pp 29–48

Blaszczynski A: Harm Minimization Strategies in Gambling: An Overview of International Initiatives and Interventions. Melbourne, Australian Gaming Council, 2001

Blaszczynski A, Silove D: Cognitive and behavioural therapies for pathological gambling. J Gambl Stud 11(2):195–220, 1995

Blinn-Pike L, Worthy S, Jonkman J: Adolescent gambling: a review of an emerging field of research. J Adolesc Health 47(2):223–236, 2010

Bullock S, Potenza M: Pathological gambling: neuropsychopharmacology and treatment. Curr Psychopharmacol 1(1):67–85, 2012

Calado F, Griffiths M: Problem gambling worldwide: an update and systematic review of empirical research (2000–2015). J Behav Addict 5(4):592–613, 2016

Calado F, Alexandre J, Rosenfeld L, et al: The efficacy of a gambling prevention program among high-school students. J Gambl Stud 36:573–595, 2020

Campbell C, Derevensky J, Meerkamper E, Cutajar J: Parents' perceptions of adolescent gambling: a Canadian national study. Journal of Gambling Issues 25:36–53, 2011

Carlbring P, Smit F: Randomized trial of internet-delivered self-help with telephone support for pathological gamblers. J Consult Clin Psychol 76(6):1090–1094, 2008

Castren S, Temcheff C, Derevensky J, et al: Teacher awareness and attitudes regarding adolescent risk behaviours: a sample of Finnish middle and high school teachers. Int J Ment Health Addict 15(2):295–311, 2017

Celio M, Lisman S: Examining the efficacy of a personalized normative feedback intervention to reduce college student gambling. J Am Coll Health 62(3):154–164, 2014

Delfabbro P, King D, Derevensky J: Adolescent gambling and problem gambling: prevalence, current issues and concerns. Curr Addict Rep 3(3):268–274, 2016

Derevensky J: Teen Gambling: Understanding a Growing Epidemic. New York, Rowman & Littlefield, 2012

Derevensky J: 24-Hour Problem Gambling Helpline Report (July 1, 2018–June 30, 2019). Sanford, FL, Florida Council on Compulsive Gambling, 2019

Derevensky J: The prevention and treatment of gambling disorders: some art, some science, in Cambridge Handbook of Substance and Behavioral Addictions. Edited by Sussman S. Cambridge, UK, Cambridge University Press, 2020, pp 241–253

Derevensky J, Gilbeau L: Adolescent gambling: another risky behavior, in Treating and Preventing Adolescent Mental Health Disorders: What We Know and What We Don't Know: A Research Agenda for Improving the Mental Health of Our Youth, 2nd Edition. Edited by Evans D, Foa E, Gur R, et al. New York, Oxford University Press, 2017, pp 571–584

Derevensky J, Gilbeau L: Preventing adolescent gambling problems, in Gambling Disorder. Edited by Heinz A, Romanczuk-Seiferth N, Potenza M. Berlin, Springer, 2019, pp 297–311

Derevensky J, Gupta R: Youth gambling prevention initiatives: a decade of research, in Youth Gambling Problems: The Hidden Addiction. Edited by Derevensky J, Shek D, Merrick J. Berlin, De Gruyter, 2011, pp 213–230

Derevensky J, Temcheff C, Gupta R: Treatment of adolescent gambling problems: more art than science? in Youth Gambling Problems: The Hidden Addiction. Edited by Derevensky J, Shek D, Merrick J. Berlin, De Gruyter, 2011, pp 167–186

Derevensky J, Gainsbury S, Gupta R, Ellery M: Play-for-Fun/Social Casino Gambling: An Examination of Our Current Knowledge. Winnipeg, MB, Canada, Manitoba Gambling Research Program, 2013

Dickson L, Derevensky J, Gupta R: The prevention of gambling problems in youth: a conceptual framework. J Gambl Stud 18(2):97–159, 2002

Dickson L, Derevensky J, Gupta R: Harm reduction for the prevention of youth gambling problems: lessons learned from adolescent high-risk behavior prevention programs. J Adolesc Res 19(2):233–263, 2004

Dickson-Gillespie L, Rugle L, Rosenthal R, Fong T: Preventing the incidence and harm of gambling problems. J Prim Prev 29(1):37–55, 2008

DiClemente C, Prochaska J: Self-change and therapy change of smoking behavior: a comparison of processes of change in cessation and maintenance. Addict Behav 7(2):133–42, 1982

DiClemente C, Story M, Murray K: On a roll: the process of initiation and cessation of problem gambling among adolescents. J Gambl Stud 16:289–313, 2000

Donati M, Primi C, Chiesi F: Prevention of problematic gambling behavior among adolescents: testing the efficacy of an integrative intervention. J Gambl Stud 30(4):803–818, 2014

Dowling N, Brown M: Commonalities in the psychological factors associated with problem gambling and Internet dependence. Cyberpsychol Behav Soc Netw 13(4):437–441, 2010

Emerson PV, Andes S, Bernhard B, et al: Call to Action—Addressing College Gambling: Recommendations for Science-Based Policies and Programs. Cambridge, MA, Task Force on College Gambling Policies, Cambridge Health Alliance, 2009

Engwall D, Hunter R, Steinberg M: Gambling and other risk behaviors on university campuses. J Am Coll Health 52(6):245–256, 2004

Ernst M, Nelson E, Jazbec S, et al: Amygdala and nucleus accumbens in responses to receipt and omission of gains in adults and adolescents. Neuroimage 25(4):1279–1291, 2005

Fisher S: Developing the DSM-IV-MR-J criteria to identify adolescent problem gambling in non-clinical populations. J Gambl Stud 16(2–3):253–273, 2000

Floros G: Gambling disorder in adolescents: prevalence, new developments and treatment challenges. Adolesc Health Med Ther 9:43–51, 2018

Gainsbury S: Internet Gambling: Current Research Findings and Implications. New York, Springer, 2012

Gainsbury S, Blaszczynski A: Online self-guided interventions for the treatment of problem gambling. Int Gambl Stud 11:289–308, 2012

Gainsbury S, King D, Delfabbro P, et al: The Use of Social Media in Gambling. Victoria, Australia, Gambling Research Australia, 2015

Galvan A, Hare T, Parra C, et al: Earlier development of the accumbens relative to orbitofrontal cortex might underlie risk-taking behavior in adolescents. J Neurosci 26(25):6885–6892, 2006

Grande-Gosende A, López-Núñez C, García-Fernández G, et al: Systematic review of preventive programs for reducing problem gambling behaviors among young adults. J Gambl Stud 36(1):1–22, 2019

Grant J, Kim S: Demographic and clinical features of 131 adult pathological gamblers. J Clin Psychiatry 62(12):957–962, 2001

Grant J, Kim S, Odlaug B: N-acetyl cysteine, a glutamate-modulating agent in the treatment of pathological gambling: a pilot study. Biol Psychiatry 62(6):652–657, 2007

Grant J, Odlaug B, Schreiber L: Pharmacological treatments in pathological gambling. Br J Clin Pharmacol 77:375–381, 2012

Gupta R, Derevensky J: Adolescent gambling behavior: a prevalence study and examination of the correlates associated with problem gambling. J Gambl Stud 14(4):319–345, 1998

Hansen M, Rossow I: Adolescent gambling and problem gambling: does the total consumption model apply? J Gambl Stud 24(2):135–149, 2008

Hardoon K, Gupta R, Derevensky J: Empirical vs perceived measures of gambling severity: why adolescents don't present themselves for treatment. Addict Behav 28:933–946, 2003

Hodgins D, Currie S, el-Guebaly N: Motivational enhancement and self-help treatments for problem gambling. J Consult Clin Psychol 69(1):50–57, 2001

Hodgins D, Stea J, Grant J: Gambling disorders. Lancet 378:1874–1884, 2011

Hollingshead S, Kim A, Wohl M, Derevensky J: The social casino gaming-gambling link: motivation for playing social casino games determines whether gambling increases or decreases. Journal of Gambling Issues 33:52–67, 2016

Hopper R: Brief electronic personalized normative feedback intervention for the prevention of problematic gambling among college students. Doctoral dissertation, Oklahoma State University, Stillwater, OK, 2008

Karlsson A, Håkansson A: Gambling disorder increased mortality suicidality and associated comorbidity: a longitudinal nationwide register study. J Behav Addict 7(4):1091–1099, 2018

Keen B, Blaszczynski A, Anjoul F: Systematic review of empirically evaluated school-based gambling education programs. J Gambl Stud 33(1):301–325, 2017

Kessler R, Hwang I, LaBrie R, et al: The prevalence and correlates of DSM-IV pathological gambling in the National Comorbidity Survey Replication. Psychol Med 38(9):1351–1360, 2008

Kim H, Wohl M, Salmon M, et al: Do social casino gamers migrate to online gambling: an assessment of migration rate and potential predictors. J Gambl Stud 31(4):1819–1831, 2015

Kourgiantakis T, Stark S, Lobo D, Tepperman L: Parent problem gambling: a systematic review of prevention programs for children. Journal of Gambling Issues 33:8–29, 2016

Ladouceur R, Boisvert J, Dumont J: Cognitive-behavioral treatment for adolescent pathological gambling. Behav Modif 18:230–242, 1994

Ladouceur R, Goulet A, Vitaro F: Prevention programmes for youth gambling: a review of the empirical evidence. Int Gambl Stud 13(2):141–159, 2013

Larimer M, Neighbors C, Lostutter T, et al: Brief motivational feedback and cognitive behavioral interventions for prevention of disordered gambling: a randomized clinical trial. Addiction 107(6):1148–1158, 2012

Ledgerwood D, Petry N: Gambling and suicidality in treatment-seeking pathological gamblers. J Nerv Ment Dis 192(10):711–714, 2004

Lewis M, Neighbors C: Social norms approaches using descriptive drinking norms education: a review of the research on personalized normative feedback. J Am Coll Health 54(4):213–218, 2006

Marchica L, Mills D, Derevensky J, Montreuil T: The role of emotion regulation in the etiology of video game and gambling disorders: a systematic review. Can J Addict 10(4):19–29, 2019

Melville K, Casey L, Kavanagh D: Psychological treatment dropout among pathological gamblers. Clin Psychol Rev 27(8):944–958, 2007

Messerlian C, Derevensky J: Youth gambling: a public health perspective. Journal of Gambling Issues 14:97–116, 2005

Messerlian C, Derevensky J, Gupta R: A public health perspective for youth gambling: a prevention and harm minimization framework. Int Gambl Stud 4:147–160, 2004

Miller W, Rollnick S: Motivational Interviewing: Preparing People for Change. New York, Guilford, 2002

Molinaro S, Canale N, Vieno A, et al: Country- and individual-level determinants of probable problematic gambling in adolescence: a multi-level cross-national comparison. Addiction 109(12):2089–2097, 2014

National Gambling Impact Study Commission: National Gambling Impact Study Commission Final Report. Chicago, National Opinion Research Center, 1999

National Research Council: Pathological Gambling: A Critical Review. Washington, DC, National Academies Press, 1999

Neighbors C, Rodriguez L, Rinker D, et al: Efficacy of personalized normative feedback as a brief intervention for college student gambling: a randomized controlled trial. J Consult Clin Psychol 83(3):500–511, 2015

Nordin C, Gupta R, Sjödin I: Cerebrospinal fluid amino acids in pathological gamblers and healthy controls. Neuropsychobiology 56(2–3):152–158, 2007

Nowak D, Aloe A: A meta-analytical synthesis and examination of pathological and problem gambling rates and associated moderators among college students, 1987–2016. J Gambl Stud 34(2):465–498, 2018

Oh B, Ong Y, Loo J: A review of educational-based gambling prevention programs for adolescents. Asian J Gambl Issues Public Health 7(1):4, 2017

Parke J, Wardle H, Rigbye J, Parke A: Exploring Social Gambling: Scoping Classification and Evidence Review. Technical Report, Birmingham, UK, Gambling Commission, 2012

Petry N, Ammerman Y, Bohl J, et al: Cognitive behavioral therapy for pathological gamblers. J Consult Clin Psychol 74:555–567, 2006

Petry N, Weinstock J, Morasco B, Ledgerwood D: Brief motivational interventions for college student problem gamblers. Addiction 104(9):1569–1578, 2009

Pew Research Center: Teens, social media & technology. Washington, DC, Pew Research Center, 2018. Available at: www.pewresearch.org/internet/2018/05/31/teens-social-media-technology-2018. Accessed May 3, 2020.

Potenza M, Balodis I, Derevensky J, et al: Gambling disorder. Nat Rev Dis Primers 5(1):1–21, 2019

Productivity Commission: Gambling. Productivity Commission Inquiry Report No 50. Canberra, ACT, Australia, Australian Government Productivity Commission, 2010

Sander W, Peters A: Pathological gambling: influence of quality of life and psychological distress on abstinence after cognitive-behavioral inpatient treatment. J Gambl Stud 25(2):253–262, 2009

Sansanwal R, Derevensky J, Gavriel-Fried B: What mental health professionals in Israel know and think about adolescent problem gambling. Int Gambl Stud 16:67–84, 2016

Scherrer J, Xian H, Shah K, et al: Effect of genes, environment, and lifetime co-occurring disorders on health-related quality of life in problem and pathological gamblers. Arch Gen Psychiatry 62(6):677–683, 2005

Schwartz DG: Roll the Bones: The History of Gambling. New York, Gotham Books, 2006)

Shaffer H, Hall M: Updating and refining prevalence estimates of disordered gambling behaviour in the United States and Canada. Can J Public Health 92:168–172, 2001

Shek D, Sun R: Prevention of gambling problems in adolescents: the role of problem gambling assessment instruments and positive youth development programs, in Youth Gambling Problems: The Hidden Addiction. Edited by Derevensky J, Shek D, Merrick J. Berlin, De Gruyter, 2011, pp 231–243

Slutske W: Natural recovery and treatment-seeking in pathological gambling: results of two U.S. national surveys. Am J Psychiatry 163:297–302, 2006

Slutske W, Blaszczynski A, Martin N: Sex differences in the rates of recovery treatment-seeking and natural recovery in pathological gambling: results from an Australian community-based twin survey. Twin Res Hum Genet 12:425–432, 2009

St-Pierre R, Derevensky J: Youth gambling behavior: novel approaches to prevention and intervention. Curr Addict Rep 3(2):157–165, 2016

St-Pierre R, Derevensky J, Temcheff C, et al: Evaluation of a school-based gambling prevention program for adolescents: efficacy of using the Theory of Planned Behaviour. Journal of Gambling Issues 36(6):113–137, 2017

Suurvali H, Hodgins D, Cunningham J, Toneatto T: Treatment seeking among Ontario problem gamblers: results of a population survey. Psychiatr Serv 59:1343–1346, 2008

Temcheff C, Derevensky J, St-Pierre R, et al: Beliefs and attitudes of mental health professionals with respect to gambling and other high risk behaviors in schools. Int J Ment Health Addict 12:716–729, 2014

Todirita R, Lupu V: Gambling prevention program among children. J Gambl Stud 29(1):161–169, 2013

Turner N, Macdonald J, Somerset M: Life skills, mathematical reasoning and critical thinking: a curriculum for the prevention of problem gambling. J Gambl Stud 24(3):367–380, 2008

U.K. Gambling Commission: Young People and Gambling. London, UK Gambling Commission, 2019

Volberg R, Nysse-Carris K, Gerstein D: California Problem Gambling Prevalence Survey: Final Report. Chicago, IL, University of Chicago, National Opinion Research Center, 2006

Volberg R, Gupta R, Griffiths M, et al: An international perspective on youth gambling prevalence studies. Int J Adolesc Med Health 22(1):3–38, 2010

Welte J, Barnes G, Tidwell M, Hoffman J: The prevalence of problem gambling among U.S. adolescents and young adults: results from a national survey. J Gambl Stud 24:119–133, 2008

Williams R, West B, Simpson R: Prevention of Problem Gambling: A Comprehensive Review of the Evidence and Identified Best Practices. Guelph, ONT, Canada, Ontario Problem Gambling Research Centre, 2012

Williams R, Hann R, Schopflocher D, et al: Quinte Longitudinal Study of Gambling and Problem Gambling 2015. Guelph, ONT, Canada, Ontario Problem Gambling Research Centre, 2015

Yakovenko I, Quigley L, Hemmelgarn B, et al: The efficacy of motivational interviewing for disordered gambling: systematic review and meta-analysis. Addict Behav 43:72–82, 2015

Zendle D: Is real-money video gaming just a form of gambling? Gaming Law Review 23(9):658–660, 2019

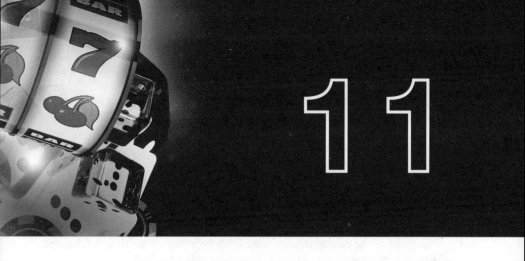

Psychosocial Treatments

Brad W. Brazeau, B.Sc.
David C. Hodgins, Ph.D.

Despite its high prevalence, as many as 85%–90% of individuals with gambling disorder do not seek or receive professional treatment (Petry et al. 2017), for reasons such as shame, stigma, and a desire to solve the problem independently (Hodgins 2005; Hodgins and el-Guebaly 2000). However, treatment-seeking behavior does tend to increase with problem gambling severity (Toneatto et al. 2008). Although approximately one-third of this population recovers naturally (Slutske 2006), the rest requires some form of treatment. Importantly, gamblers who do eventually seek treatment usually report having made previous attempts to change on their own, albeit unsuccessfully (Suurvali et al. 2009). This common change strategy, whereby gamblers address the problem independently before seeking professional treatment, serves as a guiding framework for stepped-care models.

Consistent with a stepped-care model of treatment for problem gambling (Figure 11-1; Hodgins and Schluter 2020), a multitude of interventions that vary in intensity have been developed. Lower-intensity interventions are intended to be minimally intrusive on gamblers' lifestyles yet allow for increasing intensity if necessary (Hodgins 2005). For example, if natural recovery fails (i.e., no intervention), gamblers have the option to progress to self-guided interventions (e.g., workbooks) or brief professional interventions (e.g., motivational interviews) before more intensive interventions (e.g., weekly cognitive-behavioral therapies) or inpatient programs are necessarily required. This model allows for treatment to be tailored to problem gamblers' individual needs without being overly intrusive or costly.

In addition to guiding treatment regimens of varying intensity, this model accounts for a number of other individual factors (Hodgins and Schluter 2020). For example, awareness messages, brief screening, and web-based advice can be targeted toward those who experience problem gambling as secondary to another issue (e.g., other mental health or addictive disorders). Similarly, awareness and support can be directed toward gamblers who are not ready to make changes even if it is their primary concern. Moreover, when individuals are ready to change, they can be matched to treatment based on factors other than problem severity. Such factors include self-efficacy, concurrent mental health and substance use disorders, and treatment goals, among others.

Although the "gold standard" of professional gambling treatment remains cognitive-behavioral therapy (CBT), a number of interventions continue to be developed and improved. A systematic search was conducted of multiple databases (e.g., PsycARTICLES, PubMed, Web of Science) based on PRISMA (Preferred Reporting Items for Systematic Reviews and Meta-Analyses) guidelines (Moher et al. 2009) using the MeSH terms and key words gambl* AND (treatment OR intervention OR therapy) AND random*. This search yielded 242 articles published within the previous 6 years (2014–2020). After text reviews, 26 articles were retained and are described throughout this chapter in combination with less recent but notable clinical trials.

Self-Directed Approaches

Considering the large proportion of gamblers who need but do not receive treatment, research into means of reaching this population without requiring face-to-face clinician contact has proliferated in recent years. These self-directed interventions generally take principles and strategies of established treatment approaches (e.g., CBT) and apply them to workbooks or online programs. Ironically, although gamblers tend to endorse these solutions for reasons such as confidentiality and accessibility (Rodda et al. 2013), their dropout rates remain much higher than for professional face-to-face interventions (van der Maas et al. 2019).

Bibliotherapy

Several self-directed workbooks for gambling disorder have been established (Petry and Hodgins 1999). Notably, Hodgins and Makarchuk (2002) developed a self-help workbook for gamblers based on CBT principles. The activities within the workbook are organized into four modules: self-assessment, goal set-

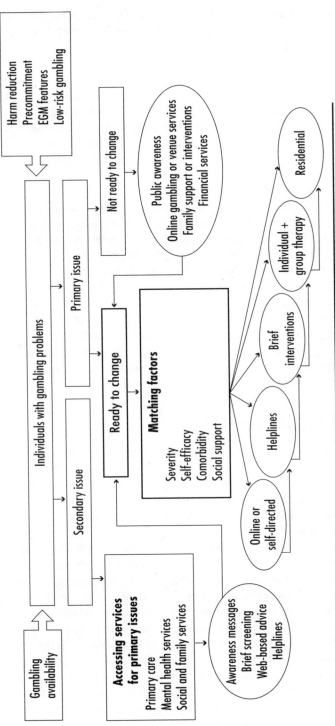

FIGURE 11–1. Stepped-care model of problem gambling interventions.

EGM = electronic gaming machine.

Source. Adapted from Hodgins and Schluter 2020.

ting, goal implementation, and goal maintenance. This particular workbook has demonstrated efficacy in multiple trials (e.g., Abbott et al. 2017; Hodgins et al. 2001, 2009). The efficacy of this workbook is maintained even without any therapist contact (e.g., motivational interviewing), although the effects are not as strong.

In the first trial examining the efficacy of Hodgins and Makarchuk's (2002) workbook, Hodgins and colleagues (2001, 2004) randomized 102 Canadian participants to one of three groups: workbook only, workbook plus telephone motivational interview, or a 4-week wait-list control condition. Follow-up assessments were conducted at 1, 3, 6, and 24 months. Results indicated that both the workbook-only and workbook plus motivational interview groups experienced reductions in gambling frequency and severity compared with the wait-list control group at all time points. These improved outcomes were more substantial for the workbook plus motivational interview group. Although still significant, group differences were smaller at 6- and 24-month follow-ups compared with 1- and 3-month follow-ups (Hodgins et al. 2001, 2004).

More recently, in Australia, Oei and colleagues (2018) conducted a trial with a different CBT-based workbook that they developed. Fifty-five community problem gamblers were randomized to either the workbook treatment group or the wait-list control group, with follow-up assessments occurring at 6 weeks. Posttreatment results for the workbook group demonstrated significant reductions in both gambling frequency and severity. Moreover, those in the workbook condition also experienced improvements in psychological well-being (i.e., declines in symptoms of depression, anxiety, and general distress).

Online Interventions

Access to the internet continues to expand, and with that comes the growth of internet gambling. MacKay (2011) estimated that more than 2,400 gambling websites were created between 1995 and 2011 and suggested that online gambling would, in turn, proliferate as well. However, the internet has also served as an important platform through which to offer a variety of new self-directed gambling interventions.

In Italy, Canale and colleagues (2016) randomly assigned 168 adolescents to either a control condition (personalized feedback) or an experimental condition (personalized feedback plus online training). The online training consisted of interactive educational activities such as games, quizzes, and trivia related to gambling issues (i.e., prevalence, cognitive distortions, myths and facts) that were designed to increase engagement and awareness. Results indicated decreases in gambling problems, but not gambling frequency or expenditures, for the experimental condition at 2 months. For frequent gamblers in particular, those in the intervention group experienced a reduction in gambling problems and frequency compared with the control group. Additionally, frequent gamblers in the control group reported significantly less realistic attitudes regarding the profitability of gambling compared with the intervention group at 2 months. Although the authors concluded that web-based interventions appear effective, they cautioned against providing personalized feedback in isolation to frequent gamblers.

In a pilot trial, Cunningham et al. (2019a) examined the efficacy of a self-guided online CBT-based gambling intervention compared with no intervention. The online intervention was based on previously developed workbook modules (Hodgins and Makarchuk 2002) that had been demonstrated to be efficacious in several trials (e.g., Abbott et al. 2017; Hodgins et al. 2001, 2009). A large sample of American and Canadian participants ($n=321$) was recruited via Mechanical Turk and individuals were randomly assigned to either the intervention or control group, with follow-up assessments conducted at 6 weeks and 6 months. Unexpectedly, both the intervention and control groups showed large improvements, and no improvements were observed in the intervention group above and beyond those observed in the control group. However, the authors posited that the null findings could have resulted from a number of issues, such as the choice to recruit from a crowdsourcing platform and the power analysis calculations based on a targeted medium effect size difference between the groups.

In a subsequent trial, Hodgins et al. (2019) compared the efficacy of the same online intervention used by Cunningham et al. (2019a) with a brief online self-assessment tool. The online assessment tool provided both personalized and normative feedback in addition to suggestions for gambling reduction or abstinence. Hodgins et al. (2019) recruited 181 Canadians who were not interested in formal treatment via advertisements and randomly assigned them to one of the two online conditions. Follow-up assessments were conducted at 3, 6, and 12 months postbaseline. Although both groups demonstrated reductions in gambling frequency and severity, no differential improvements were observed between the two groups. The authors encourage future research to examine attractiveness, uptake, and effectiveness of similar online interventions, both in isolation and with supplemental therapist guidance.

Taken together, the results of these recent online clinical trials show promise. However, some questions have yet to be answered. For example, it is unclear whether certain types of online interventions are superior to others (e.g., personalized or normative feedback, CBT-based interventions). Additionally, the optimal role of professional guidance and support, and the degree to which it should be utilized, have yet to be determined. Finally, future research should also explore what characteristics of problem gamblers facilitate behavioral change in different types of online interventions.

Brief Approaches

When self-guided interventions are not enough, gambling problems can often be effectively addressed with brief treatment approaches. Brief interventions aim to minimize the intensity of treatment and tend to consist of a single session. At first glance, it might be assumed that more sessions would be superior to a single session. However, this is not always the case. In an effort to compare brief treatments with extended treatments, Toneatto (2016) randomly assigned 99 problem gamblers from the community to receive one of four treatments: six sessions of either cognitive therapy, behavioral therapy, or motivational therapy or a single-session intervention consisting of nonspecific practical advice and support. Results at the 12-month follow-up demonstrated improvement for all treatment groups but no differential improvement between groups in terms of gambling frequency, severity, and expenditures. These preliminary findings suggest that brief interventions may be as successful as more extensive interventions.

Motivational Interviewing

A popular approach to the treatment of addictive disorders is motivational interviewing. This treatment strategy is grounded in the stages of change model (Miller and Rollnick 2012), which posits that behavioral changes are facilitated by motivational states. With problem gambling, the goal of motivational interventions is to encourage gamblers' commitment to change by raising awareness of consequences, reducing ambivalence, clarifying core values, and analyzing the pros and cons of changing (Toneatto 2016). This type of intervention can be extended over multiple sessions but is most often provided in the context of a single session.

Diskin and Hodgins (2009) examined the efficacy of a brief motivational intervention by randomly assigning 81 Canadian participants to one of two groups: a single-session motivational interview or a control standard clinical assessment interview. The motivational interview was based on the principles described earlier, while the face-valid control interview included assessment with the Structured Clinical Interview for DSM-IV (SCID-II; First et al. 1997). Both the treatment and control groups experienced reductions in gambling severity. More important, 12-month follow-up data indicated that those in the motivational treatment condition reported more reductions in gambling frequency, expenditures, and psychological distress than those in the control group. The results of this study indicate that a single-session motivational interview can serve as a beneficial brief intervention for problem gamblers.

Although motivational interviews show promise when provided in isolation, they are commonly and effectively provided to supplement other treatment strategies. For example, a trial described earlier in this chapter (Hodgins et al. 2001, 2004) compared the efficacy of a CBT-based workbook with the same workbook plus a single-session motivational interview. The findings demonstrated greater improvement for those in the workbook plus motivational interview group in terms of gambling frequency, severity, and expenditures. Moreover, these differential gains appear to have been maintained at 2 years postbaseline. The results of this trial imply that although the use of self-directed workbooks can be successful, their benefits can be enhanced with the addition of a single motivational interview.

Considering the incremental benefit of a single motivational interview when provided in addition to a self-directed CBT-based workbook, Hodgins et al. (2009) examined whether the provision of multiple booster interviews would be more beneficial than a single interview. They randomly assigned 314 Canadian problem gamblers to one of four groups: wait-list control, CBT-based workbook only, workbook plus motivational interview (BT), or workbook plus motivational interview plus six booster interviews (BBTs). Although results for the original three treatment conditions resembled the earlier trial (Hodgins et al. 2001, 2004), no incremental improvement was observed in the BBT group at 12 months compared with the BT group that did not receive booster interviews. This study provides further evidence that brief treatment (e.g., a single motivational interview) can be just as efficacious as more prolonged treatments (e.g., several motivational interviews).

As outlined in the stepped-care model (Hodgins and Schluter 2020), different subpopulations of problem gamblers may benefit from different degrees of treatment intensity. In contrast to Hodgins et al. (2009), Abbott and colleagues (2018) found that the provision of booster motivational interviews did improve outcomes over and above those of a self-directed workbook and a single motivational interview session, but only for certain subgroups. Specifically, the group in this trial that received booster interviews had greater treatment goal success if their baseline problem gambling severity and psychological distress were high. Additionally, the same subgroups in this treatment condition experienced differential reductions in days gambled and dollars lost compared with the other treatment conditions when they had a goal of gambling reduction rather than abstinence. These findings emphasize the need to consider gamblers' baseline characteristics when matching them to appropriate interventions.

Gambler Helplines

Until recently, the effectiveness of gambler helplines has not been evaluated despite their availability in many countries. In New Zealand, Abbott et al. (2018) randomly assigned 462 problem gamblers to one of four conditions: a single motivational interview (MI), a single motivational interview plus a cognitive-behavioral self-help workbook (MI + W), a single motivational interview plus a cognitive-behavioral self-help workbook plus four booster follow-up telephone interviews (MI + W + B), or a gamblers' helpline treatment-as-usual (TAU) control condition. Overall results indicated significant reductions in days gambled per month across all groups at the 3-month follow-up, with these reductions generally maintained at 6- and 12-month follow-ups. Reductions in proportion of gamblers meeting criteria for problem gambling were observed as well, with 95%–97% meeting criteria at baseline and 55%–67% meeting criteria at 12 months. Abbott et al. (2018) also found that TAU performed as well as MI in terms of reductions in days gambled. Importantly, they also found that MI + W did not perform better than MI or TAU. However, there was evidence for the superiority of MI + W + B with certain subgroups, as described earlier. These findings imply that helpline interventions may be as effective as other brief approaches, depending on the gambler subpopulation receiving treatment.

Personalized Feedback

A number of trials have examined the effectiveness of interventions that provide gamblers with personalized feedback. This feedback usually entails a summary of the gambler's current problem severity and often includes comparisons with a normative sample. In one trial, Celio and Lisman (2014) randomly assigned 136 American college students to receive either an intervention providing personalized normative feedback about their gambling (PNF) or to complete an attention-control task. Risk-taking behavior tasks were administered to measure outcomes. At the 1-week follow-up, those in the PNF group demonstrated significantly reduced risk-taking performance compared with the control group. The authors suggested that personalized normative feedback interventions may serve as an effective standalone strategy to combat problem gambling in the short term. Similar findings were observed by multiple subsequent trials (e.g., Martens et al. 2015; Neighbors et al. 2015).

More recently, Jonsson et al. (2019, 2020) compared data from 1,788 Norwegian high-expenditure problem gamblers offered personalized feedback by either letter or telephone to those in a control condition. Follow-up results at 12 months demonstrated a reduction in theoretical loss of 30% in the telephone group compared with 13% in the letter group and 7% in the control group. These findings imply that although personalized written feedback may be beneficial, these effects can be enhanced by providing personalized feedback over the phone instead.

Interestingly, the provision of individualized feedback may be as effective as more extensive professional treatments for some gamblers (Yakovenko and Hodgins 2016). In a trial mentioned earlier, Toneatto (2016) found that gamblers who received assessment feedback via telephone, in combination with provided handouts describing practical advice and strategies, improved just as much as those in the other, extended treatment conditions (cognitive, behavioral, or motivational therapy). Improvements were observed across a number of outcomes, including frequency of gambling, symptom severity, and expenditures. Taken together, the findings of these trials show promise in terms of offering personalized feedback as a brief standalone intervention for problem gambling.

Mindfulness-Based Interventions

A relatively new approach to treating problematic gambling is mindfulness-based intervention. These treatments, although unique in many aspects, all focus on the reduction of experiential avoidance via meditation and relaxation techniques. Experiential avoidance occurs when an individual is reluctant or unwilling to experience unpleasant internal events, such as bodily sensations, thoughts, or emotions. To avoid these experiences, problem gamblers often take steps to escape or dissociate from them by engaging in gambling behaviors (Riley 2014). Although the number of studies in this domain is limited, a recent systematic review and meta-analysis (Maynard et al. 2018) demonstrated promising results in terms of reducing gambling symptoms, behaviors, and expenditures.

In Australia, McIntosh et al. (2016) compared the efficacy of a standard CBT-based treatment carried out in isolation with the same treatment administered in combination with a four-session mindfulness-based intervention. Seventy-seven problem gamblers were randomly assigned to one of the treatment groups. Although no group differences in gambling behavior per se were observed, those who also received mindfulness-based treatment did experience a greater improvement in subjective quality of life and greater decrease in thought suppression and rumination. The authors suggest that mindfulness-based approaches can serve as a useful adjunct to traditional gambling therapies to improve transdiagnostic factors such as ruminative tendencies.

Cognitive and Behavioral Approaches

Cognitive Therapy

Cognitive models of gambling disorder view the condition as stemming from a combination of fallacies and erroneous beliefs. These cognitive distortions are particularly evident in slot machine players, whose verbalizations while gambling are irrational at least 80% of the time (Walker 1992). Such verbalizations directed at the slot machines often include statements such as "You owe me!" and "I'm due for a win." These statements, among others, are evidence of significant cognitive distortions present in problem gamblers.

According to Toneatto (2002), a number of cognitive distortions are commonly observed in problem gamblers. These distortions include a sense of magnified gambling skill (e.g., exaggerated confidence despite losses), superstitious beliefs (e.g., belief that mental states or rituals can increase chances of winning), attributional biases (e.g., viewing losses as indications that a win is imminent), selective memory (e.g., selective recall of wins), sense of control over luck (e.g., belief that luck can be enhanced in certain settings), probability biases (e.g., faulty beliefs about randomness), and illusory correlations (e.g., belief that wins are causally related to external unrelated events). To summarize, Joukhador et al. (2003) classified gambling-related cognitive distortions as either primary illusory control (i.e., beliefs that gambling outcomes can be controlled) or secondary illusory control (i.e., beliefs that gambling outcomes can be predicted).

Cognitive interventions place primary emphasis on addressing erroneous beliefs as a means of reducing problem gambling behavior. These interventions operate by first raising awareness of cognitive distortions and then challenging and restructuring irrational thought patterns. To raise awareness, Toneatto (2002) suggested asking gamblers Socratic questions such as how they explain their wins and losses. When challenging irrational thoughts, therapists can help gamblers question the accuracy of their beliefs. It can help to provide educational information as well, such as principles of probability (e.g., each outcome is independent of the previous outcomes on a slot machine).

Toneatto and Gunaratne (2009) reviewed a number of trials examining the efficacy of cognitive therapies compared with other interventions for problem gambling. Although significant improvements were found across the board in terms of gambling frequency and severity, there was no evidence for the superiority of an explicit focus on cognitive distortions. In fact, brief and multimodal interventions were found to be just as effective as, if not more effective than, cognitive therapy in isolation. The results of this review suggest that although cognitive therapies do benefit problem gamblers, other interventions may be more justifiable when expanding their focus beyond cognitive distortions alone.

Cognitive-Behavioral Therapy

CBT remains the most commonly studied professional approach for problematic gambling (Cowlishaw et al. 2012; Petry et al. 2017; van der Maas et al. 2019). This model builds on cognitive therapies and conceptualizes gambling addiction as a combination of thought distortions, maladaptive behaviors, and inappropriate coping strategies (Sharpe and Tarrier 1993). According to Sharpe (2002), problem gambling is triggered by internal and external cues, which lead to physiological arousal and gambling-related cognitive distortions. The presence of healthy coping skills can inhibit gambling behaviors despite urges to gamble and thus serves as a primary focus of cognitive-behavioral interventions.

A central tenet of cognitive-behavioral therapies is the emphasis on triggers that precede gambling episodes. Such triggers can be internal (e.g., negative affect or boredom) or external (e.g., available cash or interpersonal conflict), and gamblers are encouraged to increase awareness of their common personal triggers and to develop strategies to avoid or cope with them. Coping includes cognitive strategies (e.g., cognitive restructuring, challenging cognitive distortions, self-talk) and behavioral strategies (e.g., assertiveness, controlling easy access to money). Gamblers learn to plan ahead for high-risk situations and to learn and deploy new skills.

Although most CBT interventions are delivered using a combination of cognitive and behavioral techniques, Smith and colleagues (2015) sought to examine the differential efficacy of cognitive and behavioral components in isolation. They randomly assigned 99 treatment-seeking Australian gamblers to receive either a cognitive intervention or a behavioral (exposure-based) intervention. Findings indicated that both groups experienced a reduction in gambling symptoms at 1, 3, and 6 months, but no significant differences between groups were observed. The authors concluded that both cognitive and behavioral therapies in isolation appear equally effective. Importantly, however, it remains unclear if the benefits of these therapies alone persist for the long term. Additionally, comparison of these two therapies to an integrated CBT is warranted.

More recently, Casey and colleagues (2017) examined the effectiveness of an internet-based CBT program compared with monitoring, feedback, and support for Australian problem gamblers. Participants (n = 174) were randomly assigned to one of three conditions: 1) internet-based CBT (I-CBT); 2) internet-based monitoring, feedback, and support (I-MFS); or 3) a wait-list control condition. Both the I-CBT and I-MFS groups experienced a significant reduction in gambling severity compared with the wait-list control group. However, those in the I-CBT group demonstrated benefits above and beyond both other groups, including reductions in gambling urges, cognitive distortions, and psychological distress. Additionally, the I-CBT group reported higher treatment satisfaction and overall life satisfaction. The authors concluded that CBT's incremental benefit over nonspecific feedback and support also translates to online media.

Despite the clear success of many gambling-focused CBT trials, few studies have examined whether these benefits translate to real-world clinical practice. One such study (Smith et al. 2018) compared the outcomes of 51 gamblers in a CBT randomized controlled trial (RCT) with those of 269 gamblers receiving routine CBT in the community. Their findings suggest that, on the whole, CBT delivered in clinical practice results in outcomes equally as robust as those in controlled trials.

Other Approaches

In addition to professional interventions, other solutions are available to problem gamblers, such as Gamblers Anonymous (GA), voluntary self-exclusion, and couples therapy.

Gamblers Anonymous

Since 1957, GA has served as the most popular intervention for problem gambling internationally (Petry 2005). Generally speaking, it mirrors similar 12-step programs (e.g., Alcoholics Anonymous) in that it provides social, moral, and practical support in a group setting. This support typically involves positive reinforcement for abstaining from gambling (e.g., encouragement, certificates). Although it is not theoretically grounded or delivered by clinicians, gamblers frequently endorse

GA for its accessibility and provision of social support. The fact that attendance is free serves as another attractive feature. However, despite its popularity, the efficacy of GA remains unclear because of the lack of RCTs (Schuler et al. 2016).

In the trials that have been conducted, GA does appear to successfully encourage abstinence for gamblers that have high attendance and engagement (Schuler et al. 2016). A major barrier to this success is that many gamblers, even when referred, do not attend more than a single session of GA. Petry et al. (2006) randomly assigned 231 gamblers to one of three conditions: GA referral only, GA referral plus CBT workbook, or GA referral plus eight sessions of individual face-to-face CBT. At the 12-month follow-up, results indicated that approximately half of the participants in all groups did not attend even one GA session. Importantly, higher attendance in all groups was associated with greater improvements in gambling symptom severity. Those in the GA-only group did not experience symptom improvements as large or long-lasting as those in the other two groups. However, no group differences were observed in proportion of gamblers deemed abstinent or showing substantially reduced gambling at 12 months. Taken together, the findings of this trial suggest that GA may be as effective as CBT in reducing frequency of gambling behaviors but not severity of symptoms.

Voluntary Self-Exclusion

In France, Caillon and colleagues (2019) randomly assigned 60 problem gamblers to either an experimental or control condition. Those in the experimental condition were asked to engage in voluntary self-exclusion from internet gambling sites for one week. Although no differences in gambling-related behaviors or cognitions were observed at 15 days, the authors noted declines in specific gambling-related cognitions (illusion of control, perceived inability to stop gambling, desire to gamble) at 2 months for the experimental condition only. Caillon et al. (2019) concluded that although some cognitive distortions were successfully addressed, voluntary self-exclusion may serve better as a treatment supplement than as a standalone strategy. Additionally, they suggest that longer self-exclusion periods may be more beneficial. However, further research is necessary to solidify these results.

Couples Therapy

Few gambling intervention trials have expanded to include gamblers' concerned significant others (CSOs). In one such trial, Nilsson et al. (2019) randomly assigned 136 couples to receive either CBT or behavioral couples therapy (BCT). Both treatments were provided online and entailed self-help modules along with telephone and email support from a therapist. Whereas the CBT intervention was provided exclusively to the problem gamblers, the BCT intervention included both gamblers and CSOs. The BCT intervention, though grounded in cognitive-behavioral principles, also focused on strategies for healthy relationship functioning. Although no significant differences in gambling outcomes were observed between the two groups, Nilsson et al. (2019) did find that commencement of and adherence to treatment was higher for the BCT group. These findings suggest that although the inclusion of a CSO may not improve gambling outcomes per se, this may be a way of increasing treatment adherence.

Unresolved Issues

Although interventions for gambling disorder continue to develop and expand, a number of unresolved issues remain. These include 1) whether self-directed treatment should be professionally guided, 2) how gambling disorder should be addressed when comorbid conditions are present, 3) whether group or individual treatment is more efficacious or effective, 4) whether treatments should focus on abstinence or reduction of gambling as a treatment goal, and 5) whether there are common elements underlying addictive disorders and associated treatments.

Guided vs. Unguided Self-Directed Treatment

Whether or not self-directed treatments should be guided by a professional continues to be debated. On one hand, treatment dropout rates tend to be higher when no clinician contact is involved (Goslar et al. 2017). On the other hand, problem gamblers often endorse a preference for little to no interaction with a professional during the recovery process (Gainsbury and Blaszczynski 2011). It is likely that the relative success of guided versus unguided self-directed interventions is dependent on certain gambler characteristics (e.g., symptom severity, individual preferences, whether or not they are actively seeking treatment).

In France, Luquiens and colleagues (2016) recruited 992 non-treatment-seeking gamblers from the gambling website Winamax. Participants were randomly assigned to one of four groups: a wait-list control group, a personalized feedback group, a CBT workbook group, or a group receiving the same CBT workbook plus personalized guidance via email from a trained psychologist. Follow-up data were assessed at 6 weeks (i.e., the end of treatment) and 12 weeks (i.e., maintenance period). Although all groups demonstrated extremely high attrition rates, the group receiving the workbook plus guidance experienced significantly higher dropout than the other groups. Notably, all groups showed decreases in problem gambling severity, but no groups improved significantly more than any others. Luquiens et al. (2016) concluded that for non-treatment-seeking gamblers, the drawbacks of therapist guidance may actually outweigh the intended benefits.

In contrast to Luquiens et al. (2016), a number of trials examining self-directed workbooks either alone or in combination with motivational interviewing have demonstrated that therapist guidance can have an incremental benefit. As described earlier in this chapter, multiple trials (e.g., Hodgins et al. 2001, 2004, 2009) have compared the efficacy of Hodgins and Makarchuk's (2002) workbook in isolation with the same workbook paired with a motivational interview. All of these trials have demonstrated that although the self-directed intervention is efficacious, the benefits can be enhanced with the provision of brief therapist support. Taken together, the findings of Luquiens et al. (2016) and Hodgins et al. (2001, 2004, 2009) stress that more research is warranted in this area. Specifically, future research should examine which subgroups of problem gamblers benefit from the provision of professional guidance and which do not.

Treatment in the Context of Concurrent Disorders

Problem gambling often manifests in combination with other psychological disorders. The most common comorbid disorders among those with gambling disorder are mood disorders (49%–56%), anxiety disorders (41%–60%), alcohol use disorder (73%), and drug use disorder (38%; Rash et al. 2016). Notably, the onset of comorbid psychiatric illnesses precedes problem gambling approximately 74% of the time (Kessler et al. 2008). Moreover, among people with gambling disorder, individuals with comorbid disorders tend to have greater problem gambling severity than those without comorbid disorders (Yakovenko and Hodgins 2018). This underscores the importance of appropriately responding to comorbidities in the context of gambling treatments. A recent scoping review (Yakovenko and Hodgins 2018) revealed that surprisingly few randomized trials of gambling treatment report either rates of comorbid disorders in their participants or the impact of comorbid disorders on outcomes. Our review uncovered a few exceptions.

In Germany, Bucker and colleagues (2018) randomly allocated 140 participants with comorbid problem gambling and mood dysfunction to one of two conditions: an online cognitive-behavioral depression-focused intervention or a wait-list control condition. Results indicated that those in the intervention experienced a greater reduction in gambling severity as well as gambling-related cognitive distortions compared with the wait-list control group. This study suggests that interventions targeting comorbid conditions can also improve problematic gambling.

In Canada, Cunningham et al. (2019b) randomly assigned 214 treatment-seeking problem gamblers with co-occurring mental health symptoms to one of two groups. Both groups received access to an online intervention for problem gambling, but only one group additionally received access to an online intervention for concurrent psychological distress (i.e., symptoms of depression and anxiety). The findings of this study demonstrated that participants in both groups experienced reductions in both gambling and co-occurring mental health symptoms. These results suggest that the provision of mood and anxiety interventions may not lead to benefits over and above those seen in gambling treatments alone.

In Brazil, Penna et al. (2018) randomly assigned 59 problem gamblers to either an aerobic exercise program (intervention) or an active stretching program (control). Both programs involved two sessions per week for a period of 8 weeks. Gambling symptoms, as well as psychiatric comorbidities, were assessed. Although both groups experienced a reduction in gambling symptoms at 8 weeks, no group differences were observed. However, those in the intervention group were three times more likely than those in the control group to be absent any psychiatric comorbidities after program completion. The findings of this study imply that an aerobic exercise program may serve as a useful adjunct to primary gambling treatment to reduce comorbid psychiatric symptoms.

Because alcohol use disorder is the most common comorbid disorder among those with gambling disorder (Dowling et al. 2015), it is important to examine whether the presence of this comorbidity impacts the outcome of gambling treatments. Indeed, one trial identified that gamblers with concurrent risky alcohol habits experienced a differential reduction in gambling severity with motivational interviewing compared with cognitive-behavioral group therapy (CBGT). Conversely, gamblers without comorbid alcohol use disorder had better outcomes with CBGT compared with motivational interviewing (Josephson et al. 2016). These findings highlight the need to consider concurrent disorders in the treatment of problem gambling regardless of whether treatment actually addresses comorbidities.

Group vs. Individual Treatment

Group therapy can generally be provided with fewer therapy resources per client, and it also offers clients peer support. However, relatively few studies have looked specifically at the superiority of either individual or group therapy. In one such study, Dowling et al. (2007) found that 92% of their participants in individual CBT no longer met criteria for gambling disorder at follow-up, compared with 60% in group CBT. Subsequently, Oei et al. (2010) found that although both individual- and group-delivered CBT effectively reduced gambling frequency and severity, the effect sizes were larger for those who received one-on-one therapy. Taken together, these studies suggest that although both modes of delivery are effective, individual therapy is superior to group therapy. However, they do not address the question of cost-effectiveness and whether the lower cost of group therapy compensates for its lower efficacy. Perhaps gamblers with different characteristics might be better suited to one versus the other, and this remains an area for future research.

Treatment Goals: Abstinence vs. Moderation

One of the more contentious unresolved issues in the gambling literature is whether treatment goals should focus on abstinence or moderation. Traditionally, abstinence has been favored. For example, GA requires complete cessation of all forms of gambling. However, it has been argued that strict abstinence goals may discourage gamblers from seeking treatment, and flexibility in goal selection may be desirable (Petry 2005).

Stea et al. (2015) conducted a secondary analysis of data from an RCT examining brief motivational treatments for problem gambling. In this trial, participants were asked to select their own goals (i.e., abstinence or moderation) before commencing treatment. The findings indicated that those who selected an abstinence-based goal gambled significantly fewer days than those who selected a moderation-based goal. Importantly, however, no differences in terms of total expenditures, average daily expenditures, or perceived goal achievement were observed. In sum, the results of this analysis do not provide support for the superiority of abstinence-based goals. Stea et al.'s (2015) conclusions were further supported by a more recent trial by Abbott et al. (2018), who found that those with a gambling moderation goal experienced a larger reduction in days gambled and dollars lost at 12 months compared with those with a gambling abstinence goal.

Search for Common Elements Underlying Addictive Disorders and Associated Treatments

An interesting line of research that has relevance to providing gambling treatment examines common change strategies across different types of gamblers and types of treatments. Rodda and colleagues have analyzed the content of single-session counseling transcripts (Rodda et al. 2017), posts on online support forums (Rodda et al. 2018a) and web forums (Rodda et al. 2015), and the published descriptions of treatment models (Rodda et al. 2018b). There are numerous commonalities in the processes of change among these diverse sources of information. The same authors also administered a comprehensive list of 99 change strategies abstracted from previous research to current and past problem gamblers to assess frequency of use and perceived effectiveness (Rodda et al. 2018c). The strategies represented 15 different empirically derived categories. The most effective categories were all cognitive in nature and were used by more than 90% of the gamblers. These were cognitive motivators (e.g., reminding self of negative consequences of gambling), feedback on gambling effects (e.g., calculating money and time spent gambling), advance planning (e.g., planning ahead and limiting money carried), urge management (e.g., distracting self), and well-being strategies (e.g., healthy eating). Treatment providers may wish to incorporate these strategies into their psychological interventions.

Another trend in the mental health treatment literature is the development of transdiagnostic treatment models that target underlying common elements for groups of diagnostic disorders (Fairburn et al. 2009; Wilamowska et al. 2010). The Component Model of Addiction Treatment is designed to focus on both substance use and behavioral addictions, including gambling (Kim and

Hodgins 2018, 2021). The common elements are pragmatically derived based upon the availability of evidence-based approaches to modify them and include lack of motivation, urgency, maladaptive expectancies, deficits in self-control, deficits in social support, and compulsivity, as well as their potential intervention possibilities. Although the components are established as enduring but malleable across different addictions, validation of the integrated treatment model is continuing.

Conclusion

The gambling literature has significantly evolved over the past couple of decades, but more research is warranted. Most important, future research should investigate whether guided or unguided self-directed treatment is superior, as well as which treatment goal is most conducive to successful recovery. Additionally, more research should explore which characteristics of problem gamblers impact outcomes of various interventions. No single treatment program is likely to benefit all gamblers. Thus, having a variety of evidence-based interventions available to gamblers is crucial. Grounding these treatments in a stepped-care model allows professionals to meet gamblers where they are in their recovery journeys.

References

Abbott M, Bellringer M, Vandal A, et al: Effectiveness of problem gambling in a service setting: a protocol for a pragmatic randomised controlled clinical trial. BMJ Open 7(3):e013490, 2017

Abbott M, Hodgins DC, Bellringer M, et al: Brief telephone interventions for problem gambling: a randomized controlled trial. Addiction 113:883–895, 2018

Bucker L, Bierbrodt J, Hand I, et al: Correction: Effects of a depression-focused internet intervention in slot machine gamblers: a randomized controlled trial. PLoS One 13:e0203145, 2018

Caillon J, Grall-Bronnec M, Perrot B, et al: Effectiveness of at-risk gamblers' temporary self-exclusion from internet gambling sites. J Gambl Stud 35:601–615, 2019

Canale N, Vieno A, Griffiths MD, et al: The efficacy of a web-based gambling intervention program for high school students: a preliminary randomized study. Comp Human Behav 55:946–954, 2016

Casey LM, Oei TPS, Raylu N, et al: Internet-based delivery of cognitive behaviour therapy compared to monitoring, feedback and support for problem gambling: a randomised controlled trial. J Gambl Stud 33:993–1010, 2017

Celio MA, Lisman SA: Examining the efficacy of a personalized normative feedback intervention to reduce college student gambling. J Am Coll Health 62:154–164, 2014

Cowlishaw S, Merkouris S, Dowling NA, et al: Psychological therapies for pathological and problem gambling. Cochrane Database Syst Rev 11:CD008937, 2012

Cunningham JA, Godinho A, Hodgins DC: Pilot randomized controlled trial of an online intervention for problem gamblers. Addict Behav Rep 9:100175, 2019a

Cunningham JA, Hodgins DC, Mackenzie CS, et al: Randomized controlled trial of an internet intervention for problem gambling provided with or without access to an internet intervention for co-occurring mental health distress. Internet Interv 17:100239, 2019b

Diskin KM, Hodgins DC: A randomized controlled trial of a single session motivational intervention for concerned gamblers. Behav Res Ther 47:382–388, 2009

Dowling NA, Smith DP, Thomas T: A comparison of individual and group cognitive-behavioural treatment for female pathological gambling. Behav Res Ther 45:2192–2202, 2007

Dowling NA, Cowlishaw S, Jackson AC, et al: Prevalence of psychiatric co-morbidity in treatment-seeking problem gamblers: a systematic review and meta-analysis. Aust N Z J Psychiatry 49:519–539, 2015

Fairburn CG, Cooper Z, Doll HA, et al: Transdiagnostic cognitive-behavioral therapy for patients with eating disorders: a two-site trial with 60-week follow-up. Am J Psychiatry 166:311–319, 2009

First M, Gibbon M, Spitzer R, et al: Structured Clinical Interview for DSM-IV Axis II Personality Disorders. Washington, DC, American Psychiatric Press, 1997

Gainsbury S, Blaszczynski A: Online self-guided interventions for the treatment of problem gambling. Int Gambl Stud 11:289–308, 2011

Goslar M, Leibetseder M, Muench HM, et al: Efficacy of face-to-face versus self-guided treatments for disordered gambling: a meta-analysis. J Behav Addict 6:142–162, 2017

Hodgins DC: Implications of a brief intervention trial for problem gambling for future outcome research. J Gambl Stud 21:13–19, 2005

Hodgins DC, el-Guebaly N: Natural and treatment-assisted recovery from gambling problems: a comparison of resolved and active gamblers. Addiction 95:777–789, 2000

Hodgins DC, Makarchuk K: Becoming a Winner: Defeating Problem Gambling: A Self-Help Manual for Problem Gamblers. Calgary, AB, Addictive Behaviours Laboratory, University of Calgary, 2002

Hodgins DC, Schluter MG: The role of treatment in reducing gambling-related harm, in Harm Reduction for Problem Gambling: A Public Health Approach. Edited by Bowden-Jones H, Dickson C, Dunand C, Simon OH. London, Taylor & Francis, 2020, pp 102–111

Hodgins DC, Currie SR, el-Guebaly N: Motivational enhancement and self-help treatments for problem gambling. J Cons Clin Psychol 69:50–57, 2001

Hodgins DC, Currie SR, el-Guebaly N, Peden N: Brief motivational treatment for problem gambling: a 24-month follow-up. Psychol Addict Behav 18:293–296, 2004

Hodgins DC, Currie SR, Currie G, Fick GH: Randomized trial of brief motivational treatments for pathological gamblers: more is not necessarily better. J Consult Clin Psychol 77:950–960, 2009

Hodgins DC, Cunningham JA, Murray R, Hagopian S: Online self-directed interventions for gambling disorder: randomized controlled trial. J Gambl Stud 35:635–651, 2019

Jonsson J, Hodgins DC, Munck I, Carlbring P: Reaching out to big losers: a randomized controlled trial of brief motivational contact providing gambling expenditure feedback. Psychol Addict Behav 33:179–189, 2019

Jonsson J, Hodgins DC, Munck I, Carlbring P: Reaching out to big losers leads to sustained reductions in gambling over 1 year: a randomized controlled trial of brief motivational contact. Addiction 115(8):1522–1531, 2020

Josephson H, Carlbring P, Forsberg L, Rosendahl I: People with gambling disorder and risky alcohol habits benefit more from motivational interviewing than from cognitive behavioral group therapy. PeerJ 4:e1899, 2016

Joukhador J, Maccallum F, Blaszczynski A: Differences in cognitive distortions between problem and social gamblers. Psychol Rep 92:1203–1214, 2003

Kessler RC, Hwang I, Labrie R, et al: The prevalence and correlates of DSM-IV pathological gambling in the National Comorbidity Survey Replication. Psychol Med 38:1351–1360, 2008

Kim HS, Hodgins DC: Component Model of Addiction Treatment: a pragmatic transdiagnostic treatment model of behavioral and substance addictions. Front Psychiatry 9:406, 2018

Kim HS, Hodgins DC: The transdiagnostic mechanisms of behavioral addictions and their treatment, in Textbook of Addiction Treatment: International Perspectives, 2nd Edition. Edited by el-Guebaly N, Carra G, Galanter M, Baldacchino AM. Milan, Springer, 2021, pp 911–927

Luquiens A, Tanguy M-L, Lagadec M, et al: The efficacy of three modalities of internet-based psychotherapy for non–treatment-seeking online problem gamblers: a randomized controlled trial. J Med Internet Res 18:e36, 2016

MacKay T-L: Problem Gambling Risk Factors in Internet and Non-Internet Gamblers. Calgary, Alberta, University of Calgary, 2011

Martens MP, Arterberry BJ, Takamatsu SK, et al: The efficacy of a personalized feedback-only intervention for at-risk college gamblers. J Consult Clin Psychol 83:494–499, 2015

Maynard BR, Wilson AN, Labuzienski E, Whiting SW: Mindfulness-based approaches in the treatment of disordered gambling: a systematic review and meta-analysis. Res Soc Work Pract 28:348–362, 2018

McIntosh CC, Crino RD, O'Neill K: Treating problem gambling samples with cognitive behavioural therapy and mindfulness-based interventions: a clinical trial. J Gambl Stud 32:1305–1325, 2016

Miller WR, Rollnick S: Motivational Interviewing: Helping People Change, 3rd Edition. New York, Guilford, 2012

Moher D, Liberati A, Tetzlaff J, Altman DG: Preferred reporting items for systematic reviews and meta-analyses: the PRISMA statement. Ann Intern Med 151:264–269, 2009

Neighbors C, Rodriguez LM, Rinker DV, et al: Efficacy of personalized normative feedback as a brief intervention. J Consult Clin Psychol 83:500–511, 2015

Nilsson A, Magnusson K, Carlbring P, et al: Behavioral couples therapy versus cognitive behavioral therapy for problem gambling: a randomized controlled trial. Addiction 115(7):1330–1342, 2019

Oei TPS, Raylu N, Casey LM: Effectiveness of group and individual formats of a combined motivational interviewing and cognitive behavioral treatment program for problem gambling: a randomized controlled trial. Behav Cogn Psychother 38:233–238, 2010

Oei TPS, Raylu N, Lai WW: Effectiveness of a self-help cognitive-behavioural treatment program for problem gamblers: a randomised controlled trial. J Gambl Stud 34:581–595, 2018

Penna AC, Kim HS, de Brito AMC, Tavares H: The impact of an exercise program as a treatment for gambling disorder: a randomized controlled trial. Ment Health Phys Act 15:53–62, 2018

Petry NM: Gamblers Anonymous and cognitive-behavioral therapies for pathological gamblers. J Gambl Stud 21:27–33, 2005

Petry NM, Hodgins DC: Cognitive and behavioral treatments, in Pathological Gambling: A Clinical Guide to Treatment. Edited by Grant JE, Potenza, MN. Washington, DC, American Psychiatric Publishing, 1999, pp 169–187

Petry NM, Ammerman Y, Bohl J, et al: Cognitive-behavioral therapy for pathological gamblers. J Consult Clin Psychol 74:555–567, 2006

Petry NM, Ginley MK, Rash CJ: A systematic review of treatments for problem gambling. Psychol Addict Behav 31:951–961, 2017

Rash CJ, Weinstock J, van Patten R: A review of gambling disorder and substance use disorders. Subst Abuse Rehabil 7:3–13, 2016

Riley B: Experiential avoidance mediates the association between thought suppression and mindfulness with problem gambling. J Gambl Stud 30:163–171, 2014

Rodda SN, Lubman DI, Dowling NA, et al: Web-based counseling for problem gambling: exploring motivations and recommendations. J Med Internet Res 15:e99, 2013

Rodda SN, Lubman DI, Cheetham A, et al: Single session web-based counselling: a thematic analysis of content from the perspective of the client. Br J Guid Counc 43:117–130, 2015

Rodda SN, Hing N, Hodgins DC, et al: Change strategies and associated implementation challenges: an analysis of online counselling sessions. J Gambl Stud 33:955–973, 2017

Rodda SN, Bagot KL, Cheetham A, et al: Types of change strategies for limiting or reducing gambling behaviors and their perceived helpfulness: a factor analysis. Psychol Addict Behav 32:679–688, 2018a

Rodda SN, Hing N, Hodgins DC, et al: Behaviour change strategies for problem gambling: an analysis of online posts. Int Gambl Stud 18:420–438, 2018b

Rodda SN, Merkouris SS, Abraham C, et al: Therapist-delivered and self-help interventions for gambling problems: a review of contents. J Behav Addict 7:211–226, 2018c

Schuler A, Ferentzy P, Turner NE, et al: Gamblers Anonymous as a recovery pathway: a scoping review. J Gambl Stud 32:1261–1278, 2016

Sharpe L: A reformulated cognitive-behavioral model of problem gambling: a biopsychosocial perspective. Clin Psychol Rev 22:1–25, 2002

Sharpe L, Tarrier N: Towards a cognitive-behavioural theory of problem gambling. Br J Psychiatry 162:407–412, 1993

Slutske WS: Natural recovery and treatment-seeking in pathological gambling: results of two U.S. national surveys. Am J Psychiatry 163:297–302, 2006

Smith DP, Battersby MW, Harvey PW, et al: Cognitive versus exposure therapy for problem gambling: randomised controlled trial. Behav Res Ther 69:100–110, 2015

Smith DP, Fairweather-Schmidt AK, Harvey PW, Battersby MW: How does routinely delivered cognitive–behavioural therapy for gambling disorder compare to "gold standard" clinical trial? Clin Psychol Psychother 25:302–310, 2018

Stea JN, Hodgins DC, Fung T: Abstinence versus moderation goals in brief motivational treatment for pathological gambling. J Gambl Stud 31:1029–1045, 2015

Suurvali H, Cordingley J, Hodgins DC, Cunningham JA: Barriers to seeking help for gambling problems: a review of the empirical literature. J Gambl Stud 25:407–424, 2009

Toneatto T: Cognitive therapy for problem gambling. Cogn Behav Pract 9:191–199, 2002

Toneatto T: Single-session interventions for problem gambling may be as effective as longer treatments: results of a randomized control trial. Addict Behav 52:58–65, 2016

Toneatto T, Gunaratne M: Does the treatment of cognitive distortions improve clinical outcomes for problem gambling? J Contemp Psychother 39:221–229, 2009

Toneatto T, Cunningham JA, Hodgins DC, et al: Recovery from problem gambling without formal treatment. Addict Res Theory 16:111–120, 2008

van der Maas M, Shi J, Elton-Marshall T, et al: Internet-based interventions for problem gambling: scoping review. J Med Internet Res 6:e65, 2019

Walker MB: Irrational thinking among slot machine players. J Gambl Stud 8:245–261, 1992

Wilamowska ZA, Thompson-Hollands J, Fairholme CP, et al: Conceptual background, development, and preliminary data from the unified protocol for transdiagnostic treatment of emotional disorders. Depress Anxiety 27:882–890, 2010

Yakovenko I, Hodgins DC: Latest developments in treatment for disordered gambling: review and critical evaluation of outcome studies. Curr Addict Rep 3:299–306, 2016

Yakovenko I, Hodgins DC: A scoping review of co-morbidity in individuals with disordered gambling. Int Gambl Stud 18:143–172, 2018

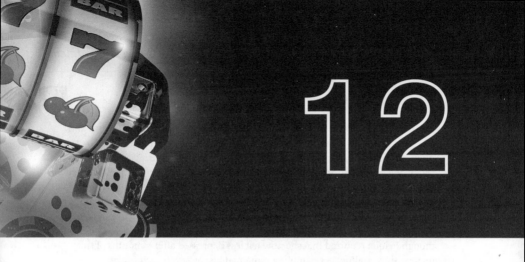

12

Pharmacological Treatments

Jon E. Grant, M.D., M.P.H., J.D.
Samuel R. Chamberlain, M.B./B.Chir., Ph.D., MRCPsych

Gambling disorder, characterized by persistent and recurrent maladaptive patterns of gambling behavior, is associated with impaired functioning and reduced quality of life (Hodgins et al. 2011). Financial and marital problems are common (Grant and Kim 2001). Many individuals with gambling disorder engage in illegal behavior, such as stealing, embezzlement, and writing bad checks, to fund their gambling (Potenza et al. 2000). Gambling disorder frequently co-occurs with other psychiatric disorders, including mood, anxiety, and substance use disorders, as well as ADHD (Lorains et al. 2011; Petry et al. 2005), and is associated with worse overall health (Pietrzak et al. 2007). Gambling disorder appears to follow a similar trajectory to substance dependence, with high rates in adolescent and young adult groups, lower rates in older adults, and periods of abstinence and relapse (Leeman and Potenza 2012). The similarities between gambling disorder and substance use disorders have led to gambling disorder's classification together with substance use disorders in DSM-5 and have in turn intimated at various pharmacological interventions for gambling disorder.

Case Vignette

Eriqua is a 29-year-old woman with a 4-year history of gambling problems and a 12-year history of cigarette smoking. Although initially reluctant to seek treatment for gambling, she was encouraged by her partner to see a psychiatrist because her gambling problem had led to large family debts. The psychiatrist noted that Eriqua was already receiving sertraline, which had been prescribed by her family doctor for depression. On closer questioning, it was found that the consequences of gambling had led to depressed mood and that Eriqua had not mentioned the gambling to her family doctor because of a sense of shame. Although Eriqua reported that she now felt less depressed after 6 months of treatment with sertraline, her gambling remained just as severe as it previously had been. After discussion of the treatment options and benefits and risks, Eriqua commenced treatment with N-acetylcysteine (NAC) as an add-on to her sertraline. After NAC treatment for 3 months and psychotherapy, including imaginal desensitization, her gambling symptoms were greatly improved. She also reported that she found herself smoking cigarettes less than before even though smoking had not been an explicit focus of the psychological treatment approach.

Pharmacological Treatment

Several medications have been investigated as treatments for gambling disorder (Table 12–1). These have included antidepressants (particularly serotonin reuptake inhibitors [SRIs]), glutamate modulators, opioid antagonists, and mood-stabilizing agents. Multiple open-label studies using various medications for short periods of time (8–14 weeks) have demonstrated efficacy in approximately 70%–75% of subjects with gambling disorder. Given the fairly high placebo response rate typically observed in gambling disorder (51%) (Grant and Chamberlain 2017), these open-label results must be viewed with caution. Double-blind, placebo-controlled studies may offer more guidance on appropriate interventions for gambling disorder. Twenty-one double-blind, placebo-controlled pharmacotherapy studies have also been performed in gambling disorder, but the results of these studies have demonstrated mixed efficacy and tolerability.

Antidepressants

Hypotheses underlying the examination of antidepressant medications for gambling are based on the neurobiology of gambling disorder and other impulse control disorders. Low levels of the serotonin metabolite 5-hydroxyindole acetic acid (5-HIAA) and blunted serotonergic response within the ventromedial prefrontal cortex (vmPFC) have been putatively associated with impulsive behaviors (Virkkunen et al. 1995). Individuals with gambling disorder demonstrate diminished activation of the vmPFC when viewing gambling-related videotapes or during the inhibition of responses when performing the Stroop color-word interference task (Potenza et al. 2003a, 2003b). Individuals with

TABLE 12–1. Double-blind, placebo-controlled pharmacotherapy trials for gambling disorder

Reference	Medication	Design/duration	Subjects	Mean daily dose (±SD)	Outcome
Antidepressants					
Hollander et al. 1992	Clomipramine	Parallel design 10 weeks	1 enrolled 1 completer	125 mg	90% improvement in gambling symptoms on medication
Saiz-Ruiz et al. 2005	Sertraline	Parallel design 6 months	60 enrolled 44 completers	95 mg	Similar improvement in both groups
Hollander et al. 2000	Fluvoxamine	Crossover 16 weeks with a 1-week placebo lead-in	15 enrolled 10 completers	195 mg (±50)	Fluvoxamine superior to placebo
Blanco et al. 2002	Fluvoxamine	Parallel design 6 months	32 enrolled 13 completers	200 mg	Fluvoxamine not statistically significantly differentiated from placebo
Kim et al. 2002	Paroxetine	Parallel design 8 weeks with 1-week placebo lead-in	53 enrolled 41 completers	51.7 mg (±13.1)	Paroxetine group significantly improved compared with placebo

TABLE 12–1. Double-blind, placebo-controlled pharmacotherapy trials for gambling disorder *(continued)*

Reference	Medication	Design/duration	Subjects	Mean daily dose (±SD)	Outcome
Antidepressants *(continued)*					
Grant et al. 2003	Paroxetine	Parallel design 16 weeks	76 enrolled 45 completers	50 mg (±8.3)	Paroxetine and placebo groups demonstrated comparable improvement
Grant and Potenza 2006	Escitalopram	Open-label (12 weeks) with responders randomized to 8 weeks parallel-design escitalopram or placebo	13 enrolled, all with co-occurring anxiety disorder and gambling disorder	25.4 mg (±6.6)	Open-label reductions in anxiety and gambling; improvements appear to persist with active but not placebo drug
Black et al. 2007	Bupropion	Parallel design 12 weeks	39 enrolled 22 completers	324 mg	Bupropion and placebo groups demonstrated similar symptom improvement

TABLE 12–1. Double-blind, placebo-controlled pharmacotherapy trials for gambling disorder *(continued)*

Reference	Medication	Design/duration	Subjects	Mean daily dose (±SD)	Outcome
Opioid antagonists					
Kim et al. 2001	Naltrexone	Parallel design 12 weeks with 1-week placebo lead-in	89 enrolled 45 completers	188 mg (±96)	Naltrexone group significantly improved compared with placebo
Grant et al. 2008a	Naltrexone	Parallel design 18 weeks with 1-week placebo lead-in (50 mg, 100 mg, 150 mg naltrexone vs. placebo)	77 enrolled 49 completers	Combined groups; no specific efficacious dose noted	Naltrexone group significantly improved compared with placebo on gambling and psychosocial function
Toneatto et al. 2009	Naltrexone	Parallel design 11 weeks Gambling with alcohol comorbidity; all subjects received cognitive-behavioral therapy	58 enrolled 32 completers	100 mg (±59.4)	No differences between groups

TABLE 12–1. Double-blind, placebo-controlled pharmacotherapy trials for gambling disorder (continued)

Reference	Medication	Design/duration	Subjects	Mean daily dose (±SD)	Outcome
Opioid antagonists (continued)					
Kovanen et al. 2016	Naltrexone as needed	Parallel design 20 weeks	101 enrolled 69 completers	50 mg, taken two to three times per week on average	No differences between groups (placebo was taken more often than naltrexone)
Grant et al. 2006	Nalmefene	Parallel design 16 weeks	207 enrolled 73 completers	Fixed-dose study	Nalmefene 25 mg and 50 mg significantly improved symptoms compared with placebo
Grant et al. 2010	Nalmefene	Parallel design 16 weeks	233 enrolled 126 completers	Fixed-dose study (20 mg, 40 mg, or placebo)	Initial analysis revealed no differences; post-hoc analysis: 40-mg group significantly improved compared with placebo group

TABLE 12–1. Double-blind, placebo-controlled pharmacotherapy trials for gambling disorder (*continued*)

Reference	Medication	Design/duration	Subjects	Mean daily dose (±SD)	Outcome
Glutamate modulators					
Grant et al. 2007	*N*-acetylcysteine (NAC)	Open-label with responders randomly assigned to 6-week, parallel-design NAC or placebo	27 enrolled 23 completers	1,476.9 mg (±311.3)	NAC group had significant gambling symptom improvement in open-label phase; sustained in double-blind phase
Grant et al. 2014	NAC with imaginal desensitization	Parallel design 12 weeks	28 individuals with gambling disorder and nicotine dependence enrolled	1,200 mg to 3,000 mg	NAC + imaginal desensitization group significantly improved compared with placebo group
Mood-stabilizing agents					
Hollander et al. 2005	Lithium carbonate SR	Parallel design 10 weeks	40 patients with bipolar spectrum disorder enrolled; 29 completers	1,170 mg (±221)	Lithium group significantly improved compared with placebo group

TABLE 12–1. Double-blind, placebo-controlled pharmacotherapy trials for gambling disorder *(continued)*

Reference	Medication	Design/duration	Subjects	Mean daily dose (±SD)	Outcome
Mood-stabilizing agents *(continued)*					
Berlin et al. 2013	Topiramate	Parallel design 14 weeks	42 enrolled 27 completers	222.5 mg (±108.5)	No differences between groups
de Brito et al. 2017	Topiramate	Parallel design 12 weeks Both groups received a brief cognitive intervention	38 enrolled 30 completers	180.7 mg (±95.5)	Topiramate > placebo in reducing gambling craving, time and money spent gambling, cognitive distortions, and social adjustment
McElroy et al. 2008	Olanzapine	Parallel design 12 weeks	42 enrolled 25 completers	8.9 mg (±5.2)	Similar reductions in gambling symptoms in olanzapine and placebo groups
Fong et al. 2008	Olanzapine	Parallel design 7 weeks	23 enrolled 21 completers	2.5 mg to 10 mg	Similar reductions in gambling symptoms in olanzapine and placebo groups

gambling disorder also show relatively diminished activation of the vmPFC during a simulated gambling task, and severity of gambling problem correlated inversely with signal intensity within this brain region (Reuter et al. 2005). In addition, levels of serotonin type 1B receptor in the ventral striatum have been associated with problem gambling severity (Potenza et al. 2013). Taken together, the findings suggest that drugs targeting serotonin neurotransmission may hold promise for the treatment of gambling disorder.

Of the 21 double-blind, placebo-controlled pharmacological studies of gambling disorder, seven have examined SRIs. Clomipramine, an SRI that also inhibits norepinephrine reuptake, was the first SRI tested in a controlled fashion for gambling. Hollander et al. (1992) reported a response to clomipramine in a single subject using a double-blind, placebo-controlled design. After receiving placebo for 10 weeks without response, the woman reported a 90% improvement in gambling symptoms after being treated with 125 mg/day of clomipramine. Interestingly, there have been no further controlled studies of clomipramine to confirm the limited results of this initial study. In addition to its more common side effects (dry mouth, constipation, sexual dysfunction), clomipramine may also cause cardiac conduction problems and has significant drug-drug interactions.

In a double-blind, placebo-controlled study using sertraline, 60 subjects with pathological gambling were treated for 6 months (mean dose=95 mg/day) (Saiz-Ruiz et al. 2005). At the end of the study, 23 sertraline-treated subjects (74%) and 21 placebo-treated subjects (72%) were rated as responders based on the primary outcome measure (Criteria for Control of Pathological Gambling Questionnaire), indicating that active treatment did not differentiate from placebo.

Only two SRIs have been examined in at least two randomized, placebo-controlled trials of gambling disorder. A double-blind, 16-week crossover study of fluvoxamine in 15 subjects demonstrated a statistically significant difference compared with placebo (Hollander et al. 2000). Interpretation of the study is complicated, however, because the medication did not separate from placebo during the first phase but did in the second phase. A later study of fluvoxamine in 32 gamblers, with a duration of 6 months, failed to show statistical significance compared with placebo. This study's results are complicated by high rates of treatment discontinuation (only three subjects on medication completed the study) (Blanco et al. 2002).

Paroxetine has similarly resulted in mixed outcomes for gambling disorder. An initial 8-week double-blind, placebo-controlled study indicated paroxetine's potential efficacy as a treatment for gambling disorder (Kim et al. 2002). A larger multicenter, double-blind, placebo-controlled trial of paroxetine for gambling disorder, however, failed to reproduce the results, as 48% of those assigned to receive placebo and 59% of those taking paroxetine were considered responders (Grant et al. 2003).

Participants with gambling disorder and co-occurring anxiety were treated with 12 weeks of open-label escitalopram followed by 8 weeks of double-blind escitalopram or placebo for those who responded during the open-label phase. Escitalopram was significantly more beneficial for both gambling and anxiety than placebo (Grant and Potenza 2006).

Although the majority of double-blind trials of antidepressants have focused on SRIs, one study examined bupropion, a dopaminergic medication, in a group of subjects ($n=18$) treated for 12 weeks (mean dose=324 mg/day) and a placebo group ($n=21$) (Black et al. 2007). Both groups showed similar reductions in gambling symptoms, with 35.7% of those on medication responding compared with 47.1% of those assigned to placebo.

In summary, the antidepressant medications have resulted in mixed outcomes for gambling disorder. What guidance do these studies provide? First, antidepressants might be useful for gamblers who have co-occurring anxiety or depressive symptoms driving their gambling behavior. Second, there might be a subtype of gambling disorder that responds to antidepressants, although it is currently unclear what that might look like. Finally, it may be that certain antidepressants with dual mechanisms, such as clomipramine, may be beneficial, but these have yet to be examined in well-powered trials.

Opioid Antagonists

Opioid receptor antagonists inhibit dopamine release in the nucleus accumbens and ventral pallidum through the disinhibition of gamma-aminobutyric acid (GABA) input to the dopamine neurons in the ventral tegmental area (Broekkamp and Phillips 1979; Phillips and LePiane 1980; van Wolfswinkel and van Ree 1985). Individuals with gambling disorder have demonstrated differences in nucleus accumbens activation during a simulated gambling task (Reuter et al. 2005), though imaging this relatively small region can be challenging. Although modulation of drive and subsequent behavioral output by dopamine, endorphin, and GABA have been investigated, the specific mechanisms underlying opioid receptor antagonism in those with gambling disorder remain poorly understood.

In the initial 12-week study of naltrexone in 45 participants with gambling disorder, the drug demonstrated superiority to placebo in reducing gambling symptoms using a mean dose of 188 mg/day (Kim et al. 2001). A separate analysis of subjects with at least moderate urges to gamble revealed that naltrexone was more effective in gamblers with more severe urges to gamble. A follow-up 18-week naltrexone study in 77 subjects confirmed the findings of the initial study (Grant et al. 2008a). Subjects assigned to take naltrexone had significantly greater reductions in gambling urges and gambling behavior compared with subjects taking placebo.

Two other studies, however, have questioned these initial naltrexone findings. One study examining cognitive-behavioral therapy plus naltrexone in gamblers with co-occurring alcohol use disorder found no extra benefit for naltrexone compared with placebo (Toneatto et al. 2009), which is not surprising as cognitive-behavioral therapy is a standard psychotherapy for both gambling and alcohol use disorder. The second study using naltrexone on an as needed basis also failed to show benefit compared with placebo (Kovanen et al. 2016). Because subjects only took naltrexone two or three times per week, this study seems to indicate that this limited use of naltrexone is not beneficial but does not detract from the findings that daily use has shown benefit.

Two multicenter studies have further demonstrated the efficacy of opioid antagonists with the examination of nalmefene (a medication with a broader antagonism of opioid receptors than naltrexone) in the treatment of individuals with gambling disorder. In a 16-week multicenter trial of 207 gamblers assigned to nalmefene at varying doses (25, 50, or 100 mg/day) or placebo, 59% of those assigned to nalmefene showed significant reductions in gambling symptoms (urges, thoughts, and behavior) compared with only 34% of those taking placebo (Grant et al. 2006). A second 16-week multicenter study of 233 gamblers using nalmefene (20 or 40 mg) or placebo failed to show benefit in the intention-to-treat population, but post hoc analyses of those who received a full titration of the medication for at least 1 week demonstrated significantly greater reductions in gambling symptoms compared with those taking placebo (Grant et al. 2010).

To summarize the findings from opioid antagonist medications, we find the most robust benefit for these medications among the medication classes reviewed in the treatment of individuals with gambling disorder. There has been no negative study of an opioid antagonist in gambling disorder compared just with placebo and analyzed with those who actually took medication at the proper dose. In addition, opioid antagonists may preferentially work for gamblers who report urges to gamble and even for those with a family history of alcoholism (Grant et al. 2008b).

Glutamate Modulators

Because improving glutamatergic tone in the nucleus accumbens has been implicated in reducing the reward-seeking behavior in substance addictions (Kalivas et al. 2006), NAC, a glutamate-modulating agent, was administered open-label to 27 subjects with gambling disorder for 8 weeks, with responders then randomly assigned to receive NAC or placebo for an additional 6 weeks. At the end of the initial 8 weeks, 59% reported significant reductions in gambling symptoms and were classified as responders. At the end of the double-blind phase, 83% of those assigned to NAC were still classified as responders, compared with 28.6% of those assigned to placebo (Grant et al. 2007). A second 12-week double-blind, placebo-controlled study combined NAC with imaginal desensitization in 28 gambling subjects who were also nicotine dependent. Imaginal desensitization is a psychotherapeutic component whereby individuals are encouraged to visualize situations involving gambling triggers and then to visualize leaving those situations while remaining relaxed throughout. NAC provided significant benefit compared with placebo in reducing nicotine dependence symptoms during treatment and reducing gambling symptoms 3 months after formal treatment ended (Grant et al. 2014).

In summary, glutamate may be a promising target for pharmacotherapy in gambling disorder. NAC is sold over the counter but may have quality control issues when not issued as a prescription medication. There is also some question as to the extent of its central nervous system penetrance. Thus, although these studies show promise, it might be that more potent glutamate agents, rather than NAC, should be examined for gambling disorder. On the other hand, NAC does have the advantage of having an excellent side-effect profile relative to other types of psychotropic medication. The most common side effects with NAC are indigestion and nausea.

Mood-Stabilizing Agents

The category of mood-stabilizing agents might be a bit of a misnomer because these agents have complex and often differing modes of action from each other. However, we have grouped them based on how they are most typically used in clinical practice.

Topiramate is a drug that is thought to influence mesolimbic dopamine transmission indirectly through GABAergic and glutamatergic mechanisms (Johnson 2004). A 14-week double-blind, placebo-controlled trial of topiramate in 42 subjects failed to show significant treatment effects for topiramate on any outcome measures (Berlin et al. 2013). A second 12-week study, however, that combined topiramate with cognitive therapy demonstrated significant improvement in gambling symptoms (de Brito et al. 2017). The second study, unlike the Berlin et al. study, retained 79% of their subjects (compared with 64%), which may have affected the results.

In a 10-week study of 40 subjects with gambling disorder and bipolar spectrum disorders, sustained-release lithium carbonate (mean lithium level=0.87 mEq/L) demonstrated superiority to placebo in reducing gambling symptoms (Hollander et al. 2005). Although a majority (83%) reported significant decreases in gambling urges, thoughts, and behaviors, no differences were found in amount of money lost, episodes of gambling per week, or time spent per gambling episode. Lithium, of course, requires careful titration and plasma dose monitoring and careful psychoeducation regarding its safety (e.g., the impact of being unwell or dehydrated; importance of seeking prompt medical attention if feeling unwell).

Two placebo-controlled studies have examined the use of olanzapine in the treatment of gambling disorder. In a 12-week trial of 42 subjects, olanzapine (mean dose=8.9 ± 5.2 mg) failed to show any benefit compared with placebo in reducing gambling behavior and gambling urges (McElroy et al. 2008). Similarly, a second 7-week study in 23 subjects reported similar reductions in gambling symptoms in both the olanzapine and placebo groups (Fong et al. 2008).

In summary, the mood-stabilizing agents have shown mixed outcomes. Topiramate and lithium may both be beneficial for select people with gambling disorder. The olanzapine studies are difficult to interpret given the extremely small sample size and the question of whether they were adequately powered.

Limitations of the Treatment Research

Several limitations should be mentioned based on gambling disorder pharmacological treatment studies published to date:

1. Many gambling disorder studies have generally lacked a large enough sample to provide adequate statistical power. Exceptions include the multicenter nalmefene studies that were adequately powered at the time of enrollment.
2. Different classes of medication seem similarly effective in people with gambling disorder. No head-to-head comparison studies of medications have been performed in a randomized, placebo-controlled design.
3. No study has examined whether certain individuals with gambling disorder would benefit differentially from specific pharmacotherapies.
4. Comparisons of treatment studies have generally been problematic because of the lack of consensus on appropriate outcome measure or measures.
5. The long-term effects of medication for gambling disorder remain largely untested. Only two studies have examined pharmacological effects for 6 months, and these studies experienced drop-out rates of 59% (Blanco et al. 2002) and 44% (Saiz-Ruiz et al. 2005). No study has examined pharmacological treatment effects for longer than 6 months or determined whether the effects of acute treatment last beyond the 8–16 weeks.
6. There are limited data concerning the effectiveness of pharmacotherapy for subjects with gambling disorder with co-occurring psychiatric conditions. Only scant preliminary data suggest that individuals with gambling disorder and bipolar symptoms respond to lithium (Hollander et al. 2005) and that individuals with gambling disorder and nicotine dependence respond to NAC (Grant et al. 2014).

Recommendations Based on Treatment Outcome Literature

In the area of gambling disorder, the systematic study of pharmacological treatment efficacy and tolerability is in its infancy. With few well-powered studies published yet, it is difficult to make treatment recommendations with a substantial degree of confidence. No drugs are currently approved by the U.S. Food and Drug Administration for gambling disorder. Nonetheless, specific drug therapies offer promise for the effective treatment of individuals with gambling disorder. Although several different classes of medication have shown efficacy in treating people with gambling disorder in individual studies, only the opiate antagonists have had successful replication in randomized, placebo-controlled studies. As highlighted by the case vignette of Eriqua, studies also report promise using the glutamate modulator NAC, including in conjunction with psychological therapy incorporating imaginal desensitization. At present, issues such as which medication to use and for whom, or the duration of pharmacotherapy, cannot be sufficiently addressed with the available data.

References

Berlin HA, Braun A, Simeon D, et al: A double-blind, placebo-controlled trial of topiramate for pathological gambling. World J Biol Psychiatry 14:121–128, 2013

Black DW, Arndt S, Coryell WH, et al: Bupropion in the treatment of pathological gambling: a randomized, double-blind, placebo-controlled, flexible-dose study. J Clin Psychopharmacol 27:143–150, 2007

Blanco C, Petkova E, Ibanez A, Saiz-Ruiz J: A pilot placebo-controlled study of fluvoxamine for pathological gambling. Ann Clin Psychiatry 14:9–15, 2002

Broekkamp CL, Phillips AG: Facilitation of self-stimulation behavior following intracerebral microinjections of opioids into the ventral tegmental area. Pharmacol Biochem Behav 11:289–295, 1979

de Brito AM, de Almeida Pinto MG, Bronstein G, et al: Topiramate combined with cognitive restructuring for the treatment of gambling disorder: a two-center, randomized, double-blind clinical trial. J Gambl Stud 33(1):249–263, 2017

Fong T, Kalechstain A, Bernhard B, et al: A double-blind, placebo-controlled trial of olanzapine for the treatment of video poker pathological gamblers. Pharmacol Biochem Behav 89:298–303, 2008

Grant JE, Chamberlain SR: The placebo effect and its clinical associations in gambling disorder. Ann Clin Psychiatry 29(3):167–172, 2017

Grant JE, Kim SW: Demographic and clinical features of 131 adult pathological gamblers. J Clin Psychiatry 62:957–962, 2001

Grant JE, Potenza MN: Escitalopram treatment of pathological gambling with co-occurring anxiety: an open-label pilot study with double-blind discontinuation. Int Clin Psychopharmacol 21:203–209, 2006

Grant JE, Kim SW, Potenza MN, et al: Paroxetine treatment of pathological gambling: a multi-center randomized controlled trial. Int Clin Psychopharmacol 18:243–249, 2003

Grant JE, Potenza MN, Hollander E, et al: A multicenter investigation of the opioid antagonist nalmefene in the treatment of pathological gambling. Am J Psychiatry 163:303–312, 2006

Grant JE, Kim SW, Odlaug BL: N-acetyl cysteine, a glutamate-modulating agent, in the treatment of pathological gambling: a pilot study. Biol Psychiatry 62:652–657, 2007

Grant JE, Kim SW, Hartman BK: A double-blind, placebo-controlled study of the opiate antagonist naltrexone in the treatment of pathological gambling urges. J Clin Psychiatry 69:783–789, 2008a

Grant JE, Kim SW, Hollander E, Potenza MN: Predicting response to opiate antagonists and placebo in the treatment of pathological gambling. Psychopharmacology (Berl) 200(4):521–527, 2008b

Grant JE, Odlaug BL, Potenza MN, et al: Nalmefene in the treatment of pathological gambling: multi-centre, double-blind, placebo-controlled study. Br J Psychiatry 197:330–331, 2010

Grant JE, Odlaug BL, Chamberlain SR, et al: A randomized, placebo-controlled trial of N-acetylcysteine plus imaginal desensitization for nicotine-dependent pathological gamblers. J Clin Psychiatry 75(1):39–45, 2014

Hodgins DC, Stea JN, Grant JE: Gambling disorders. Lancet 378:1874–1884, 2011

Hollander E, Frenkel M, Decaria C, et al: Treatment of pathological gambling with clomipramine. Am J Psychiatry 149:710–711, 1992

Hollander E, DeCaria CM, Finkell JN, et al: A randomized double-blind fluvoxamine/placebo crossover trial in pathological gambling. Biol Psychiatry 47:813–817, 2000

Hollander E, Pallanti S, Allen A, et al: Does sustained-release lithium reduce impulsive gambling and affective instability versus placebo in pathological gamblers with bipolar spectrum disorders? Am J Psychiatry 162:137–145, 2005

Johnson BA: Topiramate-induced neuromodulation of cortico-mesolimbic dopamine function: a new vista for the treatment of comorbid alcohol and nicotine dependence? Addict Behav 29:1465–1479, 2004

Kalivas PW, Peters J, Knackstedt L: Animal models and brain circuits in drug addiction. Molecular Interventions 6:339–344, 2006

Kim SW, Grant JE, Adson DE, Shin YC: Double-blind naltrexone and placebo comparison study in the treatment of pathological gambling. Biol Psychiatry 49:914–921, 2001

Kim SW, Grant JE, Adson DE, et al: A double-blind placebo-controlled study of the efficacy and safety of paroxetine in the treatment of pathological gambling. J Clin Psychiatry 63:501–507, 2002

Kovanen L, Basnet S, Castrén S, et al: A randomised, double-blind, placebo-controlled trial of as-needed naltrexone in the treatment of pathological gambling. Eur Addict Res 22(2):70–79, 2016

Leeman RF, Potenza MN: Similarities and differences between pathological gambling and substance use disorders: a focus on impulsivity and compulsivity. Psychopharmacology (Berl) 219:469–490, 2012

Lorains FK, Cowlishaw S, Thomas SA: Prevalence of comorbid disorders in problem and pathological gambling: systematic review and meta-analysis of population surveys. Addiction 106:490–498, 2011

McElroy SL, Nelson EB, Welge JA, et al: Olanzapine in the treatment of pathological gambling: a negative randomized placebo-controlled trial. J Clin Psychiatry 69(3):433–440, 2008

Petry NM, Stinson FS, Grant BF: Comorbidity of DSM-IV pathological gambling and other psychiatric disorders: results from the National Epidemiologic Survey on Alcohol and Related Conditions. J Clin Psychiatry 66:564–574, 2005

Phillips AG, LePiane FG: Reinforcing effects of morphine microinjection onto the ventral tegmental area. Pharmacol Biochem Behav 12:965–968, 1980

Pietrzak RH, Morasco BJ, Blanco C, et al: Gambling level and psychiatric and medical disorders in older adults: results from the National Epidemiologic Survey on Alcohol and Related Conditions. Am J Geriatric Psychiatry 15:301–313, 2007

Potenza MN, Steinberg MA, McLaughlin SD, et al: Illegal behaviors in problem gambling: analysis of data from a gambling helpline. J Am Acad Psychiatry Law 28:389–403, 2000

Potenza MN, Leung HC, Blumberg HP, et al: An fMRI Stroop study of ventromedial prefrontal cortical function in pathological gamblers. Am J Psychiatry 160:1990–1994, 2003a

Potenza MN, Steinberg MA, Skudlarski P, et al: Gambling urges in pathological gamblers: an fMRI study. Arch Gen Psychiatry 60:828–836, 2003b

Potenza MN, Walderhaug E, Henry S, et al: Serotonin 1B receptor imaging in pathological gambling. World J Biol Psychiatry 14:139–145, 2013

Reuter J, Raedler T, Rose M, et al: Pathological gambling is linked to reduced activation of the mesolimbic reward system. Nat Neurosci 8:147–148, 2005

Saiz-Ruiz J, Blanco C, Ibanez A, et al: Sertraline treatment of pathological gambling: a pilot study. J Clin Psychiatry 66:28–33, 2005

Toneatto T, Brands B, Selby P: A randomized, double-blind, placebo-controlled trial of naltrexone in the treatment of concurrent alcohol use disorder and pathological gambling. Am J Addict 18(3):219–225, 2009

van Wolfswinkel L, van Ree JM: Effects of morphine and naloxone on thresholds of ventral tegmental electrical self-stimulation. Naunyn Schmiedebergs Arch Pharmacol 330:84–92, 1985

Virkkunen M, Goldman D, Nielsen DA, Linnoila M: Low brain serotonin turnover rate (low CSF 5-HIAA) and impulsive violence. J Psychiatry Neurosci 20(4):271–275, 1995

Appendix A

DSM-5 Diagnostic Criteria for Gambling Disorder

A. Persistent and recurrent problematic gambling behavior leading to clinically significant impairment or distress, as indicated by the individual exhibiting four (or more) of the following in a 12-month period:

1. Needs to gamble with increasing amounts of money in order to achieve the desired excitement.
2. Is restless or irritable when attempting to cut down or stop gambling.
3. Has made repeated unsuccessful efforts to control, cut back, or stop gambling.
4. Is often preoccupied with gambling (e.g., having persistent thoughts of reliving past gambling experiences, handicapping or planning the next venture, thinking of ways to get money with which to gamble).
5. Often gambles when feeling distressed (e.g., helpless, guilty, anxious, depressed).
6. After losing money gambling, often returns another day to get even ("chasing" one's losses).
7. Lies to conceal the extent of involvement with gambling.
8. Has jeopardized or lost a significant relationship, job, or educational or career opportunity because of gambling.
9. Relies on others to provide money to relieve desperate financial situations caused by gambling.

B. The gambling behavior is not better explained by a manic episode.

Source. Reprinted from American Psychiatric Association: *Diagnostic and Statistical Manual of Mental Disorders*, 5th Edition. Arlington, VA, American Psychiatric Association, 2013. Copyright © 2013, American Psychiatric Association. Used with permission.

Appendix B

Early Intervention Gambling Health Test (EIGHT)

Source. Developed by Sean Sullivan, Ph.D., for the Compulsive Gambling Society of New Zealand Inc. and the Department of General Practice and Primary Health Care at the Auckland School of Medicine, 1999. Permission to republish granted by Dr. Sean Sullivan.

Early Intervention Gambling Health Test (EIGHT)

> Most people enjoy gambling, whether it's the lottery, sports, cards, bingo, racing, or at the casino.
>
> *Sometimes, however, it can affect our health.*
>
> To help us to check your health, please answer the questions below as truthfully as you are able from your own experience.

1. Sometimes I've felt depressed or anxious after a session of gambling.

   _____ Yes, that's true.   _____ No, I haven't.

2. Sometimes I've felt guilty about the way I gamble.

   _____ Yes, that's so.   _____ No, that isn't so.

3. When I think about it, gambling has sometimes caused me problems.

   _____ Yes, that's so.   _____ No, that isn't so.

4. Sometimes I've found it better not to tell others, especially my family, about the amount of time or money I spend gambling.

   _____ Yes, that's true.   _____ No, I haven't.

5. I often find that when I stop gambling I've run out of money.

   _____ Yes, that's so.   _____ No, that isn't so.

6. Often I get the urge to return to gambling to win back losses from a past session.

   _____ Yes, that's so.   _____ No, that isn't so.

7. I have received criticism about my gambling in the past.

   _____ Yes, that's true.   _____ No, I haven't.

8. I have tried to win money to pay debts.

   _____ Yes, that's true.   _____ No, I haven't.

Appendix C

Gambling Symptom Assessment Scale (G-SAS)

Source. Reprinted from Kim SW, Grant JE, Adson DE, et al: "Double-Blind Naltrexone and Placebo Comparison Study in the Treatment of Pathological Gambling." *Biological Psychiatry* 49:914–921, 2001. Used with permission from Society for Biological Psychiatry and Elsevier.

Gambling Symptom Assessment Scale (G-SAS)

The following questions are aimed at evaluating gambling symptoms. Please *read* the questions *carefully* before you answer.

1. If you had urges to gamble during the past WEEK, on average, how strong were your urges? Please circle the most appropriate number.

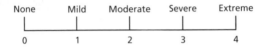

2. During the past WEEK, how many times did you experience urges to gamble? Please circle one.

0) None

1) Once

2) Two to three times

3) Several to many times

4) Constant or near constant

3. During the past WEEK, how many hours (add up hours) were you preoccupied with your urges to gamble? Please circle the most appropriate number.

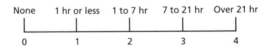

4. During the past WEEK, how much were you able to control your urges? Please circle the most appropriate number.

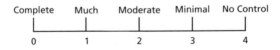

Gambling Symptom Assessment Scale (G-SAS) *(continued)*

5. During the past WEEK, how often did thoughts about gambling and placing bets come up? Please circle the most appropriate number.

   0)   None

   1)   Once

   2)   Two to three times

   3)   Several to many times

   4)   Constantly or nearly constantly

6. During the past WEEK, approximately how many hours (add up hours) did you spend thinking about gambling and thinking about placing bets? Please circle the most appropriate number.

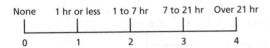

7. During the past WEEK, how much were you able to control your thoughts about gambling? Please circle the most appropriate number.

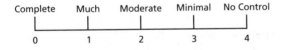

8. During the past WEEK, approximately how much total time did you spend gambling or on gambling-related activities? Please circle the most appropriate number.

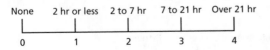

Gambling Symptom Assessment Scale (G-SAS) *(continued)*

9. During the past WEEK, on average, how much anticipatory tension and/or excitement did you have shortly before you engaged in gambling? If you did not actually gamble, please estimate how much tension and/or excitement you believe you would have experienced, if you had gambled. Please circle the most appropriate number.

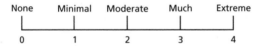

None	Minimal	Moderate	Much	Extreme
0	1	2	3	4

10. During the past WEEK, on average, how much excitement and pleasure did you feel when you won on your bet? If you did not actually win at gambling, please estimate how much excitement and pleasure you would have experienced if you had won. Please circle the most appropriate number.

None	Minimal	Moderate	Much	Extreme
0	1	2	3	4

11. During the past WEEK, how much emotional distress (mental pain or anguish, shame, guilt, embarrassment) has your gambling caused you? Please circle the most appropriate number.

None	Mild	Moderate	Severe	Extreme
0	1	2	3	4

12. During the past WEEK, how much personal trouble (relationship, financial, legal, job, medical or health) has your gambling caused you? Please circle the most appropriate number.

None	Mild	Moderate	Severe	Extreme
0	1	2	3	4

Appendix D

South Oaks Gambling Screen (SOGS)

Source.   Copyright © 1992, South Oaks Foundation, reprinted by permission. Lesieur HR, Blume SB: "The South Oaks Gambling Screen (SOGS): A New Instrument for the Identification of Pathological Gamblers." *American Journal of Psychiatry* 144:1184–1188, 1987; Lesieur HR, Blume SB: "Revising the South Oaks Gambling Screen in Different Settings." *Journal of Gambling Studies* 9:213–223, 1993.

South Oaks Gambling Screen (SOGS)

1. Please indicate which of the following types of gambling you have done in your lifetime. For each type, mark only one answer: "not at all," "less than once a week," or "once a week or more."

	Not at all	Less than once a week	Once a week or more	
a.	____	____	____	Played cards for money
b.	____	____	____	Bet on horses, dogs, or other animals (off-track betting, at the track, or with a bookie)
c.	____	____	____	Bet on sports (parlay cards, with a bookie, or at jai alai)
d.	____	____	____	Played dice games (craps, over and under, or other dice games) for money
e.	____	____	____	Went to a casino (legal or otherwise)
f.	____	____	____	Played the numbers or bet on lotteries
g.	____	____	____	Played bingo
h.	____	____	____	Played the stock and/or commodities market
i.	____	____	____	Played slot machines, poker machines, or other gambling machines
j.	____	____	____	Bowled, shot pool, played golf, or played some other game of skill for money

2. What is the largest amount of money you have ever gambled with on any one day?

____ Never have gambled   ____ More than $10, up to $100

____ $1 or less   ____ More than $100, up to $1,000

____ More than $1, up to $10   ____ More than $1,000, up to $10,000

3. Do (did) your parents have a gambling problem?

____ Both my father and mother gamble (gambled) too much.

____ My father gambles (gambled) too much.

____ My mother gambles (gambled) too much.

____ Neither parent gambles (gambled) too much.

South Oaks Gambling Screen (SOGS) *(continued)*

4. When you gamble, how often do you go back another day to win back money you lost?

   ____ Never

   ____ Some of the time (less than half the time) I lost

   ____ Most of the time I lost

   ____ Every time I lost

5. Have you ever claimed to be winning money gambling but weren't really?

   ____ Never (or never gamble)

   ____ Yes, less than half the time I lost

   ____ Yes, most of the time

6. Do you feel you have ever had a problem with gambling?

   ____ No

   ____ Yes, in the past, but not now

   ____ Yes

Check **Yes** or **No** for Questions 7–16   **Yes No**

7. Did you ever gamble more than you intended to?   ___ ___

8. Have people criticized your gambling?   ___ ___

'9. Have you ever felt guilty about the way you gamble or what happens when you gamble?   ___ ___

10. Have you ever felt like you would like to stop gambling but didn't think you could?   ___ ___

11. Have you ever hidden betting slips, lottery tickets, gambling money, or other signs of your gambling from your spouse, children, or other important people in your life?   ___ ___

12. Have you ever argued with people you live with over how you handle money?   ___ ___

13. If you answered **Yes** to Question #12: Have money arguments ever centered on your gambling?   ___ ___

South Oaks Gambling Screen (SOGS) *(continued)*

14. Have you ever borrowed from someone and not paid him or her back as a result of your gambling?　　　　　____ ____

15. Have you ever lost time from work or school due to gambling?　　　　　____ ____

16. If you borrowed money to gamble or to pay gambling debts, who or where did you borrow it from? Check **Yes** or **No** for each.

　　a.　　from household money　　　　　____ ____

　　b.　　from your spouse　　　　　____ ____

　　c.　　from other relatives or in-laws　　　　　____ ____

　　d.　　from banks, loan companies or credit unions　　　　　____ ____

　　e.　　from credit cards　　　　　____ ____

　　f.　　from loan sharks (shylocks)　　　　　____ ____

　　g.　　You cashed in stocks, bonds or other securities.　　　　　____ ____

　　h.　　You sold personal or family property.　　　　　____ ____

　　i.　　You borrowed on your checking account (passed bad checks).　　　　　____ ____

　　j.　　You have (had) a credit line with a bookie.　　　　　____ ____

　　k.　　You have (had) a credit line with a casino.　　　　　____ ____

SOGS Scoring

Scores on the South Oaks Gambling Screen itself are determined by adding up the number of questions that show an "at risk" response:

Questions 1, 2 and 3 are ***not*** counted.

__#4: Most of the time I lost *or* Every time I lost

__#5: Yes, less than half the time I lost *or* Yes, most of the time

__#6: Yes, in the past, but not now *or* Yes

__#7: Yes

__#8: Yes

South Oaks Gambling Screen (SOGS) *(continued)*

__#9: Yes

__#10: Yes

__#11: Yes

Question 12 is *not* counted.

__#13: Yes

__#14: Yes

__#15: Yes

__#16a: Yes

__#16b: Yes

__#16c: Yes

__#16d: Yes

__#16e: Yes

__#16f: Yes

__#16g: Yes

__#16h: Yes

__#16i: Yes

Questions 16j and 16k are *not* counted.

Total = _____ (20 questions are counted.)

A total score of 5 or more = probable pathological gambler.

Appendix E

Yale-Brown Obsessive Compulsive Scale Modified for Pathological Gambling (PG-YBOCS)

Source.   Reprinted from Pallanti S, DeCaria CM, Grant JE, Urpe M, Hollander E: "Reliability and Validity of the Pathological Gambling Adaptation of the Yale-Brown Obsessive-Compulsive Scale (PG-YBOCS)." *Journal of Gambling Studies* 21(4):431–443, 2005. Used with permission.

Yale-Brown Obsessive Compulsive Scale Modified for Pathological Gambling (PG-YBOCS)

1. Time occupied by urges/thoughts about gambling

How much of your time is occupied by urges/thoughts (u/t) related to gambling and/or gambling-related activities? How frequently does this occur?

0 = None

1 = Mild (less than 1 hr/day) or occasional u/t ($\leq$8x/day)

2 = Moderate (1–3 hrs/day) or frequent u/t ($\geq$8x/day but most hrs/day are free of u/t)

3 = Severe (>3 and up to 8 hrs/day) or very frequent u/t (>8x/day and occur most hrs of day)

4 = Extreme (>8 hrs/day) or near constant u/t (too numerous to count and an hour rarely passes w/o several such u/t occurring)

2. Interference due to urges/thoughts about gambling

How much do your urges/thoughts (u/t) interfere with your social or work (or role) functioning? Is there anything that you do not do because of this? (If patient is currently not working, determine how much performance would be affected if patient were employed.)

0 = None

1 = Mild, slight interference with social or occupational activity but overall performance is not impaired

2 = Moderate, definite interference with social or occupational performance, but manageable

3 = Severe, causes substantial impairment in social or occupational performance

4 = Extreme, incapacitating

3. Distress associated with urges/thoughts about gambling

How much distress do your urges/thoughts about gambling cause you? (Rate "disturbing" feeling or anxiety that seems to be triggered by these thoughts, not generalized anxiety or anxiety symptoms associated with other symptoms.)

0 = None

1 = Mild, infrequent and not too disturbing

2 = Moderate, frequent and disturbing, but still manageable

3 = Severe, very frequent and very disturbing

4 = Extreme, near constant and disabling distress

Yale-Brown Obsessive Compulsive Scale Modified for Pathological Gambling (PG-YBOCS) *(continued)*

4. Resistance against urges/thoughts of gambling

How much of an effort do you make to resist these urges/thoughts?
How often do you try to disregard them? (Only rate effort made to resist, not success or failure in actually controlling these thoughts. How much one resists the urges/thoughts may or may not correlate with ability to control them.)

0 = Makes effort always to resist; symptoms so minimal doesn't need to actively resist

1 = Tries to resist most of the time

2 = Makes some effort to resist

3 = Yields to all such urges/thoughts without attempting to control them but does so with some reluctance

4 = Completely and willingly yields to all such urges/thoughts

5. Degree of or control over urges/thoughts about gambling

How much control do you have over urges/thoughts about gambling?
How successful are you in stopping or diverting these urges/thoughts?

0 = Complete control

1 = Much control, usually able to stop/divert urges/thoughts with some effort and consideration

2 = Moderate control, sometimes able to stop/divert these urges/thoughts

3 = Little control, rarely successful in stopping these urges/thoughts, can only divert attention with difficulty

4 = No control, experienced as completely involuntary, rarely able to even momentarily divert urges/thoughts

6. Time spent in activities related to gambling

How much time do you spend in activities related to gambling? (directly related to gambling itself or activities such as negotiating financial transactions or searching for financial resources related to gambling)

0 = None

1 = Mild, spends less than 1 hr/day in these activities, or occasional involvement in these activities (≤8 times/day)

2 = Moderate, 1–3 hrs/day or >8 times/day but most hours are free of such activities

Yale-Brown Obsessive Compulsive Scale Modified for Pathological Gambling (PG-YBOCS) *(continued)*

6. Time spent in activities related to gambling *(continued)*

3 = Severe, spends >3 and up to 8 hrs/day, or very frequent involvement (>8 times/day) and activities performed most hours of the day

4 = Extreme, spends >8 hrs/day in these activities, or near-constant involvement (too numerous to count and an hour rarely passes without engaging in several such activities)

7. Interference due to activities related to gambling

How much do the above activities interfere with your social/work (or role) functioning?
Is there anything that you do not do because of them? (If patient is currently not working, determine how much performance would be affected if patient were employed.)

0 = None

1 = Mild, slight interference with social or occupational activities, but overall performance is not impaired

2 = Moderate, definite interference with social/occupational performance, but still manageable

3 = Severe, causes substantial impairment in social/occupational performance

4 = Extreme, incapacitating

8. Distress associated with behavior related to gambling

How much distress do you feel if prevented from gambling? (Pause)
How anxious would you become?

0 = None

1 = Mild, only slightly anxious if behavior is prevented or only slight anxiety during behavior

2 = Moderate, reports that anxiety would mount but remains manageable if behavior is prevented or that anxiety increases but remains manageable during such behaviors

3 = Severe, prominent and very disturbing increase in anxiety if behavior is interrupted or prominent and very disturbing increase in anxiety during the behavior

4 = Extreme, incapacitating anxiety from any intervention aimed at modifying activity or incapacitating anxiety develops during behavior related to gambling

Yale-Brown Obsessive Compulsive Scale Modified for Pathological Gambling (PG-YBOCS) *(continued)*

9. Resistance against gambling

How much of an effort do you make to resist these activities? (How much the patient resists behaviors may or may not correlate with ability to control them.)

0 = Makes an effort to always resist, or symptoms so minimal does not need to actively resist

1 = Tries to resist most of the time

2 = Makes some effort to resist

3 = Yields to almost all of these behaviors without attempting to control them but does so with some reluctance

4 = Completely and willingly yields to all behaviors related to gambling

10. Degree of control over gambling behavior

How strong is the drive to gamble?
How much control do you have over the behaviors associated with gambling-related activities?

0 = Complete control

1 = Much control, experiences pressure to gamble, but usually able to exercise voluntary control over it

2 = Moderate control, strong pressure to gamble, must be carried to completion, can only delay with difficulty

3 = Little control, very strong drive to gamble, must be carried to completion, can only delay with difficulty

4 = No control, drive to gamble experienced as completely involuntary and overpowering, rarely able to even momentarily delay gambling activity

Gambling Urge/Thought Subtotal (Q1–Q5): _____

Gambling Behavior Subtotal (Q6–Q10): _____

Overall Total: _____

Index

Page numbers printed in **boldface** type refer to tables or figures.